AF520584

SETHI'S
HPTLC

High Performance
Thin Layer Chromatography

Quantitative Analysis of Pharmaceutical Formulations

ISBN : 978-81-239-2279-9

First Edition : 2013

Published by:
Satish K. Jain and produced by Vinod K. Jain for CBS Publishers & Distributors Pvt. Ltd., 4819/XI Prahlad Street, 24 Ansari Road, Daryaganj, New Delhi - 110002 (India)
E-mail: cbspubs@airtelmail.com, delhi@cbspd.com • www.cbspd.com

Branches:
- ***Bengaluru:*** 2975, 17th Cross, K.R. Road, Bansankari 2nd Stage, Bengaluru - 560070
  Ph.: +91-80-26771678/79
  E-mail: cbsbng@gmail.com, bangalore@cbspd.com
- ***Pune:*** Bhuruk Prestige, Sr. No. 52/12/2+1+3/2, Narhe, Haveli (Near Katraj-Dehu Road By-pass), Pune - 411051
  Ph.: +91-20-64704058/59, 32342277 • E-mail: pune@cbspd.com
- ***Kochi:*** 36/14, Kalluvilakam, Lissie Hospital Road, Kochi - 682018, Kerala
  Ph.: +91-484-4059061-65 • Fax: +91-484-4059065
  E-mail: cochin@cbspd.com
- ***Chennai:*** 20, West Park Road, Shenoy Nagar, Chennai - 600030
  Ph.: +91-44-26260666, 26208620 E-mail: chennai@cbspd.com

Printed at :
Aegean Offset Printers, Greater Noida (UP)

To

The woman, USHA,
my wife, my friend
who stood by me all the time.

Life is all about aspiration, struggle, failures, triumph and achievement.

Dedicated to fellow analysts exploring wider application of TLC/HPTLC, a versatile analytical technique.

Please remember, how good analyst you may be but one can't do inspired analysis without aesthetic qualities, the gift possessed by relatively very few like skill of a musician or a painter but one can emulate their mentors, teachers/gurus.

"Guru/teacher/mentor is like a live-map; if you can read the map, you know the right path to go, without map it may take life-time to find the right path."

Preface

Quality level of any analytical work depends on appropriate analytical method, performance of analytical instruments, certified standard substances, reagents, suitable sample preparation and analysts having adequate scientific knowledge of the analytical chemistry and practical experience. The analytical data so generated for any decision-making process must be technically sound, defensive and with very low level of uncertainty. Please remember, analytical data may be dealt with computers and human intellect but intuition is exclusively human.

High performance thin layer chromatography (HPTLC) works on the same principles as other chromatographic techniques such as HPLC/GC with added advantages of fastness, high sample throughput analysis, less labour intensive sample cleanup procedures, and simultaneous parallel analysis of several samples under identical conditions avoiding system suitability test (SST), disposable stationary phase, and static detection. Now HPTLC system is fully automated thus enhancing the system reproducibility allowing reliable, accurate and precise analytical results. These advantages have made HPTLC a comprehensive analytical technique for application in different fields (pharma and herbal analysis, food, cosmetology, environmental analysis, clinical laboratories, forensic and biochemistry) providing same level of quality results as that of HPLC/GC. However, there are many challenges which the analyst shall often face while working with this technique successfully as HPTLC being an open system method, is highly affected by experimental and environmental conditions which need to be controlled and regulated for reproducible results in each chromatoplate. It need to be borne in mind that consistency of performance of each application shall squarely depend on controlling various influencing factors. This compilation is an attempt to demonstrate how HPTLC fits in a well-managed analytical laboratory as an independent analytical technique on its own merit.

There is no contemporary monograph on application of HPTLC in analysis of multi-component pharmaceutical formulations except the one authored by me in 1996. The old monograph was primarily based on experimental work carried out at CDL (now CDTL), Mumbai (Bombay) and the work was based on single point validation. Since 15 years, HPTLC is the most prevalent analytical technique in pharmaceutical analysis, it was considered appropriate to fill this gap by updating the available information to help the young and novice analysts to advance their analytical knowledge. The entire text has been written in very clear, concise and simple language avoiding scientific jargon to improve the readability and understandability for bench analysts those not possessing very advanced academic qualifications. The present text in 3 volumes series contains detailed procedures for more than 500 multi-component formulations. Each formulation contains detailed analytical procedure as protocol along with typical densitogram of the sample/standard or both, and also overlaid UV-spectra of analytes to help analysts select suitable wavelength for densitometric scanning. Efforts have been made to provide all possible details under protocols to enable the analysts to repeat the method without recourse to original literature.

In addition to comprehensive introduction and a special chapter on validation of HPTLC method, the analytical methods for different formulations have been arranged in broader pharmacological activities i.e. cardiovascular system, musculoskeletal disorders, antibiotics, central nervous system, respiratory system, alimentary system, preparations for external use, and miscellaneous formulations such as vitamins and enzymes, antidiabetic drugs, cholesterol lowering drugs, etc. The methods described may not be the only one available, better alternative may well exist in literature or one may develop in the laboratory.

Most of the methods embodied in this compilation are based on work carried out in academic institutions and are claimed to have been validated as per international guidelines by the reporting authors, however, one may experience untoward surprises as institutions rarely include vigorous validation programme. It is, therefore, suggested that the method may be optimized in the given laboratory conditions before adopting for final use. For several formulations, methods by both NP-HPTLC and RP-HPTLC have been described. Such RP-HPTLC methods can help analysts to transfer such methods to RP-HPLC with reasonable success. Please remember skill obtained during actual method development can never be obtained through written description of a method. Learn from your experience and find your own solution. Analytical methods with higher accuracy and precision are difficult to perform. It may be mentioned that for majority of methods included in this monograph authors have used pre-coated plates manufactured by Merck probably due to cost and easy availability. However, pre-coated plates from other manufacturers (Whatman, Analtech, Altech, etc.) can be used but it must be kept in mind that plates from different manufacturers are likely to vary in certain specifications such as particle size, pore distribution, amount and type of binder used, etc. which are important for reproducibility of analytical results and need to be considered while revalidating or optimizing a given method. **A word of caution:** Frequent change of brand of pre-coated plates is not advisable.

From my personal experience, I can claim with belief that when other available analytical methods do not elicit the desired analytical information due to complexity of samples, HPTLC may provide the answer. Think logically, it may be a great surprise for you to observe how well this technique provides the desired answer for a separation and quantitation problem. Chromatographers are advised to read carefully **practical tips** before starting experimental work, these will help you to be a better chromatographer.

It should not be forgotten that certain minimum amount of basic knowledge and experience is needed for effective application of this technique. Attempt has been made to provide brief, comprehensive introduction to familiarize the analysts with important steps of this technique. How far I have succeeded in this attempt is left to the analysts to judge.

New Delhi, India

P.D. Sethi, M.Pharm, Ph.D.
Pharmaceutical Analyst

After transfer of the validated method to a quality control laboratory for adopting for routine quality control work, there is still a challenge to face, as HPTLC being an open system method, is highly affected by experimental and environmental conditions, one need to check regularly the suitability of chromatographic results on each chromatoplate.

Creativity – generating an idea, and innovation – implementing the idea, both must converge to fruition (applied creativity), otherwise waste of talent.

Acknowledgement

I place on record my gratitude to analytical fraternity, students, teachers and professionals for their support and inspiration in my entire analytical career.

I am extremely obliged to all TLC/HPTLC practitioners for sharing analytical data (published and unpublished) without which this compilation would never have been possible. I am thankful to Dilip Charegaonkar, CMD, M/s Anchrom Enterprises (I) Pvt. Ltd., Mumbai, India, for extending facilities in HPTLC application laboratory for verification of several reported methods and scientific support in compilation of this monograph. Valued advice by Mr. Dilip Charegaonkar for practically-oriented presentation of the subject matter is highly appreciated.

Merck Specialities Private Limited, Mumbai, India was kind enough to provide pre-coated plates for analytical work and also permission to reproduce data and figures required. I am thankful to M/s Camag, Switzerland for permission to reproduce different figures related to their HPTLC system.

I am thankful to Prof. Nitin Dubey and his team for contributing an exhaustive chapter on validation of HPTLC method and sharing their knowledge and experience with analytical fraternity. This should help analysts in planning validation of chromatographic methods. Sharing knowledge and experience with bench-analysts for the last 35 years for ultimate successful application has been source of unmatched happiness for me. At the end, I place on record my most sincere appreciation for Mr. Dharmvir for his dedicated support not only in compilation of this monograph but also giving practical shape to many of my ideas.

New Delhi, India

P.D. Sethi, M.Pharm, Ph.D.
Pharmaceutical Analyst

"Have creative mind, evaluate critically and logically."

Brief Contents
(Volumes 1 – 3)

VOLUME 1

VOLUME 2

VOLUME 3

Contents

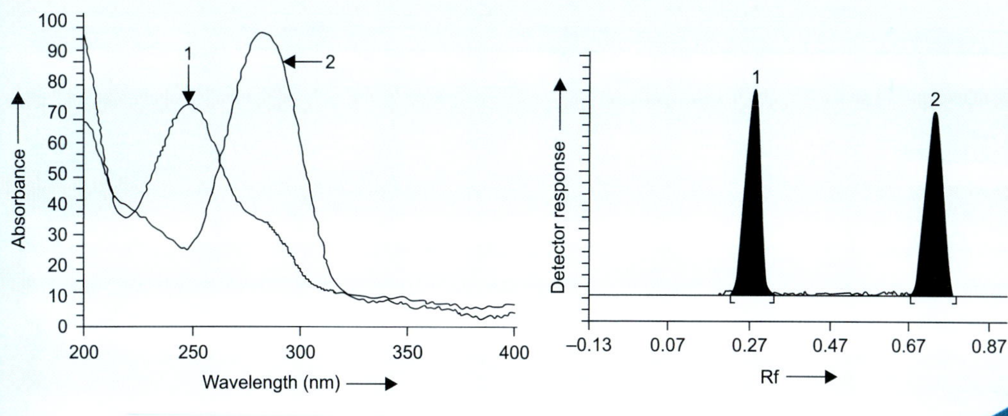

4

Musculoskeletal Disorders

- Analgesics and antipyretics
- Anti-inflammatory drugs
- Muscle relaxants

Protocols and Densitograms from 121 to 232

Measurements made without attention to why they are being made are often bad measurements.

HPTLC : High Performance Thin Layer Chromatography
HPTLC Densitogram

No. 121

Typical densitogram of the sample and standard containing aspirin, paracetamol and caffeine. For detailed experimental and chromatographic conditions, refer to Protocol No. 121. Peaks identification: 1. Paracetamol; 2. Caffeine; 3. Aspirin.

Note: This densitogram was obtained using mobile-phase-IV and scanned at UV–271 nm.

PROTOCOL FOR HPTLC ANALYSIS OF PHARMACEUTICAL FORMULATION

Protocol No. 121

Formulation: Aspirin, Paracetamol, Caffeine citrate

Classification: Musculoskeletal Disorders **Dosage form:** Tablets

Standard preparation: Dissolve 250 mg each of aspirin and paracetamol and 65 mg of caffeine separately in methanol to produce 20 ml. Further dilutions are suitably made for linearity profile.

Sample preparation: Tablets containing 250 mg of aspirin, 250 mg of paracetamol and 65 mg of caffeine dissolved in methanol to get 200 ml. For determination of aspirin and caffeine, solution was used as such; for paracetamol, 5 ml of the solution was further diluted to 10 ml with methanol.

Chromatographic equipments:

Sample applicator: Camag Linomat–IV

Development chamber: Camag twin-trough glass chamber, 10 × 10 cm

Densitometric scanner: Camag TLC Scanner–II

Chromatographic conditions:

1. Stationary phase: Silica gel $60F_{254}$ pre-coated TLC plates with pre-adsorbent spotting area, channelled, 10 × 10 cm (250 μm) – Whatman
2. Mobile phase (MP): (i) Ethyl acetate–glacial acetic acid (95 : 5 v/v); (ii) Chloroform–glacial acetic acid–ethyl acetate (36 : 24 : 1 v/v); (iii) Toluene–dioxane–glacial acetic acid (9 : 3 : 0.3 v/v); (iv) Dichloromethane–isopropanol–glacial acetic acid (21 : 3 : 0.2 v/v)
3. Standard/Sample application:
   Band length: 10 mm Volume applied: 10 μl Spacing: 10 mm
4. Chamber saturation: 10 min (MP)
5. RH (%): 55 ± 5
6. Temperature °C: 22 ± 2
7. Separation technique: Ascending
8. Quantity of mobile phase: 20 ml
9. Migration distance: 60 mm
10. Migration time: (i) 20 min; (ii) 23 min

Densitometric evaluation:

Wavelength: UV–271 nm Scanning mode: Reflectance/Absorbance

HRF:	(i)	(ii)	(iii)	(iv)
Aspirin	65	52	63	65
Paracetamol	49	21	47	10
Caffeine	18	29	54	20

Linearity (ng/band): Aspirin and Paracetamol—525–6250; Caffeine—525–3250

Recovery (%): 90–110 for all the three compounds

References: (i) Joseph Sharma and Chantel D. Rolfe, *J. Planar Chromatogr.*, **5**, 197–199, 1992; (ii) Technical Notes on TLC, Macherey-Nagel (Germany).

Comments: The proposed methods were routinely used with good reproducibility.

HPTLC : High Performance Thin Layer Chromatography
HPTLC Densitogram

No. 122

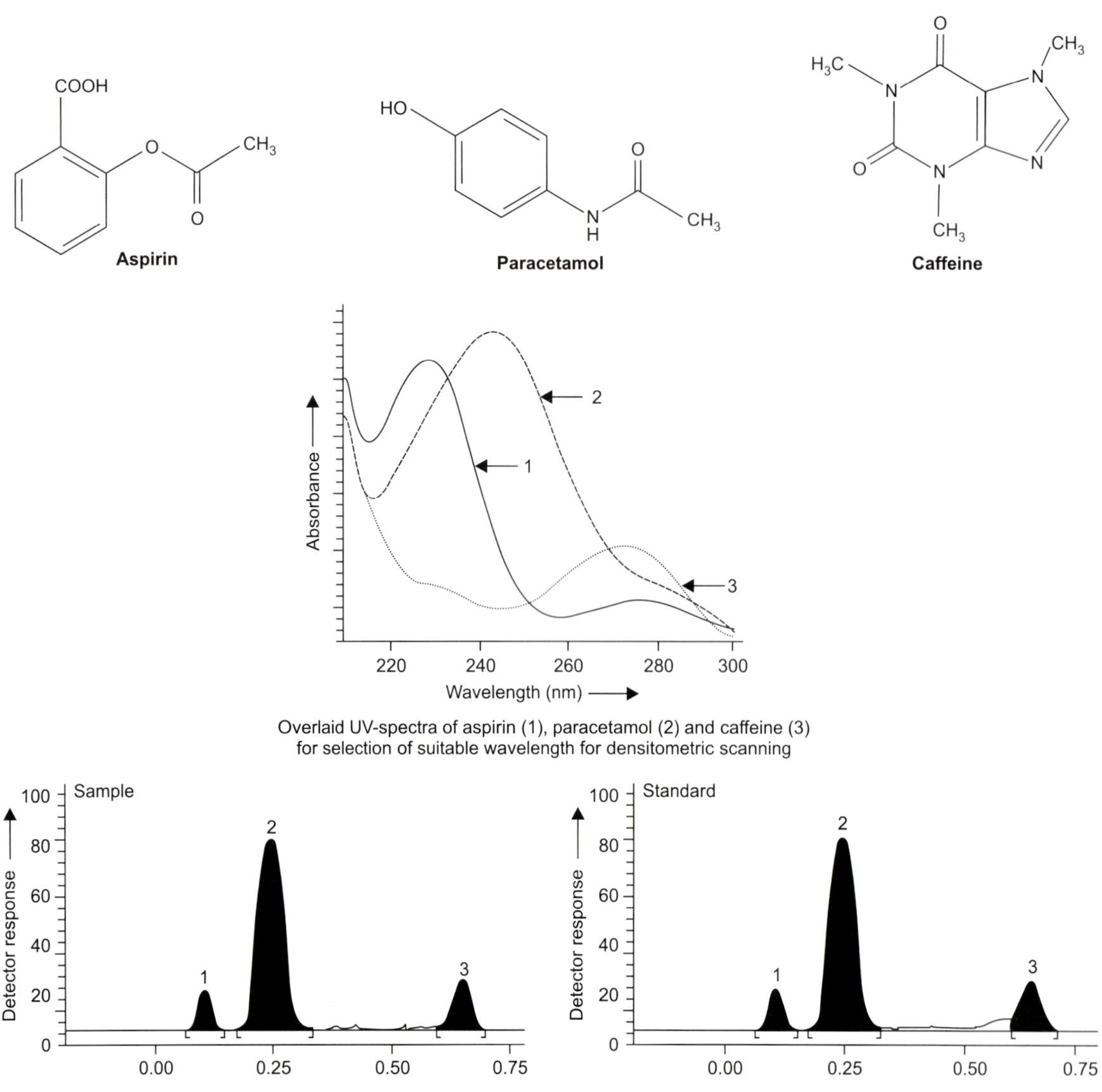

Overlaid UV-spectra of aspirin (1), paracetamol (2) and caffeine (3) for selection of suitable wavelength for densitometric scanning

Typical densitogram of the sample and standard containing aspirin, paracetamol and caffeine. For detailed experimental and chromatographic conditions, refer to Protocol No. 122. Peaks identification: 1. Caffeine; 2. Paracetamol; 3. Aspirin.

PROTOCOL FOR HPTLC ANALYSIS OF PHARMACEUTICAL FORMULATION

Protocol No. 122

Formulation: Aspirin, Paracetamol, Caffeine citrate

Classification: Musculoskeletal Disorders **Dosage form:** Tablets

Standard preparation: (a) Prepare 3 mg/ml solution of Caffeine (C) in methanol. (b) Weigh 25 mg each of aspirin (A) and paracetamol (P), add 1 ml of solution (a) and dilute to 10 ml, further dilution is done by taking 2 ml to 10 ml.

Sample preparation: Weigh powdered sample accurately equivalent to 125 mg of aspirin, suspend in methanol, sonicate for 5 min, dilute to 50 ml with methanol, filter and dilute 2 ml of the filtrate to 10 ml with methanol.

Chromatographic equipments:

Sample applicator: Camag Linomat–IV

Development chamber: Camag twin-trough glass chamber, 10 × 10 cm

Densitometric scanner: Camag TLC Scanner–II

Chromatographic conditions:

1. Stationary phase: Silica gel $60F_{254}$ pre-coated HPTLC plates, 10 × 10 cm (200 μm) – Merck
2. Mobile phase (MP): n-hexane–ethyl acetate–glacial acetic acid (4 : 6 : 0.1 v/v)
3. Standard/Sample application:
   Band length: 10 mm   Volume applied: 5 μl   Spacing: 10 mm
4. Chamber saturation: 20 min (MP)
5. RH (%): 55 ± 5
6. Temperature °C: 22 ± 2
7. Separation technique: Ascending
8. Quantity of mobile phase: 10 ml
9. Migration distance: 50 mm
10. Migration time: 12 min

Densitometric evaluation:

Wavelength: UV–254 nm or 273 nm   Scanning mode: Reflectance/Absorbance

HRF: Caffeine—10; Paracetamol—24; Aspirin—64

Linearity (ng/band): Aspirin and Paracetamol—500–3000; Caffeine—100–1000

Recovery (%): 98.41–100.73 for all the three compounds

References: —

Comments: Although the scanning has been done at 254 nm, it would be better to scan at 273 nm, the λ_{max} of caffeine, the minor component of the formulation.

HPTLC : High Performance Thin Layer Chromatography
HPTLC Densitogram

No. 123

COOH
O
CH_3
O
Aspirin

HO
O
N
H
CH_3
Paracetamol

O
H_3C
N
CH_3
N
N
O
N
CH_3
Caffeine

100
80
60
40
20
0
Absorbance
1
3
2
200 250 300 350 400
Wavelength (nm)

Overlaid UV-spectra of aspirin (1), caffeine (2) and paracetamol (3) for selection of suitable wavelength for densitometric scanning

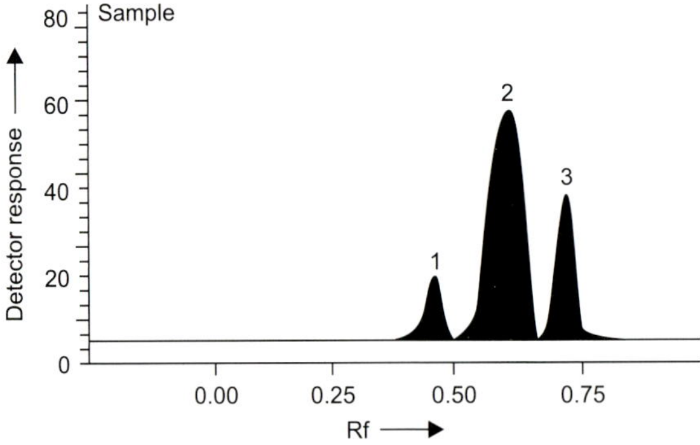

Typical densitogram of the sample and the standard containing aspirin, paracetamol and caffeine. For detailed experimental and chromatographic conditions, refer to Protocol No. 123. Peaks identification: 1. Caffeine; 2. Paracetamol; 3. Aspirin.

PROTOCOL FOR HPTLC ANALYSIS OF PHARMACEUTICAL FORMULATION

Protocol No. 123

Formulation: Aspirin, Paracetamol, Caffeine citrate

Classification: Musculoskeletal Disorders **Dosage form:** Tablets

Standard preparation: (a) Prepare 3 mg/ml solution of Caffeine (C) in methanol. (b) Weigh 25 mg each of aspirin (A) and paracetamol (P), add 1 ml of solution (a) and dilute to 10 ml, further dilution is done by taking 2 ml to 10 ml.

Sample preparation: Weigh powdered sample accurately equivalent to 125 mg of aspirin, suspend in methanol, sonicate for 5 min, dilute to 50 ml with methanol, filter and dilute 2 ml of the filtrate to 10 ml with methanol.

Chromatographic equipments:

Sample applicator: Camag Linomat–IV

Development chamber: Camag twin-trough glass chamber, 10 × 10 cm

Densitometric scanner: Camag TLC Scanner–II

Chromatographic conditions:

1. Stationary phase: Silica gel $60F_{254}$ pre-coated HPTLC plates, 10 × 10 cm (200 μm) – Merck
2. Mobile phase (MP): Ethyl acetate–toluene–methanol–glacial acetic acid (5 : 4 : 1 : 0.1 v/v)
3. Standard/Sample application:
   Band length: 10 mm Volume applied: 5 μl Spacing: 10 mm
4. Chamber saturation: 20 min (MP)
5. RH (%): 55 ± 5
6. Temperature °C: 22 ± 2
7. Separation technique: Ascending
8. Quantity of mobile phase: 10 ml
9. Migration distance: 50 mm
10. Migration time: 15 min

Densitometric evaluation:

Wavelength: UV–254 nm or 273 nm Scanning mode: Reflectance/Absorbance

HRF: Caffeine—48; Paracetamol—69; Aspirin—75

Linearity (ng/band): Aspirin—500–3000; Caffeine—100–1000

Recovery (%): 98.41–100.73 for all the three compounds

References: Anonymous

Comments: Although scanning was done at 254 nm, it would be better to scan at 273 nm, the λ_{max} of caffeine, the minor component in the formulation.

HPTLC : High Performance Thin Layer Chromatography
HPTLC Densitogram

No. 124

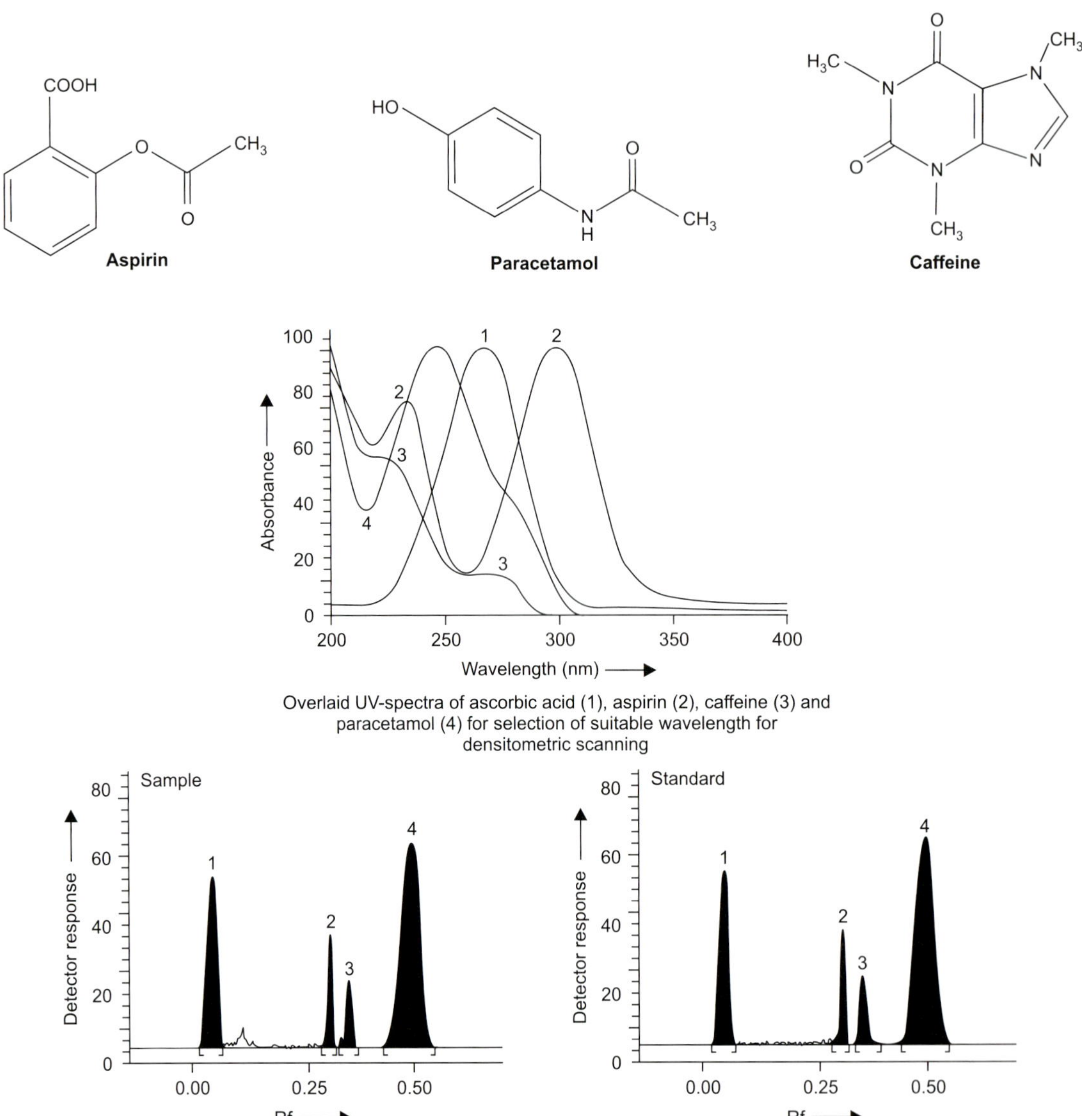

Overlaid UV-spectra of ascorbic acid (1), aspirin (2), caffeine (3) and paracetamol (4) for selection of suitable wavelength for densitometric scanning

Typical densitogram of the sample and standard containing aspirin, paracetamol, caffeine citrate and ascorbic acid. For detailed experimental and chromatographic conditions, refer to Protocol No. 124. Peaks identification: 1. Ascorbic acid; 2. Aspirin; 3. Caffeine citrate; 4. Paracetamol.

PROTOCOL FOR HPTLC ANALYSIS OF PHARMACEUTICAL FORMULATION

Protocol No. 124

Formulation: **Aspirin, Paracetamol, Caffeine citrate, Ascorbic acid**

Classification: Musculoskeletal Disorders **Dosage form:** Tablets

Standard preparation: (1) Take 10 mg each of aspirin and paracetamol (A and P), mix and dissolve in methanol and make 10 ml; (2) Prepare 1 mg/ml solution of ascorbic acid (AA) in methanol; (3) Prepare 1 mg/ml solution of caffeine (C) in methanol; (4) take 2.5 ml of solution (1), 1 ml of solution (2) and 0.3 ml of solution (3), mix and dilute to 10 with methanol.

Sample preparation: Powdered sample equivalent to 100 mg of ascorbic acid suspended in methanol to produce 100 ml, sonicate, filter and the filtrate suitably diluted for assay.

Chromatographic equipments:

Sample applicator: Camag Linomat–IV

Development chamber: Camag Horizontal glass chamber, 10 × 10 cm

Densitometric scanner: Camag TLC Scanner–II

Chromatographic conditions:

1. Stationary phase: Silica gel $60F_{254}$ pre-coated HPTLC plates, 10 × 10 cm (200 μm) – Merck
2. Mobile phase (MP): Toluene–n–propanol–formic acid (7.5 : 2.5 : 0.1 v/v)
3. Standard/Sample application:
   Band length: 10 mm Volume applied: 10 μl Spacing: 10 mm
4. Chamber saturation: 20 min (MP)
5. RH (%): 55 ± 5
6. Temperature °C: 22 ± 2
7. Separation technique: Ascending
8. Quantity of mobile phase: 10 ml
9. Migration distance: 60 mm
10. Migration time: 15 min

Densitometric evaluation:

Wavelength: UV–272 nm Scanning mode: Reflectance/Absorbance

HRF: Ascorbic acid—04; Aspirin—31; Caffeine citrate—35; Paracetamol—49

Linearity (ng/band): Aspirin and Paracetamol—500–2500; Caffeine—50–300; Ascorbic acid—200–1000

Recovery (%): 101.56–104.30 for all the three compounds

References: —

Comments:

- The method was optimized and analytical work carried out at **Anchrom's HPTLC Application Laboratory**, Mumbai, India.
- Several market samples of similar composition were analysed by the proposed method with reproducible results.

HPTLC : High Performance Thin Layer Chromatography
HPTLC Densitogram

No. 125

Aspirin

Dipyridamole

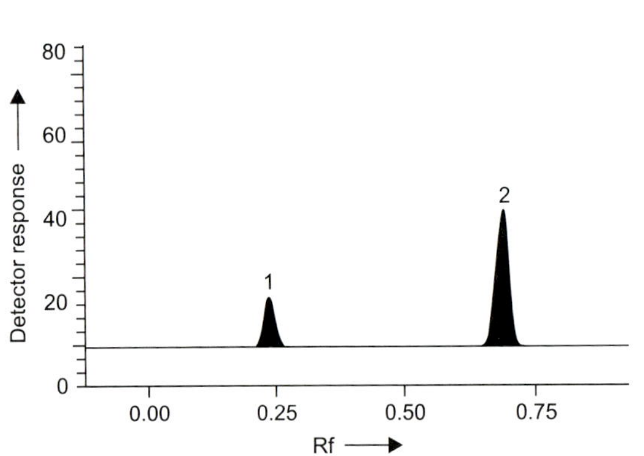

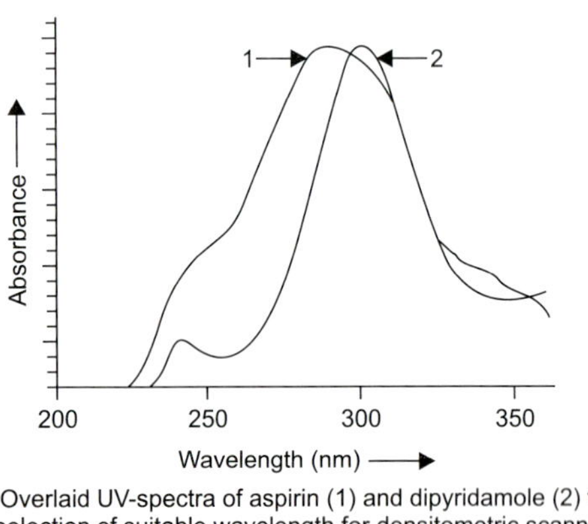

Overlaid UV-spectra of aspirin (1) and dipyridamole (2) for selection of suitable wavelength for densitometric scanning

Typical densitogram of the standard containing aspirin and dipyridamole. For detailed experimental and chromatographic conditions, refer to Protocol No. 125. Peaks identification: 1. Aspirin; 2. Dipyridamole.

PROTOCOL FOR HPTLC ANALYSIS OF PHARMACEUTICAL FORMULATION

Protocol No. 125

Formulation: Aspirin, Dipyridamole

Classification: Musculoskeletal Disorders **Dosage form:** Tablets

Standard preparation: Dissolve 65 mg of aspirin and 75 mg of dipyridamole in methanol–ethanol (1 : 1) to produce 100 ml. Dilute 5 ml of resulting solution to 50 ml with methanol and use for chromatographic analysis.

Sample preparation: Take powdered sample equivalent to 65 mg of aspirin and treat as under standard solution after sonicating for 20 min. Apply 3 μl of the final solution for chromatographic analysis.

Chromatographic equipments:

Sample applicator: Camag Linomat–IV

Development chamber: Camag twin-trough glass chamber, 10 × 10 cm

Densitometric scanner: Camag TLC Scanner–III

Chromatographic conditions:

1. Stationary phase: Silica gel $60F_{254}$ pre-coated HPTLC plates, 10 × 10 cm (200 μm) – Merck
2. Mobile phase (MP): Ethyl acetate–ethyl alcohol–13.5 M ammonia (7.5 : 1.5 : 1.5 v/v)
3. Standard/Sample application:
   Band length: 8 mm Volume applied: 3 μl Spacing: 10 mm
4. Chamber saturation: 20 min (MP)
5. RH (%): 55 ± 5
6. Temperature °C: 22 ± 2
7. Separation technique: Ascending
8. Quantity of mobile phase: 10 ml
9. Migration distance: 70 mm
10. Migration time: 15 min

Densitometric evaluation:

Wavelength: UV–290 nm Scanning mode: Reflectance/Absorbance

HRF: Aspirin—24; Dipyridamole—67

Linearity (ng/band): Aspirin—65–390; Dipyridamole—75–375

Recovery (%): 97.08–99.72 for both the compounds

References: Anant P. Argekar and Shankar S. Kunjir, *J. Planar Chromatogr.* **9(1)**, 65–67, 1996.

Comments: The method validated for accuracy, precision, linearity, LOD, LOQ, specificity, robustness and ruggedness.

HPTLC : High Performance Thin Layer Chromatography
HPTLC Densitogram

No. 126

Aspirin

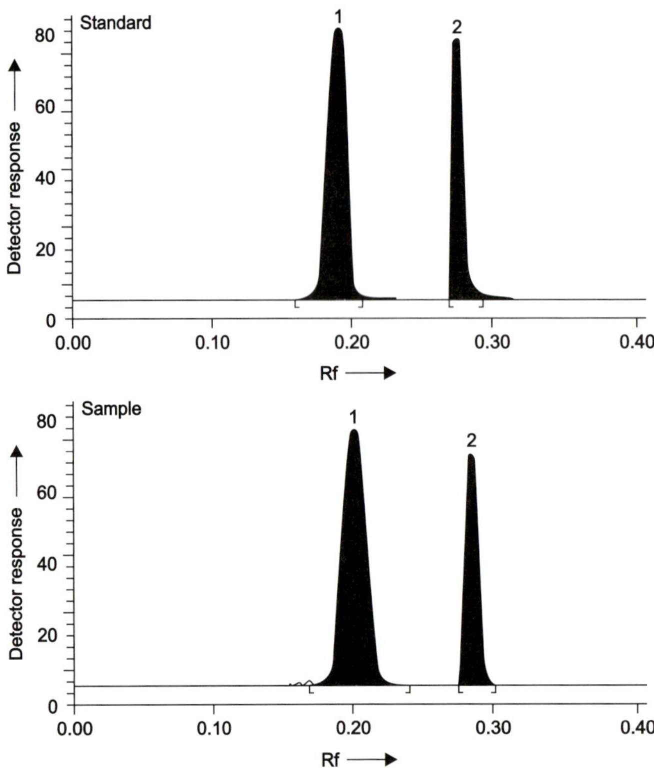

Typical densitogram of the sample and standard containing aspirin and dipyridamole. For detailed experimental and chromatographic conditions, refer to Protocol No. 126. Peaks identification: 1. Dipyridamole; 2. Aspirin.

PROTOCOL FOR HPTLC ANALYSIS OF PHARMACEUTICAL FORMULATION

Protocol No. 126

Formulation: Aspirin, Dipyridamole

Classification: Musculoskeletal Disorders **Dosage form:** Tablets

Standard preparation: Weigh accurately about 12 mg of aspirin (A) and about 15 mg of dipyridamol (D), dissolve in methanol to make 10 ml. Further dilute 1 ml to 10 ml with methanol and use for analysis.

Sample preparation: Weigh accurately powdered sample equivalent to 30 mg of aspirin, suspend in methanol, sonicate for 5 min and make up to 50 ml, filter and dilute 2 ml to 10 ml with methanol for chromatographic application.

Chromatographic equipments:

Sample applicator: Camag Linomat–IV

Development chamber: Camag twin-trough glass chamber, 10 × 10 cm

Densitometric scanner: Camag TLC Scanner–III

Chromatographic conditions:

1. Stationary phase: Silica gel $60F_{254}$ pre-coated HPTLC plates, 6 × 10 cm (200 μm) – Merck
2. Mobile phase (MP): Chloroform–methanol–glacial acetic acid (9.5 : 0.5 : 0.04 v/v)
3. Standard/Sample application:
   Band length: 10 mm Volume applied: 5 μl Spacing: 10 mm
4. Chamber saturation: 20 min (MP)
5. RH (%): 55 ± 5
6. Temperature °C: 22 ± 2
7. Separation technique: Ascending
8. Quantity of mobile phase: 10 ml
9. Migration distance: 50 mm
10. Migration time: 15 min

Densitometric evaluation:

Wavelength: UV–230 nm or 245 nm Scanning mode: Reflectance/Absorbance

HRF: Dipyridamole—19; Aspirin—29

Linearity (ng/band): Aspirin—100–600; Dipyridamole—100–750

Recovery (%): 99.70–101.60 for both the compounds

References: —

Comments:

- The method was optimized and analytical work carried out at **Anchrom's HPTLC Application Laboratory**, Mumbai, India.
- Several market samples of similar composition were analysed by the proposed method with reproducible results.

HPTLC : High Performance Thin Layer Chromatography
HPTLC Densitogram

No. 127

COOH

O

CH_3

O

Aspirin

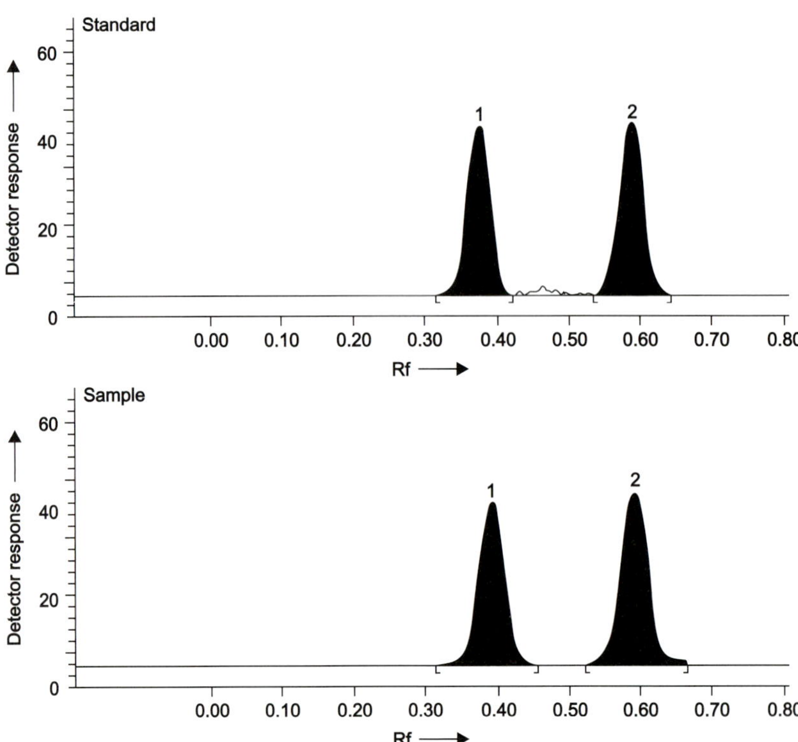

Typical densitogram of the sample and standard containing dipyridamole and aspirin. For detailed experimental and chromatographic conditions, refer to Protocol No. 127. Peaks identification: 1. Dipyridamole; 2. Aspirin.

PROTOCOL FOR HPTLC ANALYSIS OF PHARMACEUTICAL FORMULATION

Protocol No. 127

Formulation: Aspirin, Dipyridamole

Classification: Musculoskeletal Disorders **Dosage form:** Tablets

Standard preparation: Weigh accurately about 12 mg of aspirin (A) and about 15 mg of dipyridamol (D), dissolve in methanol to make 10 ml. Further dilute 1 ml to 10 ml with methanol and use for analysis.

Sample preparation: Weigh accurately powdered sample equivalent to 30 mg of aspirin, suspend in methanol, sonicate for 5 min and make up to 50 ml, filter and dilute 2 ml to 10 ml with methanol for chromatographic application.

Chromatographic equipments:

Sample applicator: Camag Linomat–IV

Development chamber: Camag twin-trough glass chamber, 10 × 10 cm

Densitometric scanner: Camag TLC Scanner–II

Chromatographic conditions:

1. Stationary phase: Silica gel 60 RP-18F_{254s} pre-coated HPTLC plates, 10 × 10 cm (200 μm) – Merck
2. Mobile phase (MP): 0.5 M sodium chloride–methanol–acetonitrile–glacial acetic acid (5 : 2 : 3 : 0.1 v/v)
3. Standard/Sample application:
   Band length: 5 mm Volume applied: 2 μl Spacing: 5 mm
4. Chamber saturation: 30 min (MP)
5. RH (%): 55 ± 5
6. Temperature °C: 22 ± 2
7. Separation technique: Ascending
8. Quantity of mobile phase: 10 ml
9. Migration distance: 50 mm
10. Migration time: 20 min

Densitometric evaluation:

Wavelength: UV–230 nm or 245 nm Scanning mode: Reflectance/Absorbance

HRF: Dipyridamole—40; Aspirin—60

Linearity (ng/band): Aspirin—100–600; Dipyridamole—100–750

Recovery (%): 98.25–101.75 for both the compounds

References: —

Comments:

- The method was optimized and analytical work carried out at **Anchrom's HPTLC Application Laboratory**, Mumbai, India.
- In NP-HPTLC, there are chances of hydrolysis of aspirin due to acidic nature of silica gel layer where as in RP-HPTLC, better stability of aspirin is assured. Further in RP-HPTLC, non chlorinated solvents are used.

HPTLC : High Performance Thin Layer Chromatography
HPTLC Densitogram

No. 128

Aspirin

Salicylic acid

Sulfosalicylic acid

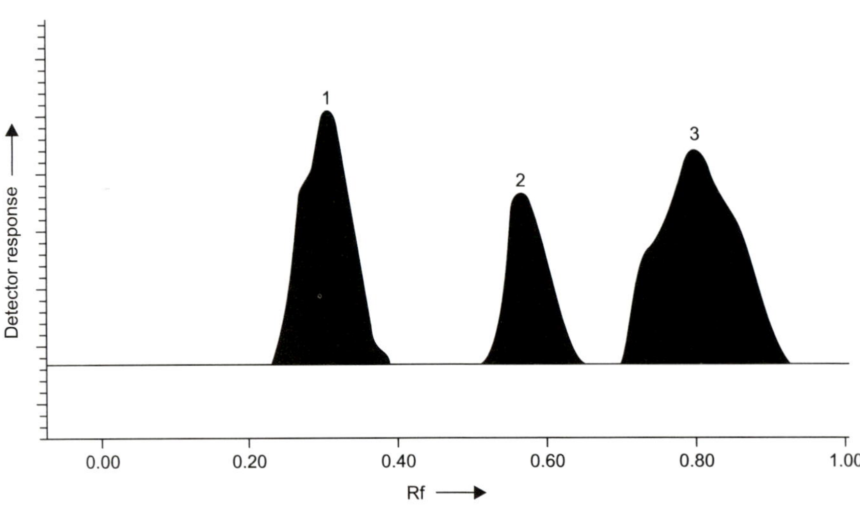

Typical densitogram of the sample containing aspirin, salicylic acid and sulfosalicylic acid. For detailed experimental and chromatographic conditions, refer to Protocol No. 128. Peaks identification: 1. Sulfosalicylic acid; 2. Salicylic acid; 3. Aspirin.

PROTOCOL FOR HPTLC ANALYSIS OF PHARMACEUTICAL FORMULATION

Protocol No. 128

Formulation: Aspirin, Salicylic acid, Sulfosalicylic acid

Classification: Musculoskeletal Disorders **Dosage form:** Tablets

Standard preparation: Prepare 1 mg/ml solution of each compound in ethanol. Further serial dilutions made to study linearity profile. Apply 10 μl of each solution.

Sample preparation: Powdered sample equivalent to 100 mg of aspirin extracted with ethanol, diluted and filtered. The filtrate suitably diluted with ethanol. Apply 10 μl of final solution for assay.

Chromatographic equipments:

Sample applicator: Camag Linomat–IV

Development chamber: Camag Flat solution glass chamber, 10 × 20 cm

Densitometric scanner: Camag TLC Scanner–II

Chromatographic conditions:

1. Stationary phase: Silica gel 60F_{254} pre-coated HPTLC plates, 10 × 20 cm (200 μm) – Merck, pre-washed with methanol–chloroform (1: 1) dried overnight, then impregnated by dipping in 2% boric acid w/v in ethanol, dried at 110°C for 60 min, prior to use
2. Mobile phase (MP): Chloroform–methanol–25% ammonia–water (12 : 7.5 : 0.2 : 0.6 v/v)
3. Standard/Sample application:
   Band length: 2 mm Volume applied: 10 μl Spacing: 10 mm
4. Chamber saturation: 30 min (MP)
5. RH (%): 55 ± 5
6. Temperature °C: 25 ± 2
7. Separation technique: Ascending
8. Quantity of mobile phase: 20 ml
9. Migration distance: 150 mm
10. Migration time: 35 min

Densitometric evaluation:

Wavelength: UV–254 nm Scanning mode: Reflectance/Absorbance

HRF: Sulfosalicylic acid—24; Salicylic acid—61; Aspirin—81

Linearity (ng/band): 100–1000 for all the three compounds

Recovery (%): 9875–101.25 for all the three compounds

References: Homayoo Ahmad Panahi, Atyeh Rahimi, Etham Moniri, Ahmad Izadi and Mohammad Mehdi Parvin, *J. Planar Chromatogr.*, **23(2)**, 137–140, 2010.

Comments:

- The method validated for accuracy, precision, linearity, LOD, LOQ, specificity, robustness and ruggedness.
- As the boric acid forms complex with α-hydroxy acids, both the acids get easily separated from aspirin.

HPTLC : High Performance Thin Layer Chromatography
HPTLC Densitogram

No. 129

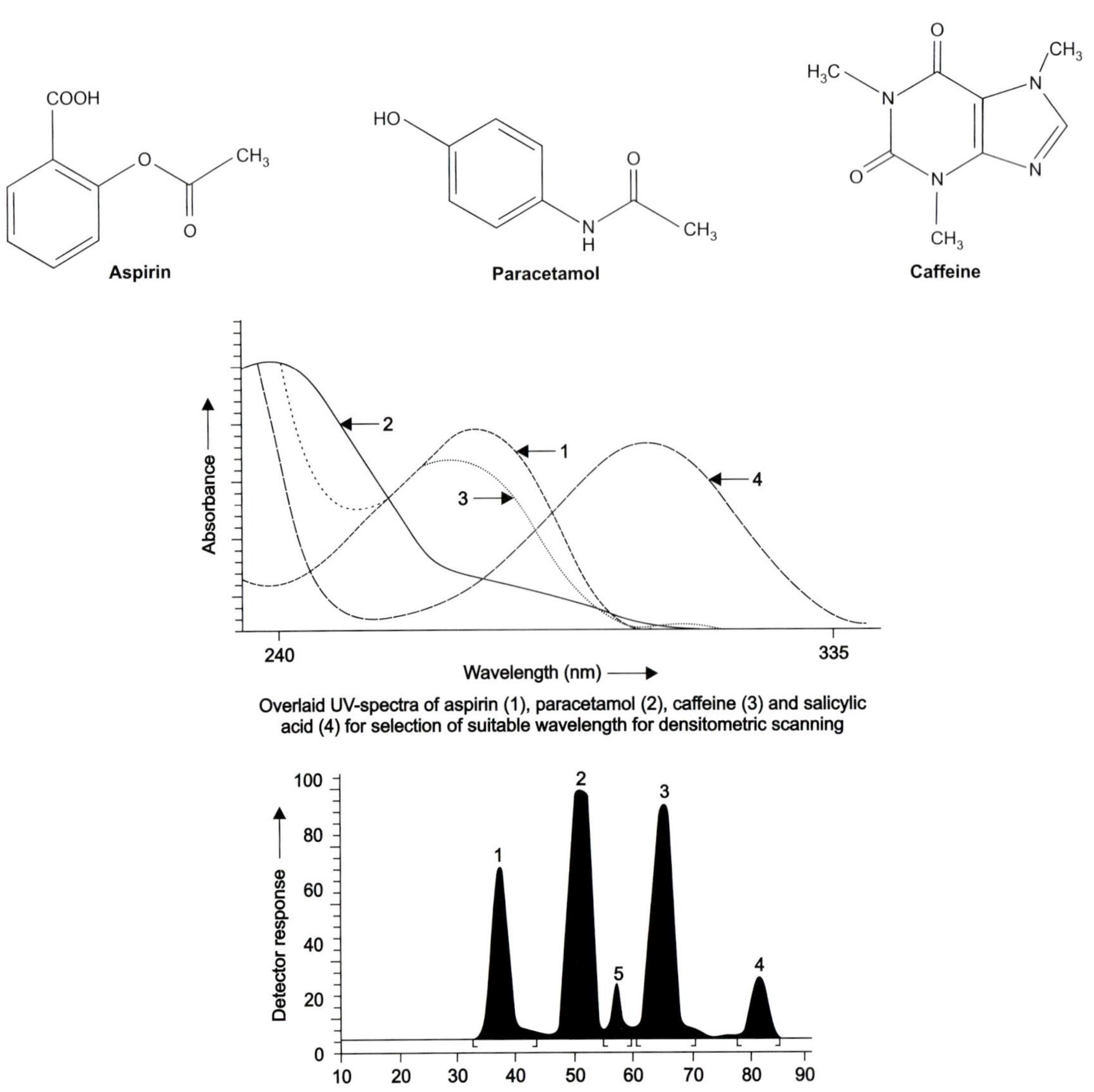

Overlaid UV-spectra of aspirin (1), paracetamol (2), caffeine (3) and salicylic acid (4) for selection of suitable wavelength for densitometric scanning

Typical densitogram of the sample containing aspirin, caffeine, paracetamol and phenobarbitone. For detailed experimental and chromatographic conditions, refer to Protocol No. 129. Peaks identification: 1. Aspirin; 2. Paracetamol; 3. Caffeine; 4. Phenobarbitone; 5. Salicylic acid.

PROTOCOL FOR HPTLC ANALYSIS OF PHARMACEUTICAL FORMULATION

Protocol No. 129

Formulation: Aspirin, Paracetamol, Caffeine, Phenobarbitone, Salicylic acid

Classification: Musculoskeletal Disorders **Dosage form:** Tablets

Standard preparation: Dissolve 25 mg of aspirin, 25 mg of paracetamol, 5 mg of caffeine and 2 mg of phenobarbitone in ethanol, make up the volume so that 1 μl of the final solution covers the linearity range as given below.

Sample preparation: Powdered sample equivalent to 250 mg of aspirin suspended in ethanol to produce 25 ml, filtered and further diluted as described under standard solution. Apply 1 μl of the solution for assay.

Chromatographic equipments:

Sample applicator: Camag nanomat–III

Development chamber: Camag flat bottom glass chamber, 20 × 20 cm

Densitometric scanner: Camag TLC Scanner–II

Chromatographic conditions:

1. Stationary phase: Silica gel $60F_{254}$ pre-coated HPTLC plates, 10 × 20 cm (200 μm) – Merck
2. Mobile phase (MP): Dichloromethane–ethyl acetate–cyclohexane–isopropanol–0.1 M HCl–fumaric acid (9 : 8 : 3 : 1.5 : 0.2 : 0.2 v/v)
3. Standard/Sample application:
   Band length: 5 mm Volume applied: 1–5 μl Spacing: 10 mm
4. Chamber saturation: 20 min (MP)
5. RH (%): 55 ± 5
6. Temperature °C: 25 ± 1
7. Separation technique: Ascending
8. Quantity of mobile phase: 20 ml
9. Migration distance: 90 mm
10. Migration time: 25 min

Densitometric evaluation:

Wavelength: UV–207 nm Scanning mode: Reflectance/Absorbance

HRF: See densitogram

Linearity (ng/band): Aspirin—200–1000; Paracetamol—200–1000; Caffeine—40–200; Phenobarbitone—400–2000

Recovery (%): 97.48–98.14 for all the compound

References: J.T. Franeta, D.D. Agbaba, S.M. Eric, S.P. Pavkov, S.D. Vladimirov and M.B. Aleksic, *J. Pharm. Biomed. Anal.*, **24**, 1169–1173, 2001.

Comments: The method validated for accuracy, precision, linearity, LOD, LOQ, specificity, robustness and ruggedness.

HPTLC : High Performance Thin Layer Chromatography
HPTLC Densitogram

No. 130

Rofecoxib

Tizanidine

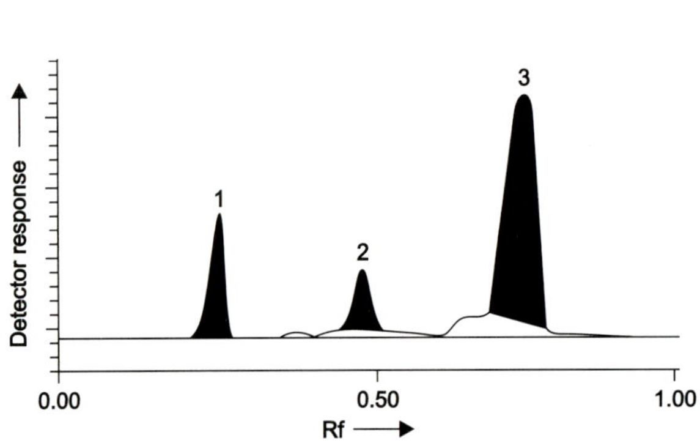

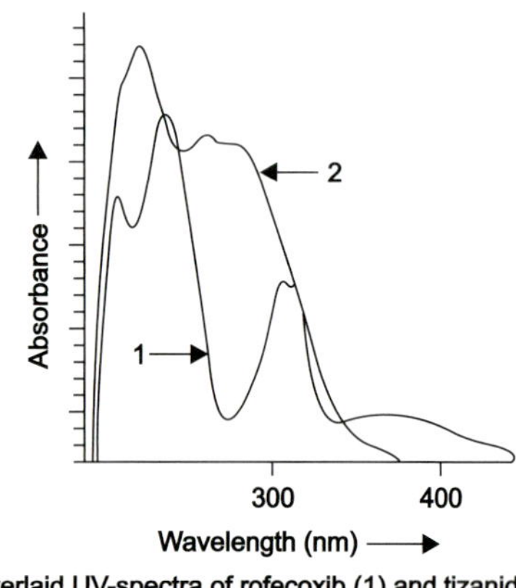

Overlaid UV-spectra of rofecoxib (1) and tizanidine (2) for selection of suitable wavelength for densitometric scanning

Typical densitogram of the standard containing rofecoxib and tizanidine. For detailed experimental and chromatographic conditions, refer to Protocol No. 130. Peaks identification: 1. Rosiglitazone (IS); 2. Tizanidine; 3. Rofecoxib.

PROTOCOL FOR HPTLC ANALYSIS OF PHARMACEUTICAL FORMULATION

Protocol No. 130

Formulation: Tizanidine hydrochloride, Rofecoxib

Classification: Musculoskeletal Disorders **Dosage form:** Tablets

Standard preparation: Prepare working standard solution of each compound separately in methanol to get 2500 μg/ml of rofecoxib and 200 μg/ml of tizanidine. The final solution should contain 500 μg/ml of (IS). Apply varying volumes for linearity profile.

Sample preparation: Accurately weighed powdered sample suspended in methanol, sonicated, add (IS) solution, dilute, filter, the filtrate used for chromatographic separation and densitometric measurements.

Chromatographic equipments:

Sample applicator: Camag Linomat–IV

Development chamber: Camag twin-trough glass chamber, 20 × 10 cm

Densitometric scanner: Camag TLC Scanner–III

Chromatographic conditions:

1. Stationary phase: Silica gel $60F_{254}$ pre-coated HPTLC plates, 10 × 10 cm (200 μm) – Merck, pre-washed with methanol, activated at 110°C prior to use
2. Mobile phase (MP): Toluene–ethyl acetate methanol–triethylamine (6 : 3 : 0.5 : 0.1 v/v)
3. Standard/Sample application:
   Band length: 5 mm Volume applied: 3 μl Spacing: 10 mm
4. Chamber saturation: 15 min (MP)
5. RH (%): 55 ± 5
6. Temperature °C: 22 ± 2
7. Separation technique: Ascending
8. Quantity of mobile phase: 20 ml
9. Migration distance: 80 mm
10. Migration time: 20 min

Densitometric evaluation:

Wavelength: UV–235 nm Scanning mode: Reflectance/Absorbance

HRF: Rosiglitazone (IS)—27; Tizanidine—49; Rofecoxib–68

Linearity (ng/band): Rofecoxib—3.75–11.25; Tizanidine—0.3–0.9

Recovery (%): 98.75–101.55 for both the compounds

References: Uttam D. Pawar, Aruna V. Sulebhavikar, Abhijit V. Naik, Satish G. Pingale and Kiran V. Mangaonkar, *E.J. Chem.*, **6(1)**, 295–302, 2009.

Comments: The method validated for accuracy, precision, linearity, LOD, LOQ, specificity, robustness and ruggedness.

HPTLC : High Performance Thin Layer Chromatography
HPTLC Densitogram

No. 131

Rofecoxib

Tizanidine

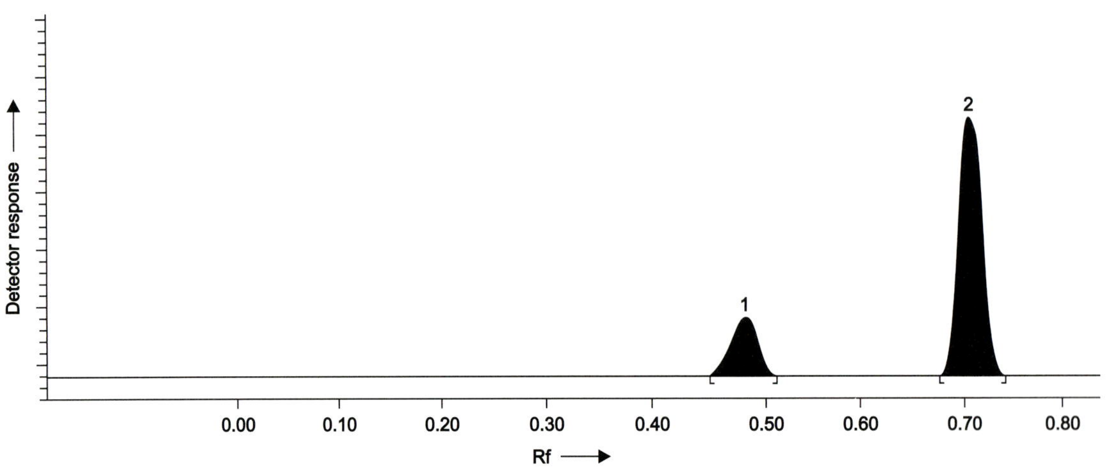

Typical densitogram of the sample containing rofecoxib and tizanidine hydrochloride. For detailed experimental and chromatographic conditions, refer to Protocol No. 131. Peaks identification: 1. Tizanidine HCl; 2. Rofecoxib.

PROTOCOL FOR HPTLC ANALYSIS OF PHARMACEUTICAL FORMULATION

Protocol No. 131

Formulation: **Tizanidine hydrochloride, Rofecoxib**

Classification: Musculoskeletal Disorders **Dosage form:** Tablets

Standard preparation: Prepare 100 μg/ml solution of each compound in methanol. Further serial dilutions are made with methanol for linearity profile. Apply 10 μl of each solution.

Sample preparation: Powdered sample equivalent to 2 mg of tizanidine HCl suspended in methanol, sonicated, diluted and filtered. The filtrate suitably diluted for assay. Apply 10 μl for chromatographic separation and assay.

Chromatographic equipments:

Sample applicator: Camag Linomat–IV

Development chamber: Camag twin-trough glass chamber, 10 × 10 cm

Densitometric scanner: Camag TLC Scanner–III

Chromatographic conditions:

1. Stationary phase: Silica gel $60F_{254}$ pre-coated HPTLC plates, 10 × 10 cm (200 μm) – Merck, pre-washed with methanol, dried prior to use
2. Mobile phase (MP): Methanol–acetone (1 : 1 v/v)
3. Standard/Sample application:
   Band length: 10 mm Volume applied: 10 μl Spacing: 10 mm
4. Chamber saturation: 20 min (MP)
5. RH (%): 55 ± 5
6. Temperature °C: 22 ± 2
7. Separation technique: Ascending
8. Quantity of mobile phase: 10 ml
9. Migration distance: 80 mm
10. Migration time: 15 min

Densitometric evaluation:

Wavelength: UV–254 nm Scanning mode: Reflectance/Absorbance

HRF: Tizanidine HCl—48; Rofecoxib—69

Linearity (ng/band): Rofecoxib—20–320; Tizanidine HCl—2–26

Recovery (%): 99.60–101.95 for both the compounds

References: C. Roosewelt, N. Harikrishnan et al., *Asian J. Chem.*, **19(6)**, 4286–4290, 2007.

Comments: The method validated for accuracy, precision, linearity, LOD, LOQ, specificity, robustness and ruggedness.

HPTLC : High Performance Thin Layer Chromatography
HPTLC Densitogram

No. 132

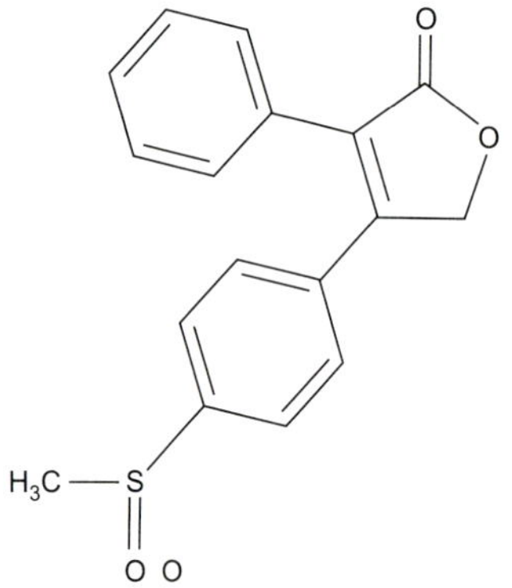

Rofecoxib

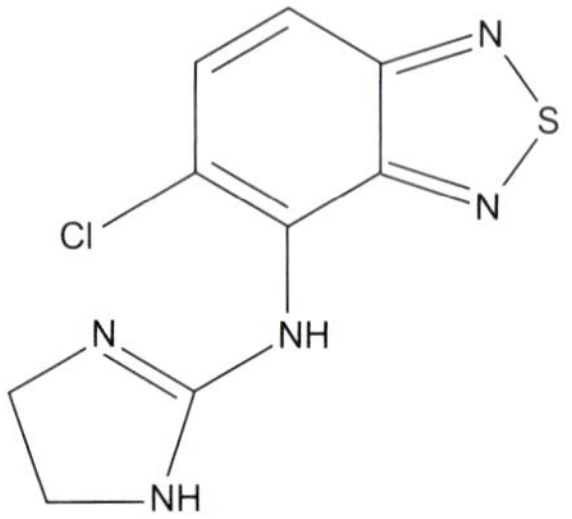

Tizanidine

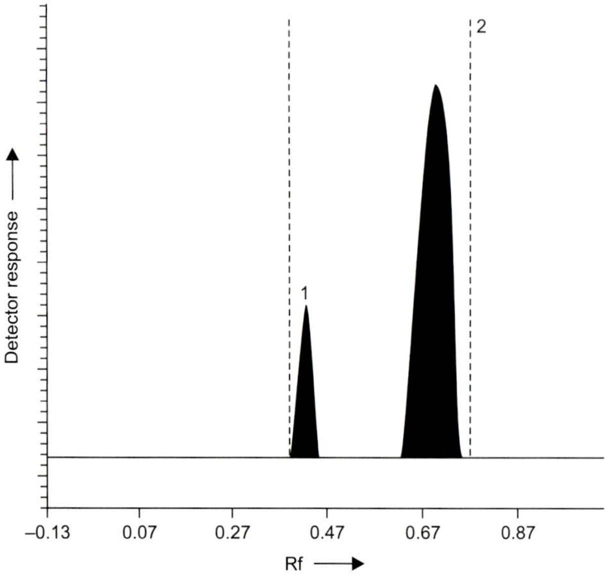

Typical densitogram of the sample containing rofecoxib and tizanidine hydrochloride. For detailed experimental and chromatographic conditions, refer to Protocol No. 132. Peaks identification: 1. Tizanidine HCl; 2. Rofecoxib.

PROTOCOL FOR HPTLC ANALYSIS OF PHARMACEUTICAL FORMULATION

Protocol No. 132

Formulation: **Tizanidine hydrochloride, Rofecoxib**

Classification: Musculoskeletal Disorders **Dosage form:** Tablets

Standard preparation: Prepare 100 μg/ml solution of each compound in methanol. Further serial dilutions are made with methanol for linearity profile. Apply 10 μl of each solution.

Sample preparation: Powdered sample equivalent to 2 mg of tizanidine HCl suspended in methanol, sonicated, diluted and filtered. The filtrate suitably diluted for assay. Apply 10 μl for chromatographic separation.

Chromatographic equipments:

Sample applicator: Camag Linomat–V

Development chamber: Camag twin-trough glass chamber, 10 × 10 cm

Densitometric scanner: Camag TLC Scanner–III

Chromatographic conditions:

1. Stationary phase: Silica gel $60F_{254}$ pre-coated TLC plates, 10 × 10 cm (250 μm) – Merck, pre-washed with methanol and heated at 115°C for 30 min, prior to use
2. Mobile phase (MP): n-Butyl acetate–formic acid–chloroform (6 : 4 : 2 v/v)
3. Standard/Sample application:
   Band length: 10 mm Volume applied: 10 μl Spacing: 10 mm
4. Chamber saturation: 20 min (MP)
5. RH (%): 55
6. Temperature °C: 22 ± 2
7. Separation technique: Ascending
8. Quantity of mobile phase: 12 ml
9. Migration distance: 70 mm
10. Migration time: 15 min

Densitometric evaluation:

Wavelength: UV–315 nm Scanning mode: Reflectance/Absorbance

HRF: Tizanidine HCl—41; Rofecoxib—69

Linearity (ng/band): Rofecoxib—16–40; Tizanidine HCl—2–10

Recovery (%): 98.4–101.0 for both the compounds

References: T.K. Ravi, M. Gandhimathi, K.R. Sireesha and Shaise Jacob, *Ind. J. Pharm. Sci.*, **68(2)**, 234–236, 2006.

Comments: The method validated for accuracy, precision, linearity, LOD, LOQ, specificity, robustness and ruggedness.

HPTLC : High Performance Thin Layer Chromatography
HPTLC Densitogram

No. 133

H$_3$C—S(=O)(=O) … O

Rofecoxib

N, S, N, Cl, NH, N, NH

Tizanidine

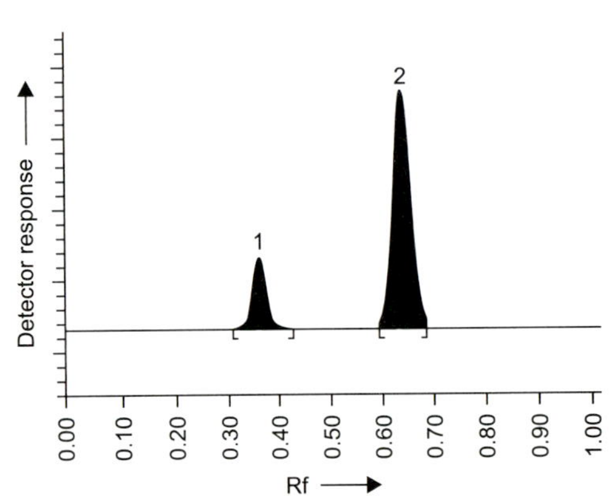

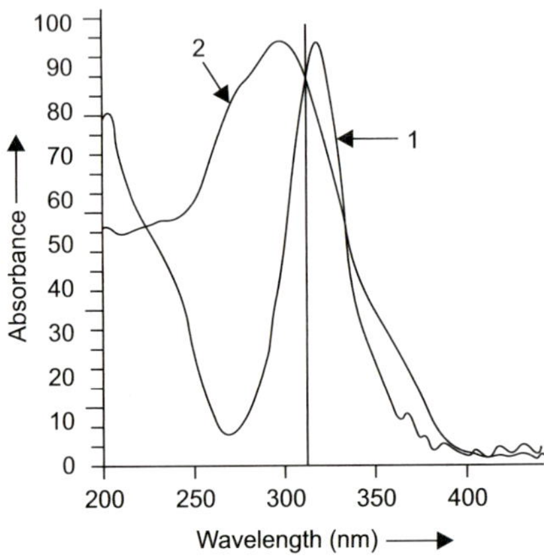

Overlaid UV-spectra of rofecoxib (1) and tizanidine (2) for selection of suitable wavelength for densitometric scanning

Typical densitogram of the sample containing tizanidine and rofecoxib. For detailed experimental and chromatographic conditions, refer to Protocol No. 133. Peaks identification: 1. Tizanidine; 2. Rofecoxib.

PROTOCOL FOR HPTLC ANALYSIS OF PHARMACEUTICAL FORMULATION

Protocol No. 133

Formulation: Tizanidine hydrochloride, Rofecoxib

Classification: Musculoskeletal Disorders **Dosage form:** Tablets

Standard preparation: Prepare 2 mg/ml solution of each compound separately in methanol. Further serial dilutions are made to get 10–100 μg/ml (tizanidine) and 100–1500 μg/ml (rofecoxib). Apply 1 μl of each solution for linearity profile.

Sample preparation: Powdered sample equivalent to 2 mg of tizanidine suspended in methanol, sonicated for 5 min, diluted, filtered and filtrate suitably diluted to get concentration of each within linearity range. Apply 2 μl for assay.

Chromatographic equipments:

Sample applicator: Camag Linomat–V

Development chamber: Camag twin-trough glass chamber, 20 × 10 cm

Densitometric scanner: Camag TLC Scanner–III

Chromatographic conditions:

1. Stationary phase: Silica gel $60F_{254}$ pre-coated TLC plates, 20 × 10 cm (250 μm) – Merck, pre-washed with methanol, dried at 110°C for 5 min prior to use
2. Mobile phase (MP): Toluene methanol–acetone (7.5 : 2.5 : 1.0 v/v)
3. Standard/Sample application:
   Band length: 6 mm Volume applied: 1–4 μl Spacing: 5 mm
4. Chamber saturation: 30 min (MP)
5. RH (%): 60 ± 5
6. Temperature °C: 25 ± 2
7. Separation technique: Ascending
8. Quantity of mobile phase: 22 ml
9. Migration distance: 90 mm
10. Migration time: 30 min

Densitometric evaluation:

Wavelength: UV–311 nm (iso-absorption point)

Scanning mode: Reflectance/Absorbance

HRF: Tizanidine HCl—36; Rofecoxib—65

Linearity (ng/band): Rofecoxib—100–1500; Tizanidine HCl—10–100

Recovery (%): Rofecoxib—99.52–101.98; Tizanidine HCl—99.41–100.57

References: Neeraj Kaul, S.R. Dhaneshwar, Himani Agrawal, Abhijit Kakad and Bharat Patil, *J. Pharm. Biomed. Anal.*, **37**, 27–38, 2005.

Comments:

- The method validated for accuracy, precision, linearity, LOD, LOQ, specificity, robustness and ruggedness.
- The analytical results were comparable with RP–HPLC method, performed separately.

HPTLC : High Performance Thin Layer Chromatography
HPTLC Densitogram

No. 134

Rofecoxib

Tizanidine

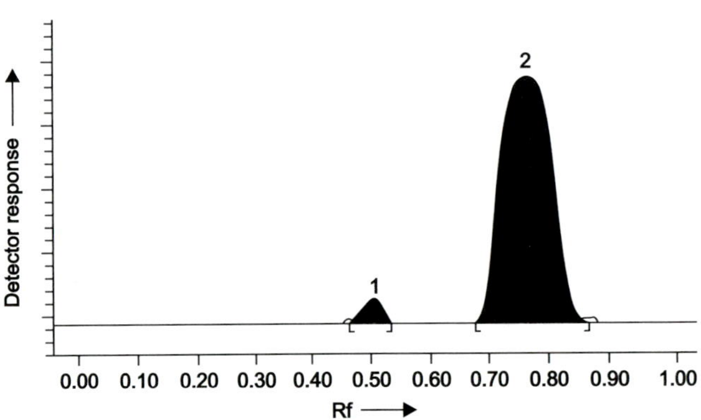

Typical densitogram of the standard containing rofecoxib and tizanidine HCl. For detailed experimental and chromatographic conditions, refer to Protocol No. 134. Peaks identification: 1. Tizanidine HCl; 2. Rofecoxib.

PROTOCOL FOR HPTLC ANALYSIS OF PHARMACEUTICAL FORMULATION

Protocol No. 134

Formulation: Tizanidine hydrochloride, Rofecoxib

Classification: Musculoskeletal Disorders **Dosage form:** Tablets

Standard preparation: Prepare 1 mg/ml solution of each compound in methanol. Further serial dilutions made for linearity profile. Apply 5 μl of each solution.

Sample preparation: Powdered sample equivalent to 25 mg of rofecoxib suspended in methanol, sonicated for 5 min, diluted, filtered and filtrate suitably diluted for assay. Apply 5 μl for separation.

Chromatographic equipments:

Sample applicator: Camag Linomat–V

Development chamber: Camag twin-trough glass chamber, 20 × 10 cm

Densitometric scanner: Camag TLC Scanner–III

Chromatographic conditions:

1. Stationary phase: Silica gel 60F_{254} pre-coated TLC plates, 20 × 10 cm (250 μm) – Merck, pre-washed with methanol, dried at 50°C for 5 min, prior to use
2. Mobile phase (MP): Methanol–acetone (1 : 1 v/v)
3. Standard/Sample application:
   Band length: 5 mm Volume applied: 5 μl Spacing: 10 mm
4. Chamber saturation: 30 min (MP)
5. RH (%): 60 ± 5
6. Temperature °C: 22 ± 2
7. Separation technique: Ascending
8. Quantity of mobile phase: 16 ml
9. Migration distance: 72 mm
10. Migration time: 15 min

Densitometric evaluation:

Wavelength: UV–254 nm Scanning mode: Reflectance/Absorbance

HRF: Tizanidine HCl—50; Rofecoxib—78

Linearity (μg/band): Rofecoxib—2.2–3; Tizanidine HCl—0.18–0.26

Recovery (%): 99.44–102.68 for both the compound

References: A. Lakshmana Rao and D. Praveena Varma, *Int. J. Chem. Sci.*, **7(2)**, 986–992, 2009.

Comments: The method validated for accuracy, precision, linearity, LOD, LOQ, specificity, robustness and ruggedness.

HPTLC : High Performance Thin Layer Chromatography
HPTLC Densitogram

No. 136

COONa H N Cl Cl

Diclofenac sodium

N S N Cl NH N NH

Tizanidine

Absorbance
2
1
200 240 280 320
Wavelength (nm)

Overlaid UV-spectra of tizanidine hydrochloride (1) and diclofenac sodium (2) in methanol for selection of suitable wavelength for densitometric scanning

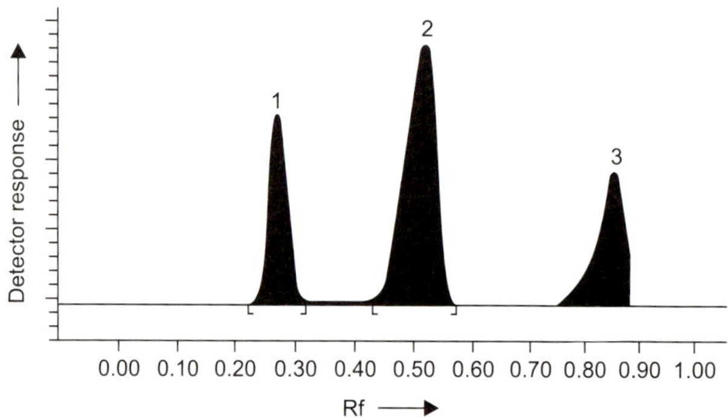

Typical densitogram of the sample containing diclofenac sodium and tizanidine HCl. For detailed experimental and chromatographic conditions, refer to Protocol No. 136. Peaks identification: 1. Tizanidine HCl; 2. Cetirizine (IS); 3. Diclofenac sodium.

PROTOCOL FOR HPTLC ANALYSIS OF PHARMACEUTICAL FORMULATION

Protocol No. 136

Formulation: **Tizanidine hydrochloride, Diclofenac sodium**

Classification: Musculoskeletal Disorders **Dosage form:** Tablets

Standard preparation: Prepare standard solution of each compound in methanol to get 100 μg/ml of diclofenac sodium and tizanidine and 1000 μg/ml of cetirizine (IS). Further dilute with methanol to get 50 μg/ml of diclofenac, 4 μg/ml of tizanidine and 50 μg/ml of (IS). Apply varying volumes for linearity profile.

Sample preparation: Powdered sample equivalent to 2 mg of tizanidine suspended in methanol, sonicated, diluted suitably and filtered. The filtrate used for chromatographic analysis.

Chromatographic equipments:

Sample applicator: Camag Linomat–IV

Development chamber: Camag twin-trough glass chamber, 10 × 10 cm

Densitometric scanner: Camag TLC Scanner–III

Chromatographic conditions:

1. Stationary phase: Silica gel $60F_{254}$ pre-coated TLC plates, 10 × 10 cm (250 μm) – Merck, pre-washed with methanol, dried at 60°C for 5 min, prior to use
2. Mobile phase (MP): Chloroform–methanol (8 : 2 v/v)
3. Standard/Sample application:
   Band length: 5 mm Volume applied: 5 μl Spacing: 5 mm
4. Chamber saturation: 30 min (MP)
5. RH (%): 60 ± 5
6. Temperature °C: 25 ± 2
7. Separation technique: Ascending
8. Quantity of mobile phase: 15 ml
9. Migration distance: 80 mm
10. Migration time: 20 min

Densitometric evaluation:

Wavelength: UV–230 nm Scanning mode: Reflectance/Absorbance

HRF: Tizanidine HCl—26; Cetirizine (IS)—52; Diclofenac sodium—86

Linearity (ng/band): Tizanidine HCl—10–40; Diclofenac sodium—125–375

Recovery (%): 99.04–99.1 for both the compounds

References: M.K. Senthil, G. Subramanian, M. Vasudevan Ravindran, *Indian Drugs*, **42(7)**, 465–468, 2006.

Comments: The method validated for accuracy, precision, linearity, LOD, LOQ, specificity, robustness and ruggedness.

HPTLC : High Performance Thin Layer Chromatography
HPTLC Densitogram

No. 137

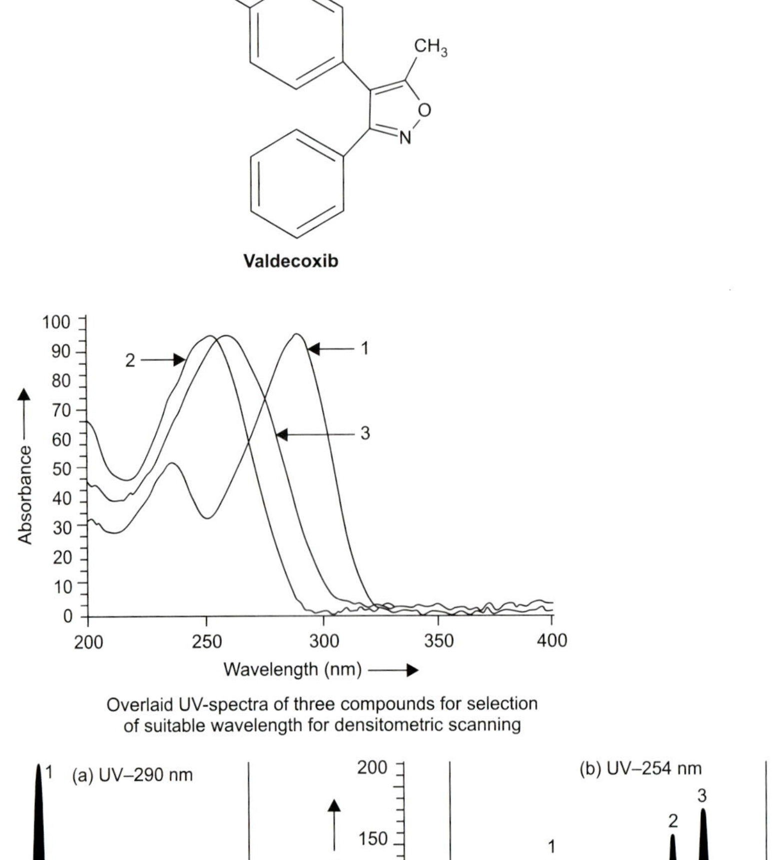

Overlaid UV-spectra of three compounds for selection of suitable wavelength for densitometric scanning

Typical densitogram (a and b) of the standard containing three different COX–2 inhibitors. For detailed experimental and chromatographic conditions, refer to Protocol No. 137. Peaks identification: 1. Etoricoxib (E); 2. Valdecoxib (V); 3. Celecoxib (C).

PROTOCOL FOR HPTLC ANALYSIS OF PHARMACEUTICAL FORMULATION

Protocol No. 137

Formulation: **Valdecoxib, Celecoxib, Etoricoxib (COX-2 inhibitors)**

Classification: Musculoskeletal Disorders **Dosage form:** Tablets

Standard preparation: Prepare 1 mg/ml solution of each compound in methanol. Further serial dilutions are made with methanol and used for analysis. Apply 5 μl of each solution.

Sample preparation: Powdered sample equivalent to 10 mg of one of the active compounds suspended in methanol, sonicated, diluted, filtered and used for analysis.

Chromatographic equipments:

Sample applicator: Camag Linomat-V

Development chamber: Flat-bottomed glass chamber, 18 × 9 × 18 cm (Sigma-Aldrich)

Densitometric scanner: Camag TLC Scanner-III

Chromatographic conditions:

1. Stationary phase: Silica gel $60F_{254}$ pre-coated TLC plates, 9 × 11 cm (250 μm) – Merck
2. Mobile phase (MP): Chloroform–acetone–toluene (12 : 5 : 2 v/v)
3. Standard/Sample application:
   Band length: 10 mm Volume applied: 5 μl Spacing: 8 mm
4. Chamber saturation: 15 min (MP)
5. RH (%): 55 ± 5
6. Temperature °C: 25 ± 2
7. Separation technique: Ascending
8. Quantity of mobile phase: 19 ml
9. Migration distance: 100 mm
10. Migration time: 30 min

Densitometric evaluation:

Wavelength: UV–254 nm and 290 nm Scanning mode: Reflectance/Absorbance

HRF: Etoricoxib—32; Valdecoxib—57; Celecoxib—65

Linearity (ng/band): Etoricoxib—20–600; Valdecoxib—40–500; Celecoxib—40–600

Recovery (%): 99.16–100.48 for all the three compounds

References: Malgorzata Starck and Marck Rejdych, *J. Planar Chromatogr.*, **22(6)**, 399–403, 2009.

Comments: The method validated for accuracy, precision, linearity, LOD, LOQ, specificity, robustness and ruggedness.

HPTLC : High Performance Thin Layer Chromatography
HPTLC Densitogram

No. 138

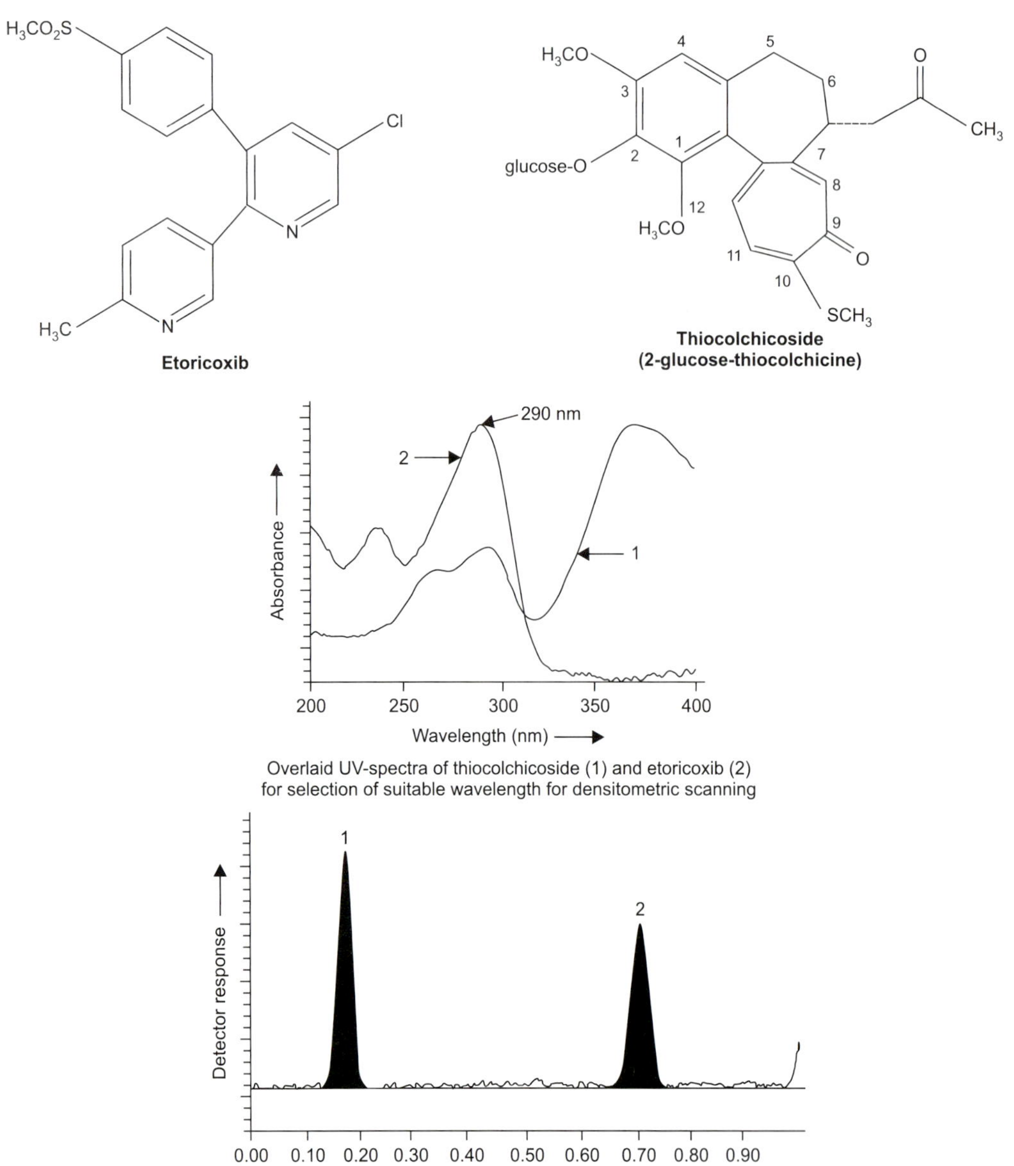

Overlaid UV-spectra of thiocolchicoside (1) and etoricoxib (2) for selection of suitable wavelength for densitometric scanning

Typical densitogram of the standard containing thiocolchicoside and etoricoxib. For detailed experimental and chromatographic conditions, refer to Protocol No. 138. Peaks identification: 1. Thiocolchicoside; 2. Etoricoxib.

PROTOCOL FOR HPTLC ANALYSIS OF PHARMACEUTICAL FORMULATION

Protocol No. 138

Formulation: Thiocolchicoside, Etoricoxib

Classification: Musculoskeletal Disorders **Dosage form:** Tablets

Standard preparation: Prepare 1 mg/ml solution of each compound separately in methanol. Further dilute to get 25 μg/ml of etoricoxib and 50 μg/ml of thiocolchicoside. Apply varying volumes (1–10 μl) for linearity profile.

Sample preparation: Powdered sample equivalent to 10 mg of etoricoxib suspended in methanol, sonicated, diluted to 10 ml, filtered and the filtrate applied for chromatographic evaluation.

Chromatographic equipments:

Sample applicator: Camag Linomat–IV

Development chamber: Camag twin-trough glass chamber, 20 × 10 cm

Densitometric scanner: Camag TLC Scanner–III

Chromatographic conditions:

1. Stationary phase: Silica gel $60F_{254}$ pre-coated TLC plates, 20 × 10 cm (250 μm) – Merck, pre-washed with methanol, dried at 110°C for 5 min prior to use
2. Mobile phase (MP): Ethyl acetate–methanol (8 : 2 v/v)
3. Standard/Sample application:
   Band length: 6 mm Volume applied: 1–10 μl Spacing: 6 mm
4. Chamber saturation: 20 min (MP)
5. RH (%): 55 ± 2
6. Temperature °C: 22 ± 2
7. Separation technique: Ascending
8. Quantity of mobile phase: 20 ml
9. Migration distance: 90 mm
10. Migration time: 20 min

Densitometric evaluation:

Wavelength: UV–290 nm Scanning mode: Reflectance/Absorbance

HRF: Thiocolchicoside—17; Etoricoxib—70

Linearity (ng/band): Thiocolchicoside—100–500; Etoricoxib—50–250

Recovery (%): 98.66–101.10 for both the compounds

References: Vivek S. Pajmane, Santosh V. Gandhi, Upasana P. Patil and Mahima R. Sengar, *J. AOAC. Int.*, **93(3)**, 783–786, 2010.

Comments:

- The method validated for accuracy, precision, linearity, LOD, LOQ, specificity, robustness and ruggedness.
- Santosh V. Gandhi et. al have reported HPTLC method for analysis of thiocolchicoside and etodolac using toluene-methanol (7.5 : 2.5 v/v) as mobile phase (Pharma Review, Oct., 2012–accpted).

HPTLC : High Performance Thin Layer Chromatography
HPTLC Densitogram

No. 139

Etoricoxib

Thiocolchicoside (2-glucose-thiocolchicine)

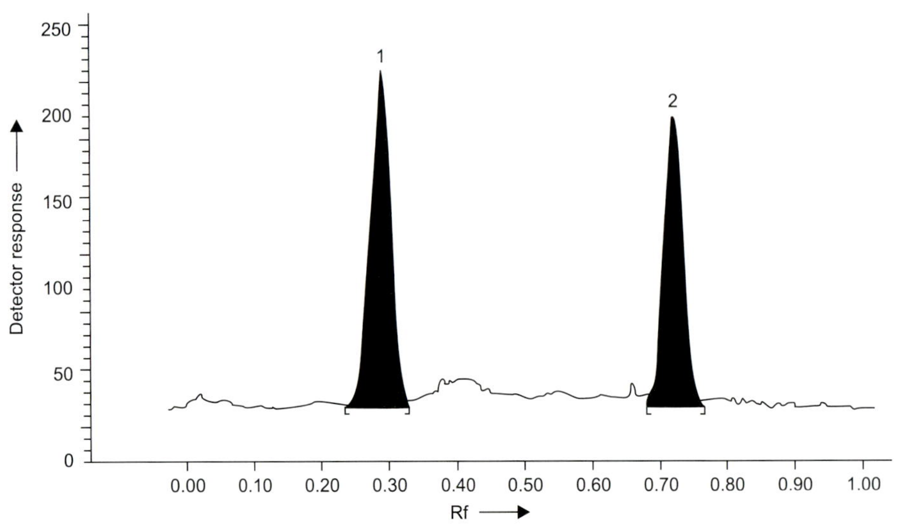

Typical densitogram of the sample containing thiocolchicoside and etoricoxib. For detailed experimental and chromatographic conditions, refer to Protocol No. 139. Peaks identification: 1. Thiocolchicoside; 2. Etoricoxib.

PROTOCOL FOR HPTLC ANALYSIS OF PHARMACEUTICAL FORMULATION

Protocol No. 139

Formulation: Thiocolchicoside, Etoricoxib

Classification: Musculoskeletal Disorders **Dosage form:** Tablets

Standard preparation: Prepare 1 mg/ml solution of each compound in methanol. Further dilute each solution with methanol to get 10 μg/ml. Apply varying volumes (5–10 μl) of each solution for linearity profile.

Sample preparation: Powdered sample equivalent to 10 mg of etoricoxib suspended in 5 ml of methanol, sonicated for 10 min, diluted to 10 ml, centrifuged for 5 min and supernatant suitably diluted with methanol and used for assay.

Chromatographic equipments:

Sample applicator: Camag Linomat–V

Development chamber: Camag twin-trough glass chamber, 10 × 10 cm

Densitometric scanner: Camag TLC Scanner–III

Chromatographic conditions:

1. Stationary phase: Silica gel $60F_{254}$ pre-coated TLC plates, 10 × 10 cm (250 μm) – Merck
2. Mobile phase (MP): Toluene–chloroform–methanol (3 : 6 : 2 v/v)
3. Standard/Sample application:
   Band length: 5 mm Volume applied: 5 μl Spacing: 5 mm
4. Chamber saturation: 30 min (MP)
5. RH (%): 60 ± 5
6. Temperature °C: 25 ± 2
7. Separation technique: Ascending
8. Quantity of mobile phase: 11 ml
9. Migration distance: 80 mm
10. Migration time: 20 min

Densitometric evaluation:

Wavelength: UV–314 nm Scanning mode: Reflectance/Absorbance

HRF: Thiocolchicoside—32; Etoricoxib—70

Linearity (ng/band): 50–100 for both the substances

Recovery (%): 98.86–100.22 for both the substances

References: K.R. Ambad and S.R. Dhaneshwar, Abstract No. F 281, 63rd IPC, 2011. Courtesy Prof. S.R. Dhaneshwar.

Comments: The method validated for accuracy, precision, linearity, LOD, LOQ, specificity, robustness and ruggedness.

HPTLC : High Performance Thin Layer Chromatography
HPTLC Densitogram

No. 140

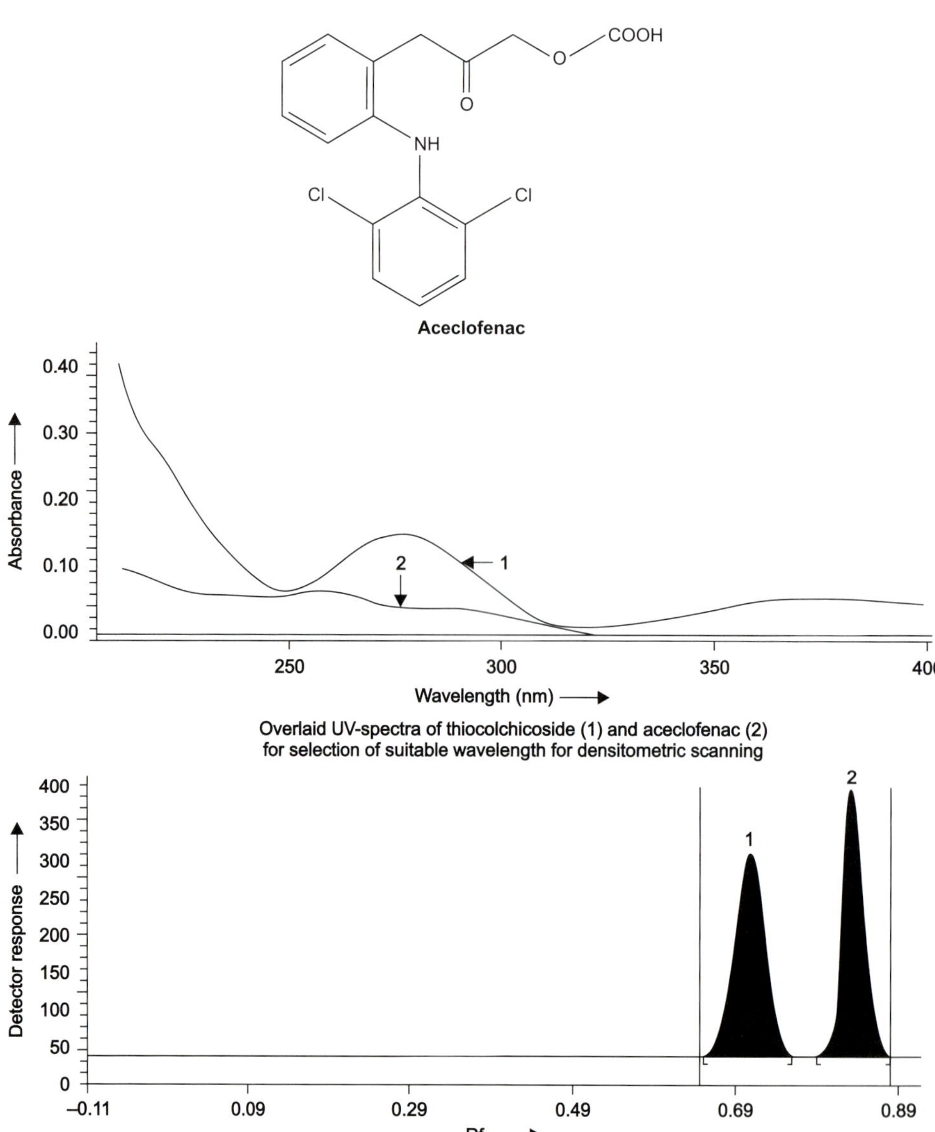

Typical densitogram of the standard containing thiocolchicoside and aceclofenac. For detailed experimental and chromatographic conditions, refer to Protocol No. 140. Peaks identification: 1. Thiocolchicoside; 2. Aceclofenac.

PROTOCOL FOR HPTLC ANALYSIS OF PHARMACEUTICAL FORMULATION

Protocol No. 140

Formulation: Thiocolchicoside, Aceclofenac

Classification: Musculoskeletal Disorders **Dosage form:** Tablets

Standard preparation: Prepare 1 mg/ml solution of each compound in methanol. Further dilutions made with methanol to get 100 μg/ml. Apply varying volumes of standard solutions for linearity studies.

Sample preparation: Powdered sample equivalent to 4 mg of thiocolchicoside was suspended in 40 ml of methanol, sonicated for 10 min, filtered and diluted to 50 ml with methanol. Further dilute with methanol to get 4 μg/ml of thiocolchicoside and 100 μg/ml of aceclofenac. Apply adequate volume for chromatographic analysis.

Chromatographic equipments:

Sample applicator: Camag Linomat–V

Development chamber: Camag twin-trough glass chamber, 10 × 10 cm

Densitometric scanner: Camag TLC Scanner–III

Chromatographic conditions:

1. Stationary phase: Silica gel $60F_{254}$ pre-coated TLC plates, 10 × 10 cm (250 μm) – Merck
2. Mobile phase (MP): Methanol–chloroform–water (9.6 : 0.2 : 0.2 v/v)
3. Standard/Sample application:
   Band length: 6 mm Volume applied: 5 μl Spacing: 12 mm
4. Chamber saturation: 30 min (MP)
5. RH (%): 60 ± 5
6. Temperature °C: 25 ± 2
7. Separation technique: Ascending
8. Quantity of mobile phase: 10 ml
9. Migration distance: 85 mm
10. Migration time: 20 min

Densitometric evaluation:

Wavelength: UV–254 nm Scanning mode: Reflectance/Absorbance

HRF: Thiocolchicoside—70; Aceclofenac—83

Linearity (ng/band): Thiocolchicoside—30–180; Aceclofenac—750–4500

Recovery (%): 98.7–101.2 for both the drugs

References: Pratima Syal, Madhusmita Sahoo, Rahul P. Raut, Asawaree A. Hable, Amruta S. Battewar, Vishnu P. Choudhari and Bhanudas S. Kuchekar, *J. Planar Chromatogr.*, **25(2)**, 133–137, 2012.

Comments: The method validated for accuracy, precision, linearity, LOD, LOQ, specificity, robustness and ruggedness.

HPTLC : High Performance Thin Layer Chromatography
HPTLC Densitogram

No. 141

Thiocolchicoside
(2-glucose-thiocolchicine)

Aceclofenac

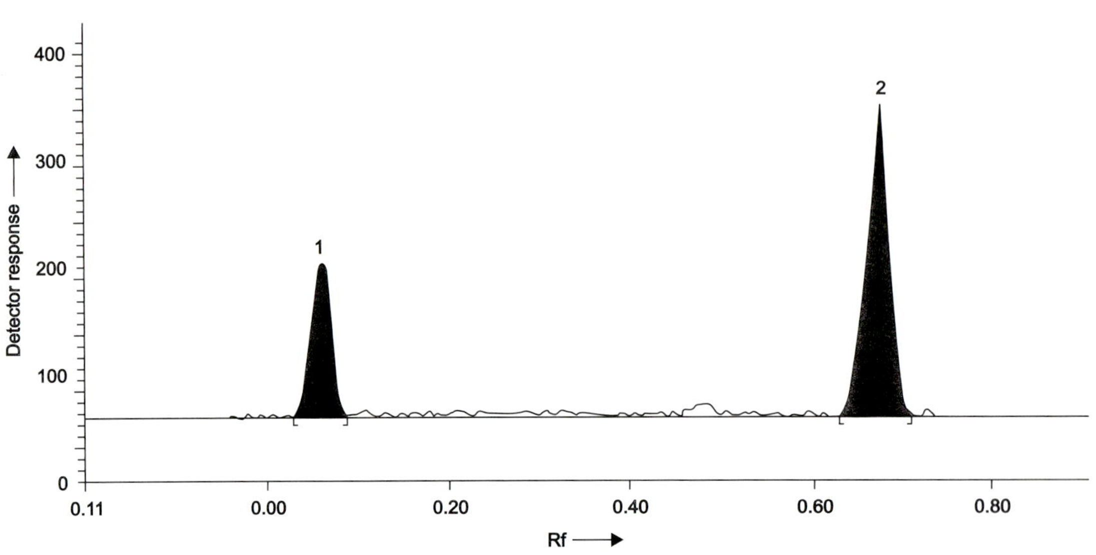

Typical densitogram of the standard containing thiocolchicoside and aceclofenac. For detailed experimental and chromatographic conditions, refer to Protocol No. 141. Peaks identification: 1. Thiocolchicoside; 2. Aceclofenac.

PROTOCOL FOR HPTLC ANALYSIS OF PHARMACEUTICAL FORMULATION

Protocol No. 141

Formulation: Thiocolchicoside, Aceclofenac

Classification: Musculoskeletal Disorders **Dosage form:** Tablets

Standard preparation: Prepare 1000 µg/ml solution of aceclofenac and 40 µg/ml solution of thiocolchicoside. Dilute appropriately with methanol to get 5 µg/ml of aceclofenac and 3 µg/ml of thiocolchicoside. Apply 2–7 µl for linearity profile.

Sample preparation: Powdered sample equivalent to 0.4 mg of thiocolchicoside suspended in 30–35 ml of methanol, sonicated for 30 min, diluted to 50 ml, centrifuged (3000 rpm) for 5 min and supernatant suitably diluted to get 40 µg/ml of thiocolchicoside. Apply 2 µl for assay.

Chromatographic equipments:

Sample applicator: Camag Linomat–V

Development chamber: Camag twin-trough glass chamber, 20 × 10 cm

Densitometric scanner: Camag TLC Scanner–III

Chromatographic conditions:

1. Stationary phase: Silica gel $60F_{254}$ pre-coated TLC plates, 20 × 10 cm (250 µm), pre-washed with methanol and activated at 110°C for 5 min, prior to use
2. Mobile phase (MP): Toluene–ethyl acetate–methanol–glacial acetic acid (4 : 6 : 2.0 : 0.5 v/v)
3. Standard/Sample application:
   Band length: 6 mm Volume applied: 2 µl Spacing: 5 mm
4. Chamber saturation: 20 min (MP)
5. RH (%): 60 ± 5
6. Temperature °C: 25 ± 2
7. Separation technique: Ascending
8. Quantity of mobile phase: 25 ml
9. Migration distance: 80 mm
10. Migration time: 20 min

Densitometric evaluation:

Wavelength: UV–255 nm Scanning mode: Reflectance/Absorbance

HRF: Thiocolchicoside—07; Aceclofenac—68

Linearity (ng/band): Thiocolchicoside—6–21; Aceclofenac—10–35

Recovery (%): Thiocolchicoside—99.31–101.12; Aceclofenac—98.16–101.66

References: Sunita T. Patel, Vidya K. Bhusari and Sunil R. Dhaneshwar, *Int. J. Pharm. Biosci.*, **2(2)**, 482–490, 2011.

Comments: The method validated for accuracy, precision, linearity, LOD, LOQ, specificity, robustness and ruggedness.

HPTLC : High Performance Thin Layer Chromatography
HPTLC Densitogram

No. 143

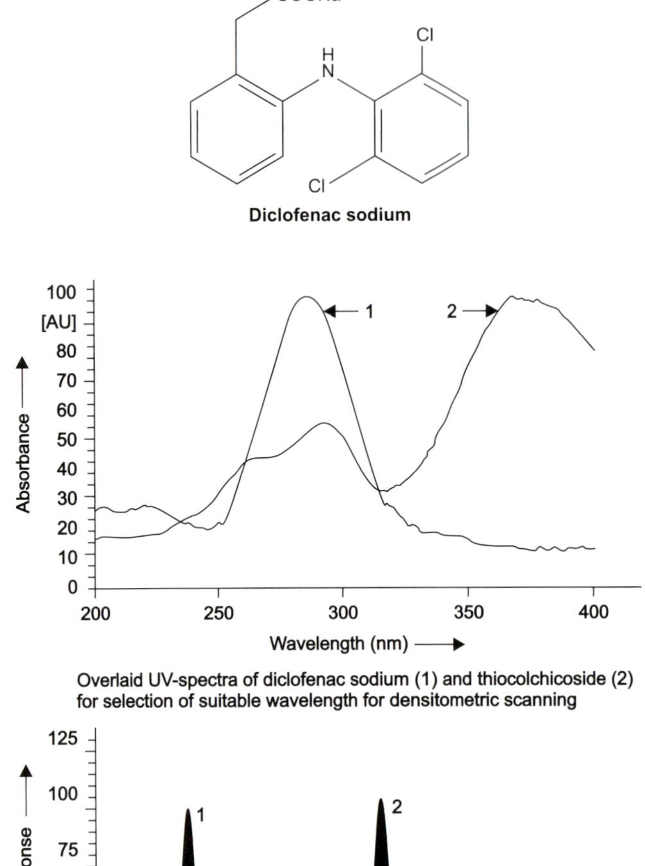

Typical densitogram of the standard containing diclofenac sodium and thiocolchicoside. For detailed experimental and chromatographic conditions, refer to Protocol No. 143. Peaks identification: 1. Thiocolchicoside; 2. Diclofenac sodium.

PROTOCOL FOR HPTLC ANALYSIS OF PHARMACEUTICAL FORMULATION

Protocol No. 143

Formulation: Thiocolchicoside, Diclofenac sodium

Classification: Musculoskeletal Disorders **Dosage form:** Tablets/Capsules

Standard preparation: Prepare 1 mg/ml solution of each compound in methanol. Further dilute 0.5 ml of each solution to 10 ml to get 50 μg/ml. Apply varying volumes of each solution for linearity profile.

Sample preparation: Quantity of the sample equivalent to 10 mg of diclofenac sodium suspended in 5 ml of methanol, sonicated for 5 min, diluted to 10 ml with methanol. Filter and dilute 0.5 ml of the filtrate to 10 ml with methanol. Apply 2 μl for chromatographic analysis.

Chromatographic equipments:

Sample applicator: Camag Linomat–V

Development chamber: Camag twin-trough glass chamber, 10 × 10 cm

Densitometric scanner: Camag TLC Scanner–III

Chromatographic conditions:

1. Stationary phase: Silica gel $60F_{254}$ pre-coated TLC plates, 10 × 10 cm (250 μm) – Merck, pre-washed with methanol and dried at 110°C for 5 min prior to use
2. Mobile phase (MP): (i) Toluene–ethyl acetate–methanol (5 : 3 : 2 v/v); (ii) Toluene–acetone–methanol–formic acid (5 : 2 : 2 : 0.01 v/v)
3. Standard/Sample application:
   Band length: 6 mm Volume applied: 2–10 μl Spacing: 5 mm
4. Chamber saturation: 15 min (MP)
5. RH (%): 55 ± 5
6. Temperature °C: 22 ± 2
7. Separation technique: Ascending
8. Quantity of mobile phase: 10 ml
9. Migration distance: 90 mm
10. Migration time: 30 min

Densitometric evaluation:

Wavelength: UV–285 nm Scanning mode: Reflectance/Absorbance

HRF: Thiocolchicoside—17; Diclofenac sodium—53

Linearity (ng/band): Diclofenac sodium—1000–5000; Thiocolchicoside—160–800

Recovery (%): 99.20–100.90 for both the compounds

References: Santosh Gandhi, Padmanabh Deshpande, Mahima Sengar, *Int. Res. J. Pharm.*, **1(1)**, 220–224, 2010.

Comments: The method validated for accuracy, precision, linearity, LOD, LOQ, specificity, robustness and ruggedness.

HPTLC : High Performance Thin Layer Chromatography
HPTLC Densitogram

No. 144

Ketoprofen

Thiocolchicoside (2-glucose-thiocolchicine)

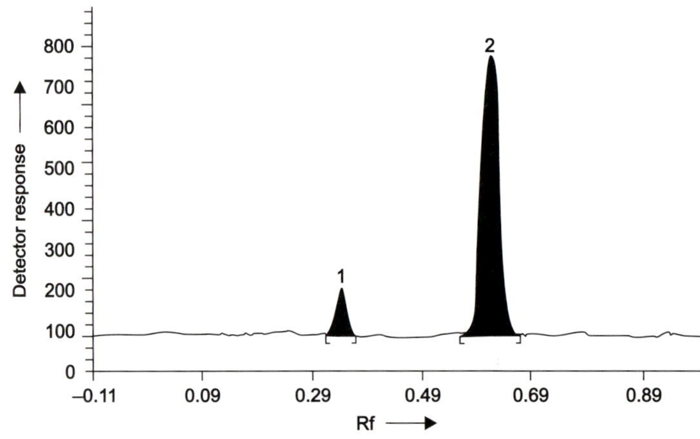

Typical densitogram of the sample containing thiocolchicoside and ketoprofen. For detailed experimental and chromatographic conditions, refer to Protocol No. 144. Peaks identification: 1. Thiocolchicoside; 2. Ketoprofen.

PROTOCOL FOR HPTLC ANALYSIS OF PHARMACEUTICAL FORMULATION

Protocol No. 144

Formulation: Thiocolchicoside, Ketoprofen

Classification: Musculoskeletal Disorders **Dosage form:** Tablets

Standard preparation: Prepare 1 mg/ml solution of thiocolchicoside in methanol. Weigh 25 mg of ketoprofen, add 2 ml of 1 mg/ml solution of thiocolchicoside, add 10 ml of methanol, sonicate for 10 min and dilute to 25 ml with methanol. Further dilute 5 ml to 10 ml with methanol and use for chromatographic separation and analysis.

Sample preparation: Powdered sample equivalent to 25 mg of ketoprofen suspended in methanol, sonicated for 20 min, diluted to 25 ml with methanol. Filtered and diluted 5 ml of the filtrate to 10 ml and used for analysis.

Chromatographic equipments:

Sample applicator: Camag Linomat–V
Development chamber: Camag twin-trough glass chamber, 10 × 10 cm
Densitometric scanner: Camag TLC Scanner–III

Chromatographic conditions:

1. Stationary phase: Silica gel $60F_{254}$ pre-coated TLC plates, 10 × 10 cm (250 μm) – Merck
2. Mobile phase (MP): Toluene–methanol–benzene (3.5 : 2.5 : 4.0 v/v)
3. Standard/Sample application:
   Band length: 6 mm Volume applied: 5 μl Spacing: 5 mm
4. Chamber saturation: 30 min (MP)
5. RH (%): 55 ± 5
6. Temperature °C: 25 ± 2
7. Separation technique: Ascending
8. Quantity of mobile phase: 10 ml
9. Migration distance: 80 mm
10. Migration time: 20 min

Densitometric evaluation:

Wavelength: UV–260 nm Scanning mode: Reflectance/Absorbance
HRF: Thiocolchicoside—34; Ketoprofen—65
Linearity (ng/band): Thiocolchicoside—125–750; Ketoprofen—1000–6000
Recovery (%): 99.25–101.15 for both the compounds

References: S.B. Wankhede, Poonam S. Boite, Somnath S. Zambare and Sohan S. Chitlange, Abstract No. F 272, 63rd IPC, 2011. Personal correspondence with Prof. S.B. Wankhede.

Comments:

- The method was validated as per ICH guidelines.
- The method is stability indicating (acid, alkali, thermal, oxidative and photolytic).

HPTLC : High Performance Thin Layer Chromatography
HPTLC Densitogram

No. 145

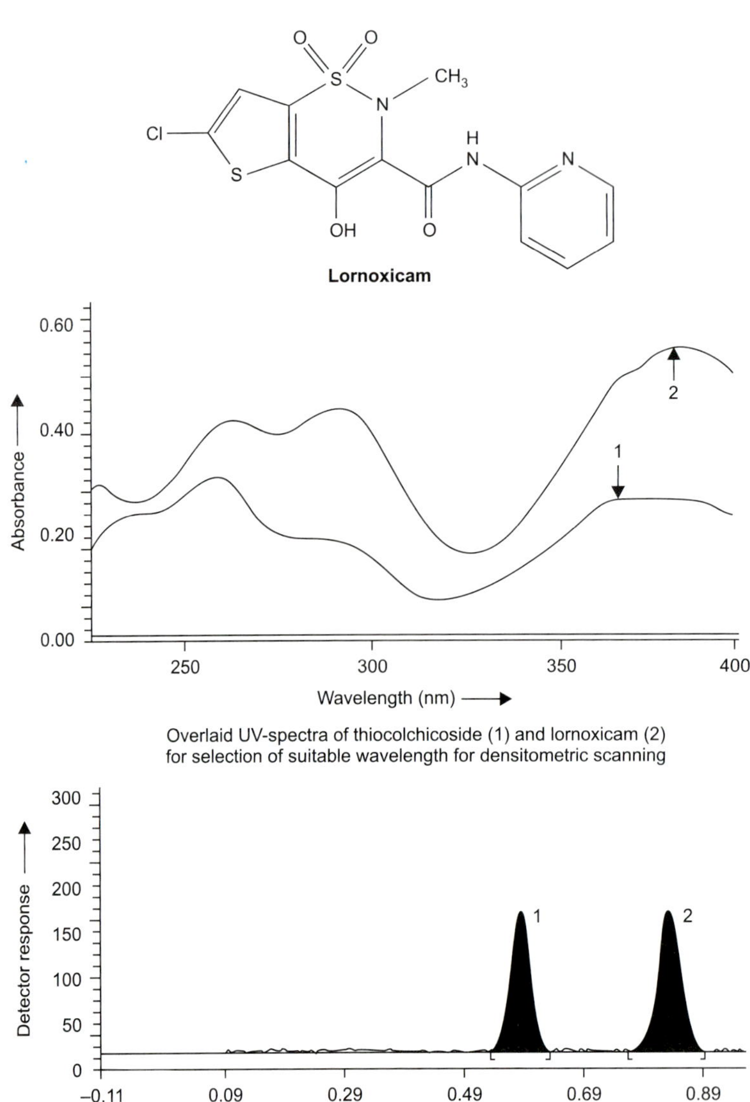

Overlaid UV-spectra of thiocolchicoside (1) and lornoxicam (2) for selection of suitable wavelength for densitometric scanning

Typical densitogram of the standard containing thiocolchicoside and lornoxicam. For detailed experimental and chromatographic conditions, refer to Protocol No. 145. Peaks identification: 1. Thiocolchicoside; 2. Lornoxicam.

PROTOCOL FOR HPTLC ANALYSIS OF PHARMACEUTICAL FORMULATION

Protocol No. 145

Formulation: Thiocolchicoside, Lornoxicam

Classification: Musculoskeletal Disorders **Dosage form:** Tablets

Standard preparation: Prepare 1 mg/ml solution of each drug in methanol. Further dilutions made to get 100 μg/ml. Apply varying volumes of each solution to establish linearity range.

Sample preparation: Powdered sample equivalent to 8 mg of thiocolchicoside suspended in 40 ml of methanol, sonicated for 10 min, filtered, diluted to 50 ml with methanol. The filtrate further diluted to get 20 μg/ml of the colchicoside and 40 μg/ml of lornoxicam. Apply 5 μl for chromatographic analysis.

Chromatographic equipments:

Sample applicator: Camag Linomat–V

Development chamber: Camag twin-trough glass chamber, 10 × 10 cm

Densitometric scanner: Camag TLC Scanner–III

Chromatographic conditions:

1. Stationary phase: Silica gel $60F_{254}$ pre-coated TLC plates, 10 × 10 cm (250 μm) – Merck
2. Mobile phase (MP): Methanol–chloroform–water (9.6 : 0.2 : 0.2 v/v)
3. Standard/Sample application:
   Band length: 6 mm Volume applied: 5 μl Spacing: 12 mm
4. Chamber saturation: 45 min (MP)
5. RH (%): 60 ± 5
6. Temperature °C: 25 ± 2
7. Separation technique: Ascending
8. Quantity of mobile phase: 10 ml
9. Migration distance: 80 mm
10. Migration time: 15 min

Densitometric evaluation:

Wavelength: UV–377 nm Scanning mode: Reflectance/Absorbance

HRF: Thiocolchicoside—58; Lornoxicam—84

Linearity (ng/band): Thiocolchicoside—30–180; Lornoxicam—60–360

Recovery (%): Thiocolchicoside—99.39–101.08; Lornoxicam—99.96–100.96

References: Personal communication, Prof. B.S. Kuchekar, Maharashtra Institute of Pharmacy, Pune, India.

Comments: The method validated for accuracy, precision, linearity, LOD, LOQ, specificity, robustness and ruggedness.

HPTLC : High Performance Thin Layer Chromatography
HPTLC Densitogram

No. 146

Glafenine

Floctafenine

A representative densitogram of the standard mixture containing thiocolchicoside, glafenine and floctafenine. For detailed experimental and chromatographic conditions, refer to Protocol No. 146. Peaks identification: 1. Thiocolchicoside (THIO); 2. Glafenine (GFN); 3. Floctafenine (FLN).

PROTOCOL FOR HPTLC ANALYSIS OF PHARMACEUTICAL FORMULATION

Protocol No. 146

Formulation: Thiocolchicoside with Glafenine or Floctafenine (1 : 100)

Classification: Musculoskeletal Disorders **Dosage form:** Tablets

Standard preparation: 1.5 mg/ml solution of THIO, 50 mg/ml solution of GFN and FLN; all prepared in methanol. Dilute solution of THIO to get 0.1 mg, 0.5 mg and 2 mg/ml in methanol. Prepare standard mixtures in different ratios i.e. 1 : 125, 1 : 50 and 1 : 100 of THIO-GFN and THIO-FLN. Apply 2.5, 5 and 7 µl of standard solutions for linearity.

Sample preparation: Apply 5 µl of each binary mixture solutions i.e. 1 : 50, 1 : 100 and 1 : 125 and carry out the chromatographic evaluation for estimation of thiocolchicoside.

Chromatographic equipments:

Sample applicator: Hamilton 10 µl syringe

Development chamber: 15 × 20 × 50 cm glass flat bottom tank

Densitometric scanner: Shimadzu CS-9000 densitometer scanner

Chromatographic conditions:

1. Stationary phase: Silica gel $60F_{254}$ pre-coated TLC plates, 20 × 20 cm (250 µm) – Merck, pre-washed with chloroform–methanol (0.1 : 1 v/v) overnight and dried
2. Mobile phase (MP): Ethyl acetate–methanol–glacial acetic acid (8.4 : 1.3 : 0.3 v/v)
3. Standard/Sample application:
   Band length: 10 mm Volume applied: 2.5–7 µl Spacing: 15 mm
4. Chamber saturation: 60 min (MP)
5. RH (%): 55 ± 5
6. Temperature °C: Ambient
7. Separation technique: Ascending
8. Quantity of mobile phase: 20 ml
9. Migration distance: 80 mm
10. Migration time: 20 min

Densitometric evaluation:

Wavelength: UV–375 nm Scanning mode: Reflectance/Absorbance

HRF: Thiocolchicoside—19; Glafenine—40; Floctafenine—81

Linearity: 2.5–15 µg/band

Recovery (%): 99.89–101.28

References: N.A. El-Ragehy, M.M. Ellaithy and M.A. Ghobashy, *Farmaco*, **58**, 463–468, 2003.

Comments:

- The method validated for accuracy, precision, linearity, LOD, LOQ, specificity, robustness and ruggedness.
- Each tablet contains 2 mg of thiocolchicoside along with 20 mg either of the two drugs.

HPTLC : High Performance Thin Layer Chromatography
HPTLC Densitogram

No. 147

COOH, O, NH, Cl, Cl

Aceclofenac

O, COOH, H_3C, O, O, O, CH_3, O, O

Diacerein

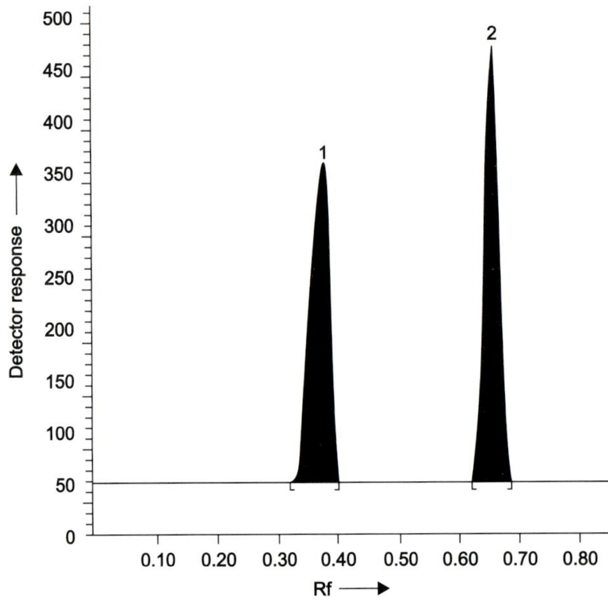

Typical densitogram of the sample containing aceclofenac and diacerein. For detailed experimental and chromatographic conditions, refer to Protocol No. 147. Peaks identification: 1. Aceclofenac; 2. Diacerein.

PROTOCOL FOR HPTLC ANALYSIS OF PHARMACEUTICAL FORMULATION

Protocol No. 147

Formulation: Aceclofenac, Diacerein

Classification: Musculoskeletal Disorders **Dosage form:** Tablets

Standard preparation: Dissolve 50 mg of aceclofenac and 25 mg of diacerein in 10 ml of DMSO, dilute to 50 ml with methanol. Apply 2–10 µl for chromatographic analysis and linearity profile.

Sample preparation: Powdered sample equivalent to 100 mg of aceclofenac suspended in 25 ml of $DMSO_4$, sonicated, diluted to 100 ml with methanol, filtered and the filtrate used for chromatographic analysis.

Chromatographic equipments:

Sample applicator: Camag Linomat–V

Development chamber: Camag twin-trough glass chamber, 10 × 10 cm

Densitometric scanner: Camag TLC Scanner–III

Chromatographic conditions:

1. Stationary phase: Silica gel $60F_{254}$ pre-coated HPTLC plates, 10 × 10 cm (200 µm) – Merck, pre-washed with methanol, activated at 115°C for 30 min prior to use
2. Mobile phase (MP): Chloroform–methanol (8 : 2 v/v)
3. Standard/Sample application:
   Band length: 5 mm Volume applied: 2–10 µl Spacing: 10 mm
4. Chamber saturation: 20 min (MP)
5. RH (%): 55 ± 5
6. Temperature °C: 22 ± 2
7. Separation technique: Ascending
8. Quantity of mobile phase: 10 ml
9. Migration distance: 85 mm
10. Migration time: 20 min

Densitometric evaluation:

Wavelength: UV–256 nm Scanning mode: Reflectance/Absorbance

HRF: Aceclofenac—38; Diacerein—66

Linearity (µg/band): Aceclofenac—10–50; Diacerein—5–25

Recovery (%): 99.22–101.54 for both the compounds

References: R. Sivakumar, N. Srisutherson, P. Kumar Nallasivan, P. Arulraj and R. Venketnaryana, *Research J. Pharm and Tech.*, **3(3)**, 825–827, 2010.

Comments: The method validated for accuracy, precision, linearity, LOD, LOQ, specificity, robustness and ruggedness.

HPTLC : High Performance Thin Layer Chromatography
HPTLC Densitogram

No. 149

Aceclofenac

Diacerein

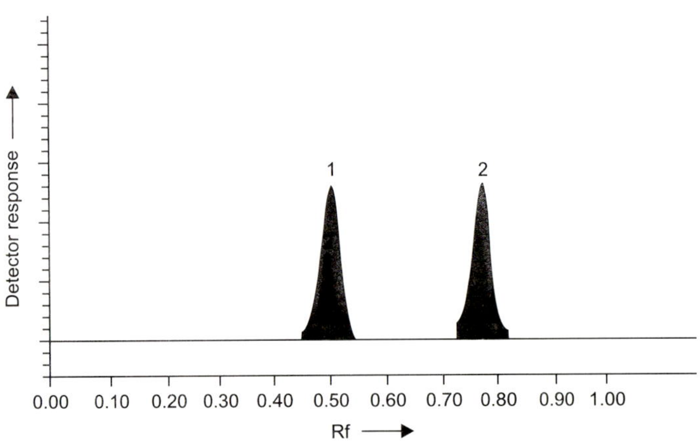

Typical densitogram of the standard containing aceclofenac and diacerein. For detailed experimental and chromatographic conditions, refer to Protocol No. 149. Peaks identification: 1. Aceclofenac; 2. Diacerein.

PROTOCOL FOR HPTLC ANALYSIS OF PHARMACEUTICAL FORMULATION

Protocol No. 149

Formulation: Aceclofenac, Diacerein

Classification: Musculoskeletal Disorders **Dosage form:** Tablets

Standard preparation: Prepare 100 μg/ml solution of each compound in methanol and apply varying volumes for linearity profile.

Sample preparation: Powdered sample equivalent to 25 mg of diacerein suspended in 25 ml of methanol, sonicated and filtered. Further dilute to get 50 μg/ml of diacerein and 100 μg/ml of aceclofenac and use for assay.

Chromatographic equipments:

Sample applicator: Camag Linomat–V

Development chamber: Camag twin-trough glass chamber, 20 × 10 cm

Densitometric scanner: Camag TLC Scanner–III

Chromatographic conditions:

1. Stationary phase: RP 18F_{254s} pre-coated HPTLC plates, 20 × 10 cm (200 μm) – Merck
2. Mobile phase (MP): Methanol–water (7 : 3 v/v)
3. Standard/Sample application:
   Band length: 10 mm Volume applied: 10 μl Spacing: 10 mm
4. Chamber saturation: 15 min (MP)
5. RH (%): 55 ± 5
6. Temperature °C: 22 ± 2
7. Separation technique: Ascending
8. Quantity of mobile phase: 20 ml
9. Migration distance: 90 mm
10. Migration time: 30 min

Densitometric evaluation:

Wavelength: UV–268 nm Scanning mode: Reflectance/Absorbance

HRF: Aceclofenac—50; Diacerein—78

Linearity (ng/band): Aceclofenac—100–1000; Diacerein—100–500

Recovery (%): 98.98–99.19 for both the compounds

References: S.P. Gandhi, M.G. Dewani, T.C. Borole and M.C. Damle, *E. J. Chem.* (accepted for publication).

Comments:

- The method validated for accuracy, precision, linearity, LOD, LOQ, specificity and ruggedness.
- The method is stability indicating (acid, base, oxidative, thermal, photolytic).

HPTLC : High Performance Thin Layer Chromatography
HPTLC Densitogram

No. 151

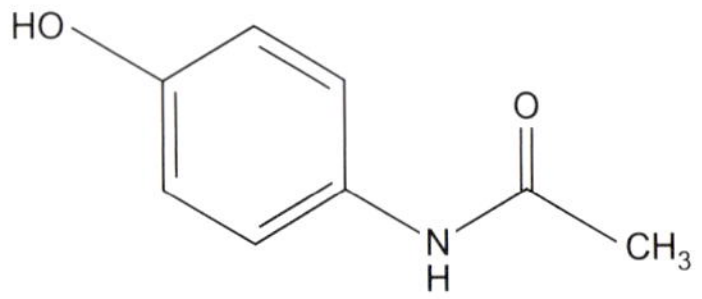

HO
N
H
O
CH_3
Paracetamol

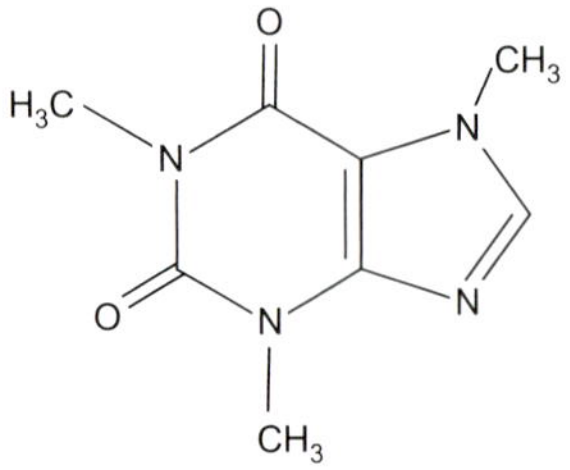

O
H_3C
N
N
CH_3
O
N
N
CH_3
Caffeine

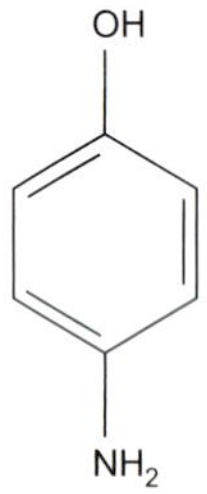

OH
NH_2
p-aminophenol

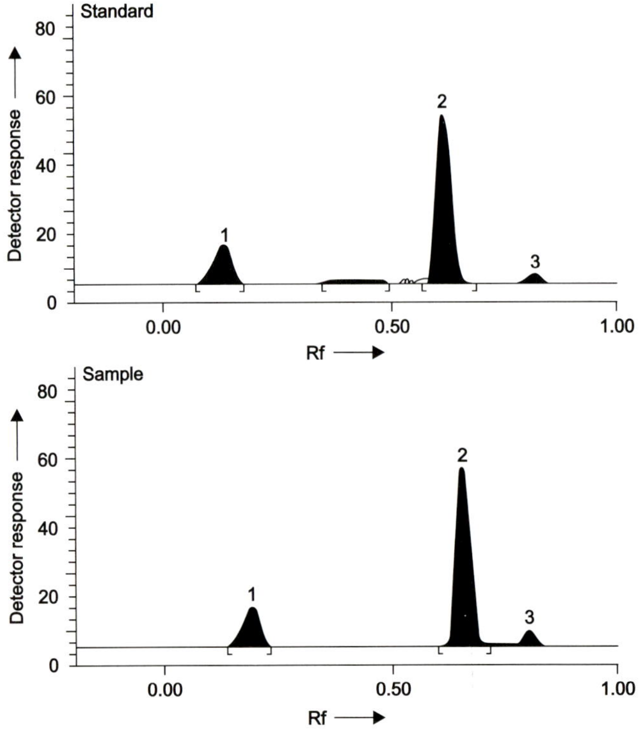

Standard
Detector response
80
60
40
20
0
1
2
3
0.00
0.50
1.00
Rf

Sample
Detector response
80
60
40
20
0
1
2
3
0.00
0.50
1.00
Rf

Typical densitogram of the sample and the standard containing paracetamol and caffeine citrate. For detailed experimental and chromatographic conditions, refer to Protocol No. 151. Peaks identification: 1. Caffeine citrate; 2. Paracetamol; 3. p-Aminophenol.

PROTOCOL FOR HPTLC ANALYSIS OF PHARMACEUTICAL FORMULATION

Protocol No. 151

Formulation: Paracetamol, Caffeine citrate

Classification: Musculoskeletal Disorders **Dosage form:** Tablets

Standard preparation: Weigh 400 mg of paracetamol and 30 mg of caffeine citrate, suspend in methanol, sonicate, dilute to 100 ml, filter and use for chromatographic separation.

Sample preparation: Powdered sample equivalent to 30 mg of caffeine citrate suspended in methanol, sonicated, diluted and filtered. The filtrate used for chromatographic analysis.

Chromatographic equipments:

Sample applicator: Camag Linomat–IV

Development chamber: Camag Horizontal glass chamber, 20 × 20 cm

Densitometric scanner: Camag TLC Scanner–II

Chromatographic conditions:

1. Stationary phase: Silica gel $60F_{254}$ pre-coated HPTLC plate, 10 × 10 cm (200 µm) – Merck
2. Mobile phase (MP): Methylene chloride–ethyl acetate–ethanol (5 : 5 : 1 v/v)
3. Standard/Sample application:
   Band length: 1 mm Volume applied: 0.5 µl Spacing: 5 mm
4. Chamber saturation: 20 min (MP)
5. RH (%): 55 ± 5
6. Temperature °C: 22 ± 2
7. Separation technique: Ascending
8. Quantity of mobile phase: 22 ml
9. Migration distance: 50 mm
10. Migration time: 20 min

Densitometric evaluation:

Wavelength: UV–254 nm Scanning mode: Reflectance/Absorbance

HRF: Caffeine citrate—22; Paracetamol—67; p-aminophenol—80

Linearity (ng/band): Paracetamol—100–1000; Caffeine citrate—10–50

Recovery (%): 100.47–102.83 for both the compounds

References: M. El Sadek, A. El Shanawany and A. Aboul Khier, *Analyst*, **115**, 1181–1184, 1990.

Comments: p-aminophenol was well separated from parent compounds.

HPTLC : High Performance Thin Layer Chromatography
HPTLC Densitogram

No. 152

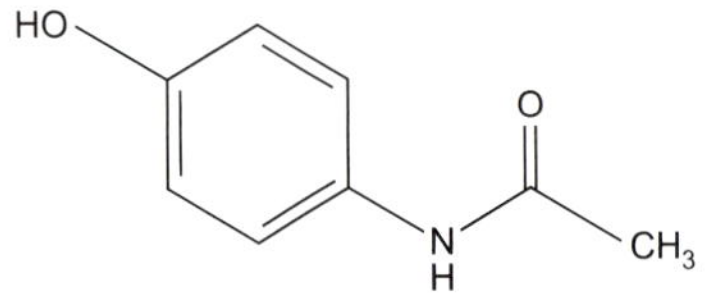

Paracetamol

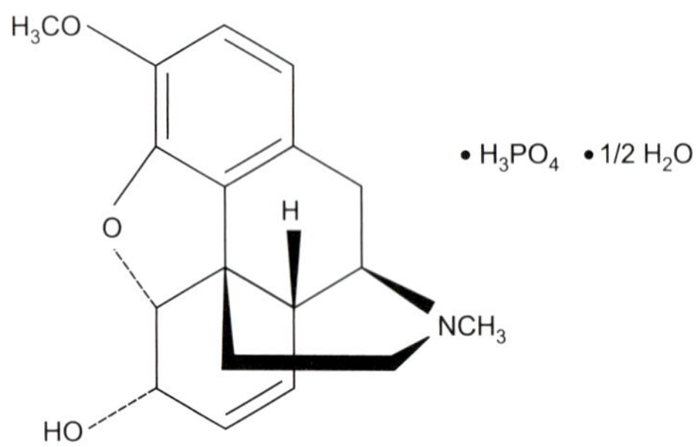

Codeine phosphate

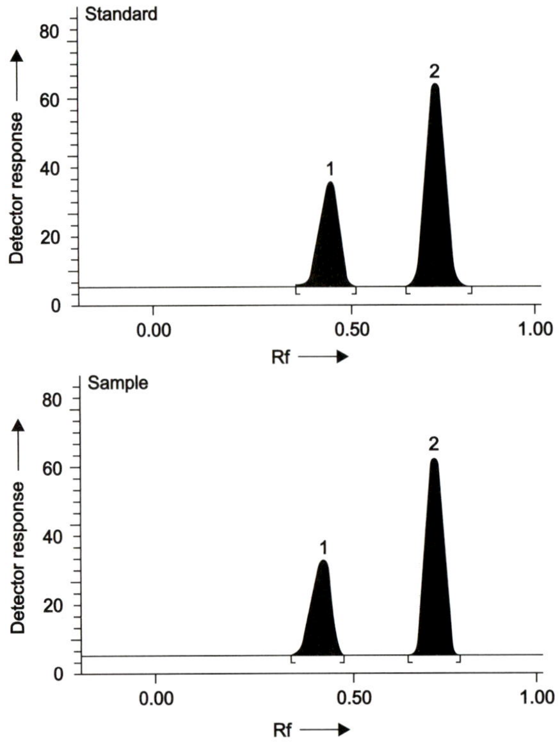

$\cdot H_3PO_4 \cdot 1/2\ H_2O$

Typical densitogram of the sample and the standard containing paracetamol and codeine phosphate. For detailed experimental and chromatographic conditions, refer to Protocol No. 152. Peaks identification: 1. Codeine phosphate; 2. Paracetamol.

PROTOCOL FOR HPTLC ANALYSIS OF PHARMACEUTICAL FORMULATION

Protocol No. 152

Formulation: Paracetamol, Codeine phosphate

Classification: Musculoskeletal Disorders **Dosage form:** Tablets

Standard preparation: Weigh accurately about 10 mg of codeine phosphate (CP) and 100 mg of paracetamol (P), dissolve in methanol to make 100 ml, dilute 0.3 ml to 100 ml with methanol and use for chromatographic separation.

Sample preparation: Weigh accurately finely powdered sample equivalent to 30 mg of codeine phosphate. Add 40–50 ml of methanol, sonicate for 5 min, dilute to 100 ml, filter and dilute 1 ml to 100 ml with methanol and use for assay.

Chromatographic equipments:

Sample applicator: Camag Linomat–IV

Development chamber: Camag twin–trough glass chamber, 10 × 10 cm

Densitometric scanner: Camag TLC Scanner–II

Chromatographic conditions:

1. Stationary phase: Silica gel $60F_{254}$ pre-coated HPTLC plates, 10 × 10 cm (200 μm) – Merck
2. Mobile phase (MP): Toluene–n-propanol–25% ammonia (6 : 4 : 0.4 v/v)
3. Standard/Sample application:
   Band length: 10 mm Volume applied: 10 μl Spacing: 10 mm
4. Chamber saturation: 20 min (MP)
5. RH (%): 55 ± 5
6. Temperature °C: 22 ± 2
7. Separation technique: Ascending
8. Quantity of mobile phase: 10.4 ml
9. Migration distance: 55 mm
10. Migration time: 14 min

Densitometric evaluation:

Wavelength: UV–244 nm or 285 nm Scanning mode: Reflectance/Absorbance

HRF: Codeine phosphate—44; Paracetamol—70

Linearity (ng/band): Paracetamol—500–500; Codeine phosphate—100–500

Recovery (%): 97.96–99.94 for both the compounds

References: —

Comments:

- The method was optimized and analytical work carried out at **Anchrom's HPTLC Application Laboratory**, Mumbai, India.
- Several market samples of similar composition were analysed by the proposed method with reproducible results.

HPTLC : High Performance Thin Layer Chromatography
HPTLC Densitogram

No. 153

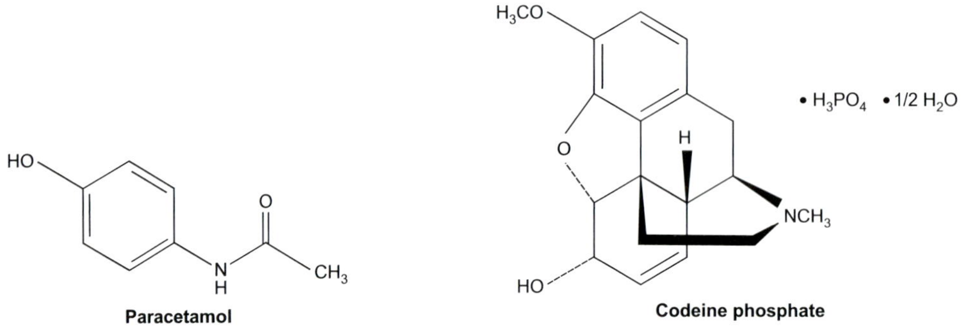

HO, N, H, O, CH_3

Paracetamol

H_3CO, O, H, NCH_3, HO, $\bullet H_3PO_4$ $\bullet 1/2\ H_2O$

Codeine phosphate

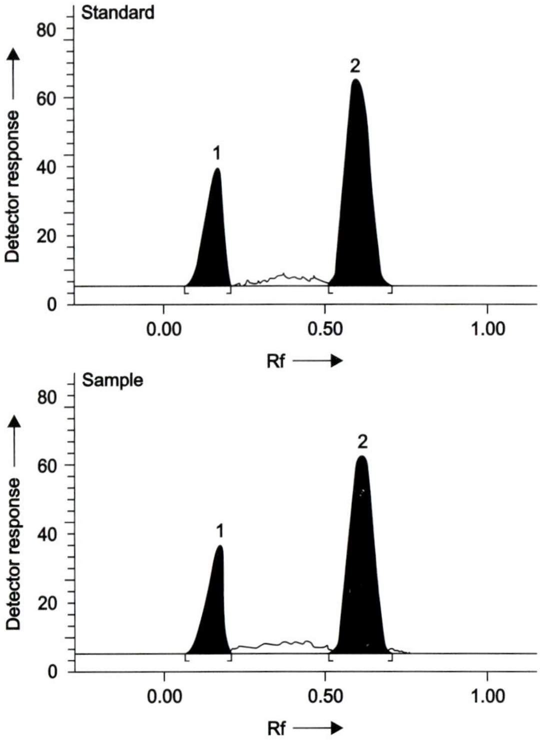

Standard

Detector response →

Rf →

Sample

Detector response →

Rf →

Typical densitogram of the sample and the standard containing paracetamol and codeine phosphate. For detailed experimental and chromatographic conditions, refer to Protocol No. 153. Peaks identification: 1. Codeine phosphate; 2. Paracetamol.

PROTOCOL FOR HPTLC ANALYSIS OF PHARMACEUTICAL FORMULATION

Protocol No. 153

Formulation: Paracetamol, Codeine phosphate

Classification: Musculoskeletal Disorders **Dosage form:** Tablets

Standard preparation: Weigh accurately about 10 mg of codeine phosphate (CP) and 100 mg of paracetamol (P), dissolve in methanol to make 100 ml, dilute 0.3 ml to 100 ml.

Sample preparation: Weigh accurately finely powdered sample equivalent to 30 mg of codeine phosphate. Add 40–50 ml of methanol, sonicate for 5 min, dilute to 100 ml, filter and dilute 1 ml to 100 ml with methanol.

Chromatographic equipments:

Sample applicator: Camag Linomat–IV

Development chamber: Camag twin–trough glass chamber, 10 × 10 cm

Densitometric scanner: Camag TLC Scanner–II

Chromatographic conditions:

1. Stationary phase: Silica gel RP-18F_{254s} pre-coated HPTLC plates, 10 × 10 cm (200 μm) – Merck
2. Mobile phase (MP): Methanol–0.5 M phosphate buffer pH 8.5 (4 : 6 v/v)
3. Standard/Sample application:
   Band length: 10 mm Volume applied: 10 μl Spacing: 10 mm
4. Chamber saturation: 30 min (MP)
5. RH (%): 55 ± 5
6. Temperature °C: 22 ± 2
7. Separation technique: Ascending
8. Quantity of mobile phase: 10 ml
9. Migration distance: 50 mm
10. Migration time: 30 min

Densitometric evaluation:

Wavelength: UV–244 nm or 285 nm Scanning mode: Reflectance/Absorbance

HRF: Codeine phosphate—16; Paracetamol—60

Linearity: —

Recovery (%): 98.50–102.80 for both the compounds

References: —

Comments:

- The method was optimized and analytical work carried out at **Anchrom's HPTLC Application Laboratory**, Mumbai, India.
- Resolution of two compounds was better with RP-HPTLC as compared to NP-HPTLC.

HPTLC : High Performance Thin Layer Chromatography
HPTLC Densitogram

No. 154

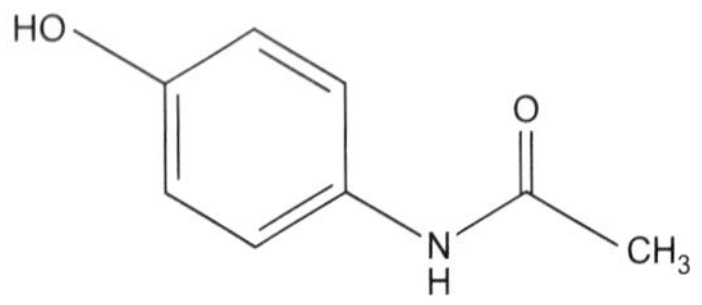

HO
O
N
H
CH_3
Paracetamol

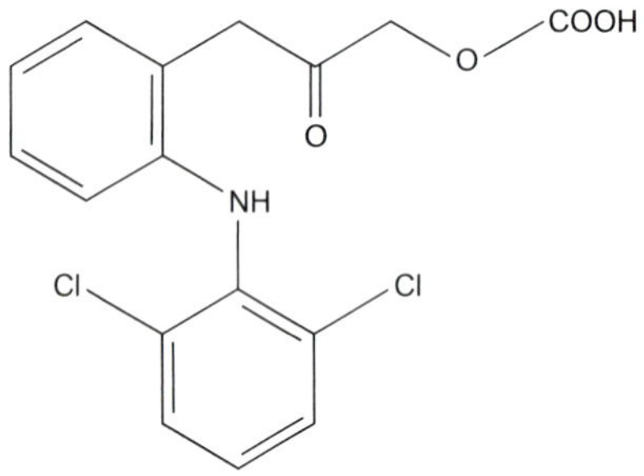

COOH
O
O
NH
Cl
Cl
Aceclofenac

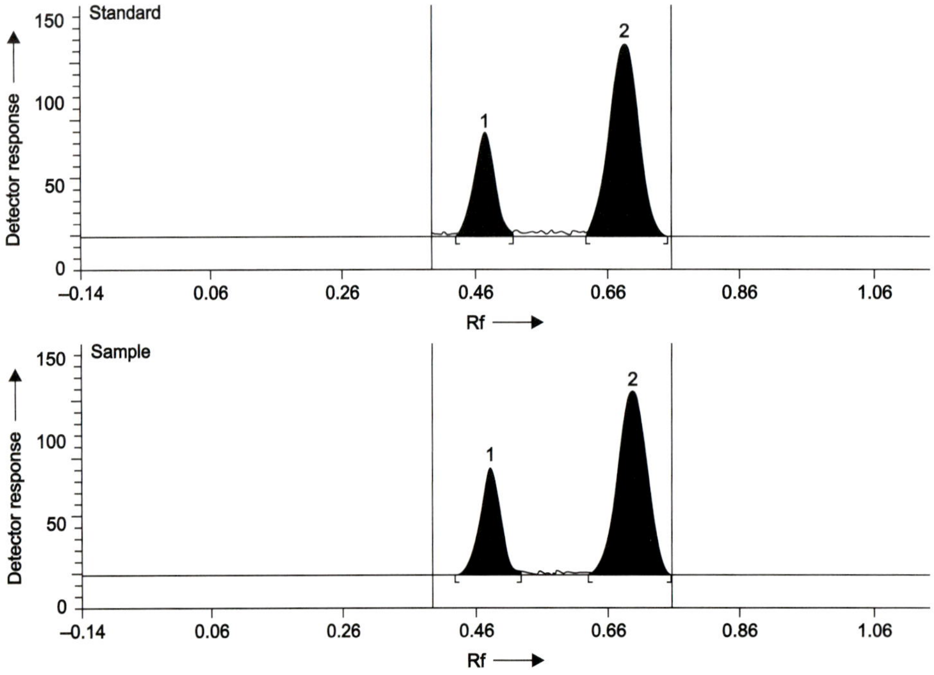

Standard
150
100
50
0
Detector response
1
2
–0.14 0.06 0.26 0.46 0.66 0.86 1.06
Rf

Sample
150
100
50
0
Detector response
1
2
–0.14 0.06 0.26 0.46 0.66 0.86 1.06
Rf

Typical densitogram of the sample and standard containing paracetamol and aceclofenac. For detailed experimental and chromatographic conditions, refer to Protocol No. 154. Peaks identification: 1. Aceclofenac; 2. Paracetamol.

PROTOCOL FOR HPTLC ANALYSIS OF PHARMACEUTICAL FORMULATION

Protocol No. 154

Formulation: Paracetamol, Aceclofenac

Classification: Musculoskeletal Disorders **Dosage form:** Tablets

Standard preparation: Prepare aceclofenac 2 mg/ml and paracetamol 5 mg/ml solution in methanol. Further serial dilutions were made with methanol for linearity studies. Prepare mixed standard solution to get 500 μg/ml and 1000 μg/ml respectively of aceclofenac and paracetamol.

Sample preparation: Powdered sample equivalent to 100 mg of aceclofenac suspended in methanol, sonicated, diluted to 100 ml, filtered, an aliquot suitably diluted with methanol to get final concentration of 500 μg/ml of aceclofenac and 1000 μg/ml of paracetamol.

Chromatographic equipments:

Sample applicator: Camag Linomat–V
Development chamber: Camag twin–trough glass chamber, 20 × 10 cm
Densitometric scanner: Camag TLC Scanner–III

Chromatographic conditions:

1. Stationary phase: Silica gel $60F_{254}$ pre-coated HPTLC plates, 10 × 10 cm (200 μm) – Merck
2. Mobile phase (MP): Toluene–isopropyl alcohol–25% ammonia (8 : 7 : 1 v/v)
3. Standard/Sample application:
   Band length: 8 mm Volume applied: 2 μl Spacing: 10 mm
4. Chamber saturation: 20 min (MP)
5. RH (%): 55 ± 5
6. Temperature °C: 24 ± 2
7. Separation technique: Ascending
8. Quantity of mobile phase: 32 ml
9. Migration distance: 80 mm
10. Migration time: 14 min

Densitometric evaluation:

Wavelength: UV–254 nm Scanning mode: Reflectance/Absorbance
HRF: Aceclofenac—48; Paracetamol—67
Linearity (ng/band): Paracetamol—500–5000; Aceclofenac—500–2000
Recovery (%): 98.75–102.25 for both the compounds

References: Hamid Khan, M. Ali, A. Ahuja, S. Ahmad and J. Ali, Abstract No. PA 218, 60th IPC, 2008.

Comments:

- The method was repeated at **Anchrom HPTLC Application Laboratory**, Mumbai using experimental conditions as described by the author. A representative densitogram is reproduced.
- The method is stability indicating (acid, base, oxidative, thermal, photolytic). The degradation products were separated from main compounds.

HPTLC : High Performance Thin Layer Chromatography
HPTLC Densitogram

No. 157

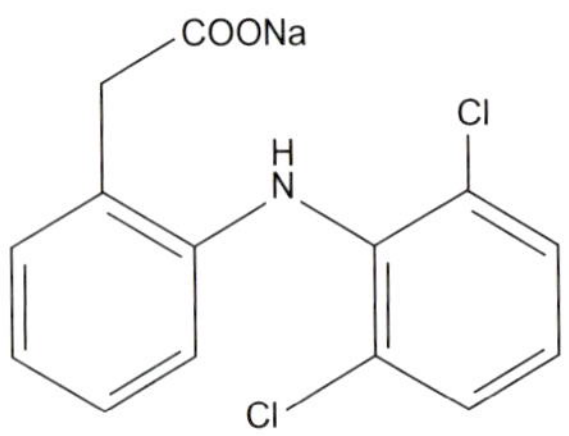

Diclofenac sodium

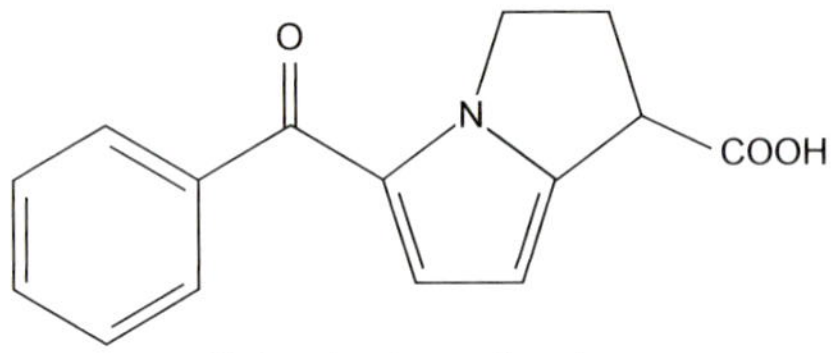

Ketorolac tromethamine

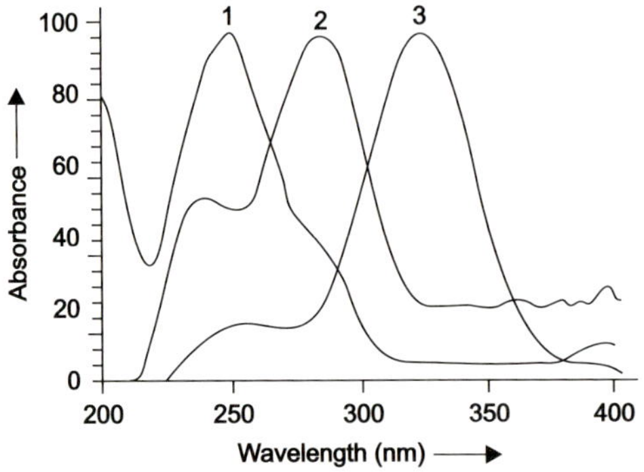

Overlaid UV-spectra of three compounds for selection of suitable wavelength for densitometric scanning

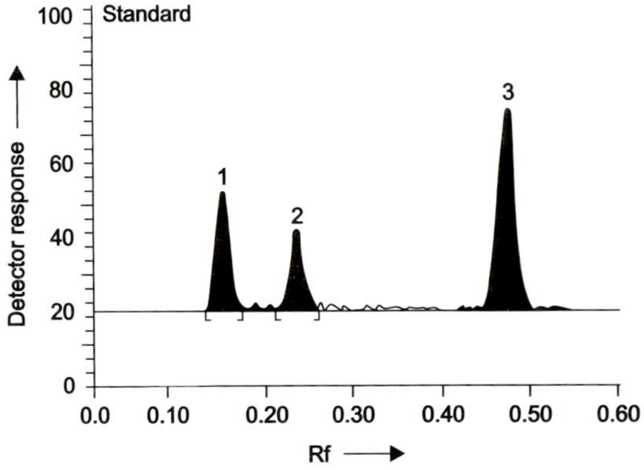

Typical densitogram of the standard containing paracetamol and diclofenac sodium. For detailed experimental and chromatographic conditions, refer to Protocol No. 157. Peaks identification: 1. Ketorolac tromethamine (IS); 2. Diclofenac sodium; 3. Paracetamol.

PROTOCOL FOR HPTLC ANALYSIS OF PHARMACEUTICAL FORMULATION

Protocol No. 157

Formulation: Paracetamol, Diclofenac sodium

Classification: Musculoskeletal Disorders **Dosage form:** Tablets

Standard preparation: Weigh accurately quantities of paracetamol, diclofenac sodium and ketorolac tromethamine (IS) and dissolve in methanol to get 20 μg/ml of paracetamol and 2 μg/ml of diclofenac. Apply 10 μl for analysis.

Sample preparation: Powdered sample equivalent to one tablet suspended in 30 ml of methanol, sonicated for 5 min, diluted to 50 ml with methanol, filtered through 0.45 μm filter. Take appropriate volume of the filtrate, add (IS) solution and dilute so that final solution contains 20 ng/μl of paracetamol and 2 ng/μl of diclofenac sodium. Apply 10 μl for chromatography.

Chromatographic equipments:

Sample applicator: Camag Linomat–IV

Development chamber: Camag twin–trough glass chamber, 10 × 10 cm

Densitometric scanner: Camag TLC Scanner

Chromatographic conditions:

1. Stationary phase: Silica gel $60F_{254}$ pre-coated TLC plate, 10 × 10 cm (250 μm) – Merck
2. Mobile phase (MP): Chloroform–methanol–25% ammonia (10 : 2.5 : 0.12 v/v)
3. Standard/Sample application:
   Band length: 10 mm Volume applied: 10 μl Spacing: 10 mm
4. Chamber saturation: 15 min (MP)
5. RH (%): 55 ± 5
6. Temperature °C: 22 ± 2
7. Separation technique: Ascending
8. Quantity of mobile phase: 12.6 ml
9. Migration distance: 70 mm
10. Migration time: 20 min

Densitometric evaluation:

Wavelength: UV–286 nm Scanning mode: Reflectance/Absorbance

HRF: Ketorolac tromethamine (IS)—15; Diclofenac Na^{+}—24; Paracetamol—48

Linearity (ng/band): Paracetamol—100–600; Diclofenac sodium—10–60

Recovery (%): 97.40–99.84 for both the compounds

References: V.M. Shinde, N.M. Tendulkar, and B.S. Desai, *J. Planar Chromatogr.*, **7**, 50–52, 1994.

Comments: 286 nm, being the absorption maxima of diclofenac sodium, minor component in the formulation, was selected for scanning.

HPTLC : High Performance Thin Layer Chromatography
HPTLC Densitogram

No. 158

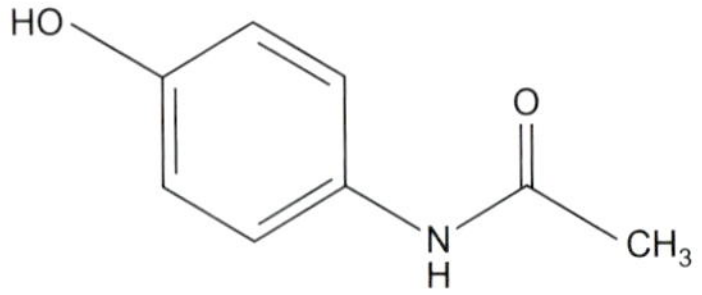

Paracetamol

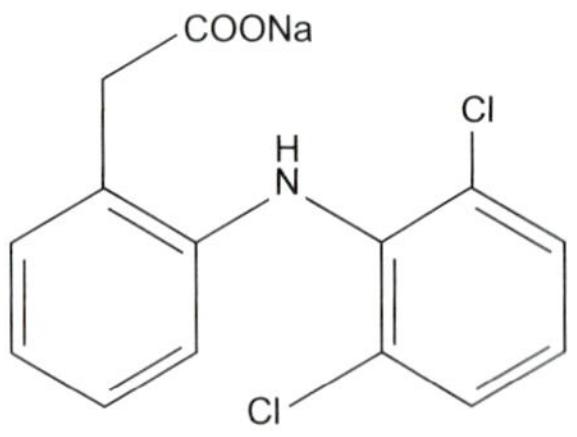

Diclofenac sodium

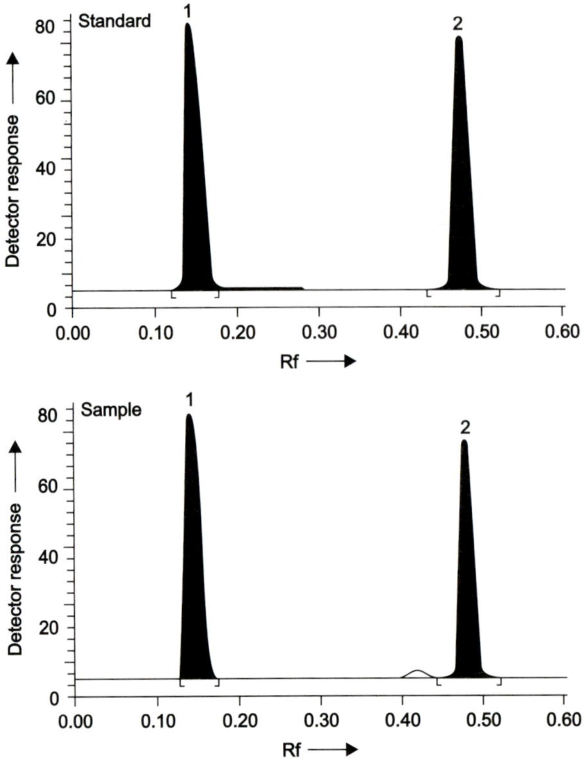

Typical densitogram of the standard and the sample containing paracetamol and diclofenac sodium. For detailed experimental and chromatographic conditions, refer to Protocol No. 158. Peaks identification: 1. Paracetamol; 2. Diclofenac sodium.

PROTOCOL FOR HPTLC ANALYSIS OF PHARMACEUTICAL FORMULATION

Protocol No. 158

Formulation: Paracetamol, Diclofenac sodium

Classification: Musculoskeletal Disorders **Dosage form:** Tablets

Standard preparation: (a) Weigh accurately about 10 mg of diclofenac sodium (D) and 65 mg of paracetamol (P), dissolve in methanol to make 100 ml and use for chromatographic evaluation.

Sample preparation: Weigh powdered sample equivalent to 10 mg of diclofenac sodium, add about 70 ml of methanol, vortex for 10 min, and make up the volume to 100 ml, filter and use the filtrate. Apply 2 µl for chromatographic separation.

Chromatographic equipments:

Sample applicator: Camag Linomat–IV

Development chamber: Camag twin–trough glass chamber, 10 × 10 cm

Densitometric scanner: Camag TLC Scanner–III

Chromatographic conditions:

1. Stationary phase: Silica gel $60F_{254}$ pre-coated HPTLC plates, 10 × 10 cm (200 µm) – Merck
2. Mobile phase (MP): n-hexane–ethyl acetate–glacial acetic acid (9 : 2.5 : 1 v/v)
3. Standard/Sample application:
   Band length: 5 mm Volume applied: 2 µl Spacing: 5 mm
4. Chamber saturation: 10 min (MP)
5. RH (%): 55 ± 5
6. Temperature °C: 22 ± 2
7. Separation technique: Ascending
8. Quantity of mobile phase: 12.5 ml
9. Migration distance: 50 mm
10. Migration time: 17 min

Densitometric evaluation:

Wavelength: UV–280 nm Scanning mode: Reflectance/Absorbance

HRF: Paracetamol—15; Diclofenac sodium—49

Linearity (ng/band): Paracetamol—100–2000; Diclofenac sodium—25–300

Recovery (%): 98.80–99.10 for both the compounds

References: —

Comments:

- The method was optimized and analytical work carried out at **Anchrom's HPTLC Application Laboratory**, Mumbai, India.
- Several market samples of similar composition were analysed by the proposed method with reproducible results.

HPTLC : High Performance Thin Layer Chromatography
HPTLC Densitogram

No. 159

Paracetamol

Diclofenac sodium

Typical densitogram of the standard and the sample containing paracetamol and diclofenac sodium. For detailed experimental and chromatographic conditions, refer to Protocol No. 159. Peaks identification: 1. Diclofenac sodium; 2. Paracetamol.

PROTOCOL FOR HPTLC ANALYSIS OF PHARMACEUTICAL FORMULATION

Protocol No. 159

Formulation: **Paracetamol, Diclofenac sodium**

Classification: Musculoskeletal Disorders **Dosage form:** Tablets

Standard preparation: (a) Weigh accurately about 10 mg of diclofenac sodium (D) and 65 mg of paracetamol (P), dissolve in methanol to make 100 ml and use for chromatographic evaluation.

Sample preparation: Weigh powdered sample equivalent to 10 mg of diclofenac sodium, add about 70 ml of methanol, vortex for 10 min, and make up the volume to 100 ml, filter and use the filtrate. Apply 2 μl for chromatographic separation.

Chromatographic equipments:

Sample applicator: Camag Linomat–IV

Development chamber: Camag twin–trough glass chamber, 10 × 10 cm

Densitometric scanner: Camag TLC Scanner–II

Chromatographic conditions:

1. Stationary phase: Silica gel 60 RP-18 F_{254s} pre-coated HPTLC plates, 10 × 10 cm (200 μm) – Merck
2. Mobile phase (MP): 0.5 M sodium chloride–methanol–glacial acetic acid (12 : 8 : 0.01 v/v)
3. Standard/Sample application:
   Band length: 5 mm Volume applied: 2 μl Spacing: 5 mm
4. Chamber saturation: 30 min (MP)
5. RH (%): 55 ± 5
6. Temperature °C: 22 ± 2
7. Separation technique: Ascending
8. Quantity of mobile phase: 20 ml
9. Migration distance: 50 mm
10. Migration time: 40 min

Densitometric evaluation:

Wavelength: UV–280 nm Scanning mode: Reflectance/Absorbance

HRF: Diclofenac sodium—20; Paracetamol—40

Linearity (ng/band): Paracetamol—100–2000; Diclofenac sodium—50–300

Recovery (%): 97.75–98.25 for both the compounds

References: —

Comments:

- The method was optimized and analytical work carried out at **Anchrom's HPTLC Application Laboratory**, Mumbai, India.
- See reversal of retention factor in RP–HPTLC as compared to NP–HPTLC.
- Several market samples of similar composition were analysed by the proposed method with reproducible results.

HPTLC : High Performance Thin Layer Chromatography
HPTLC Densitogram

No. 160

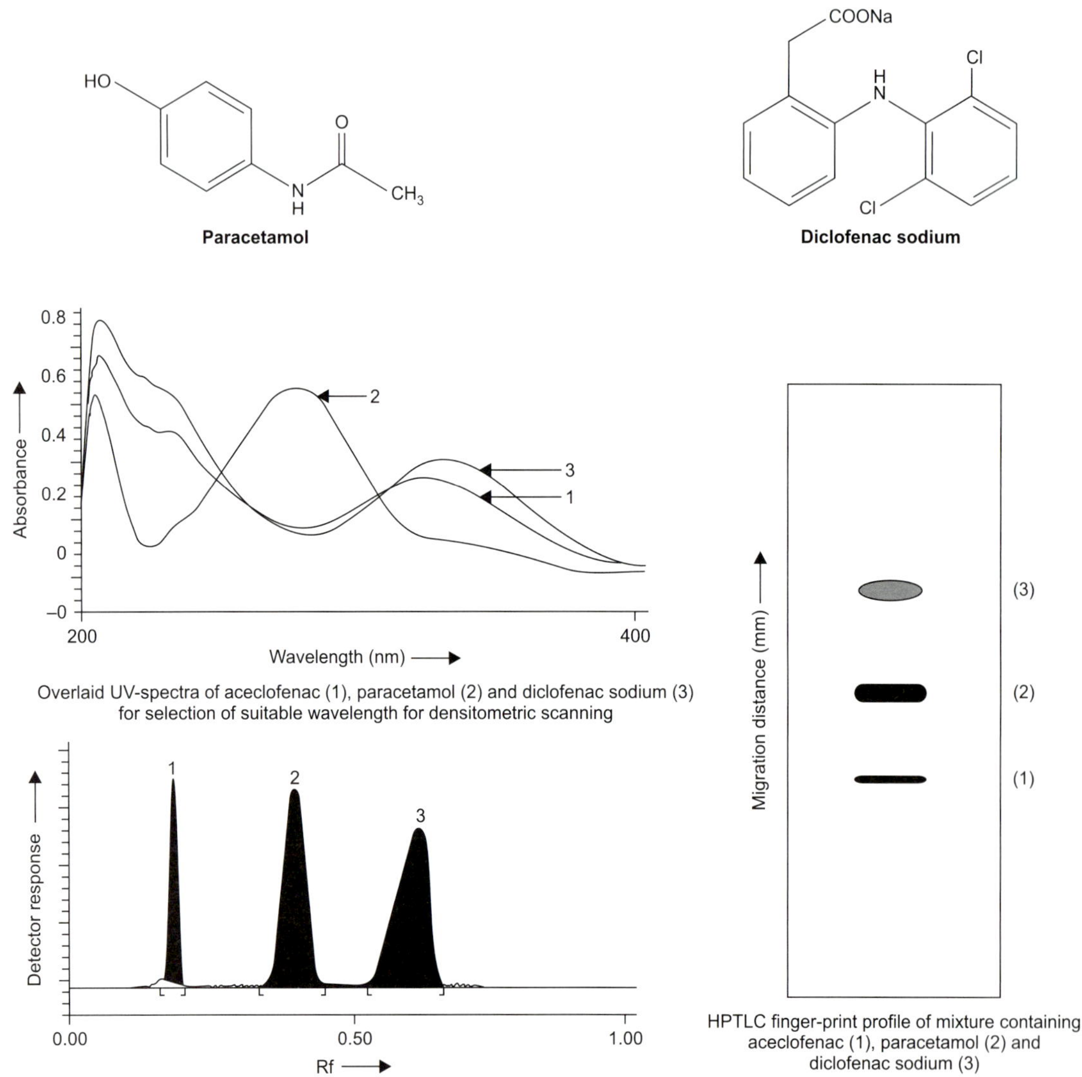

Typical densitogram of the standard containing paracetamol, diclofenac and aceclofenac (IS). For detailed experimental and chromatographic conditions, refer to Protocol No. 160. Peaks identification: 1. Aceclofenac (IS); 2. Paracetamol; 3. Diclofenac sodium.

PROTOCOL FOR HPTLC ANALYSIS OF PHARMACEUTICAL FORMULATION

Protocol No. 160

Formulation: Paracetamol, Diclofenac sodium

Classification: Musculoskeletal Disorders **Dosage form:** Tablets

Standard preparation: Prepare 1 mg/ml solution of each compound separately in methanol. Further serial dilutions are made to get different concentrations, each solution contains 500 μg/ml of aceclofenac (IS). Apply 2 μl of each solution for linearity profile.

Sample preparation: Accurately weighed quantity of powdered sample suspended in methanol, sonicated for 5 min, add 0.5 ml of (IS) solution, dilute and filter. The filtrate suitably diluted for chromatographic separation and analysis.

Chromatographic equipments:

Sample applicator: Camag Linomat–V

Development chamber: Camag twin–trough glass chamber, 10 × 10 cm

Densitometric scanner: Camag TLC Scanner–II

Chromatographic conditions:

1. Stationary phase: Silica gel $60F_{254}$ pre-coated HPTLC plates, 10 × 10 cm (200 μm) – Merck, pre-washed with methanol, dried at 100°C for 60 min prior to use
2. Mobile phase (MP): Toluene–ethyl acetate–methanol–formic acid (5 : 4 : 1 : 0.01 v/v)
3. Standard/Sample application:
   Band length: 7 mm Volume applied: 2 μl Spacing: 7 mm
4. Chamber saturation: 15 min (MP)
5. RH (%): 55 ± 5
6. Temperature °C: 25 ± 2
7. Separation technique: Ascending
8. Quantity of mobile phase: 10 ml
9. Migration distance: 80 mm
10. Migration time: 20 min

Densitometric evaluation:

Wavelength: UV–260 nm Scanning mode: Reflectance/Absorbance

HRF: Aceclofenac (IS)—22; Paracetamol—33; Diclofenac sodium—58

Linearity (ng/band): Paracetamol—300–2000; Diclofenac sodium—30–800

Recovery (%): 99.57–100/51 for both the compounds

References: Vidya V. Dighe, R.T. Sane, S.N. Menon, H.N. Tambe, Sreedevi Pillai and V.N. Gokarn, *J. Planar Chromatogr.*, **19(6)**, 443–447, 2006.

Comments: The method validated for accuracy, precision, linearity, LOD, LOQ, specificity, robustness and ruggedness.

HPTLC : High Performance Thin Layer Chromatography
HPTLC Densitogram

No. 161

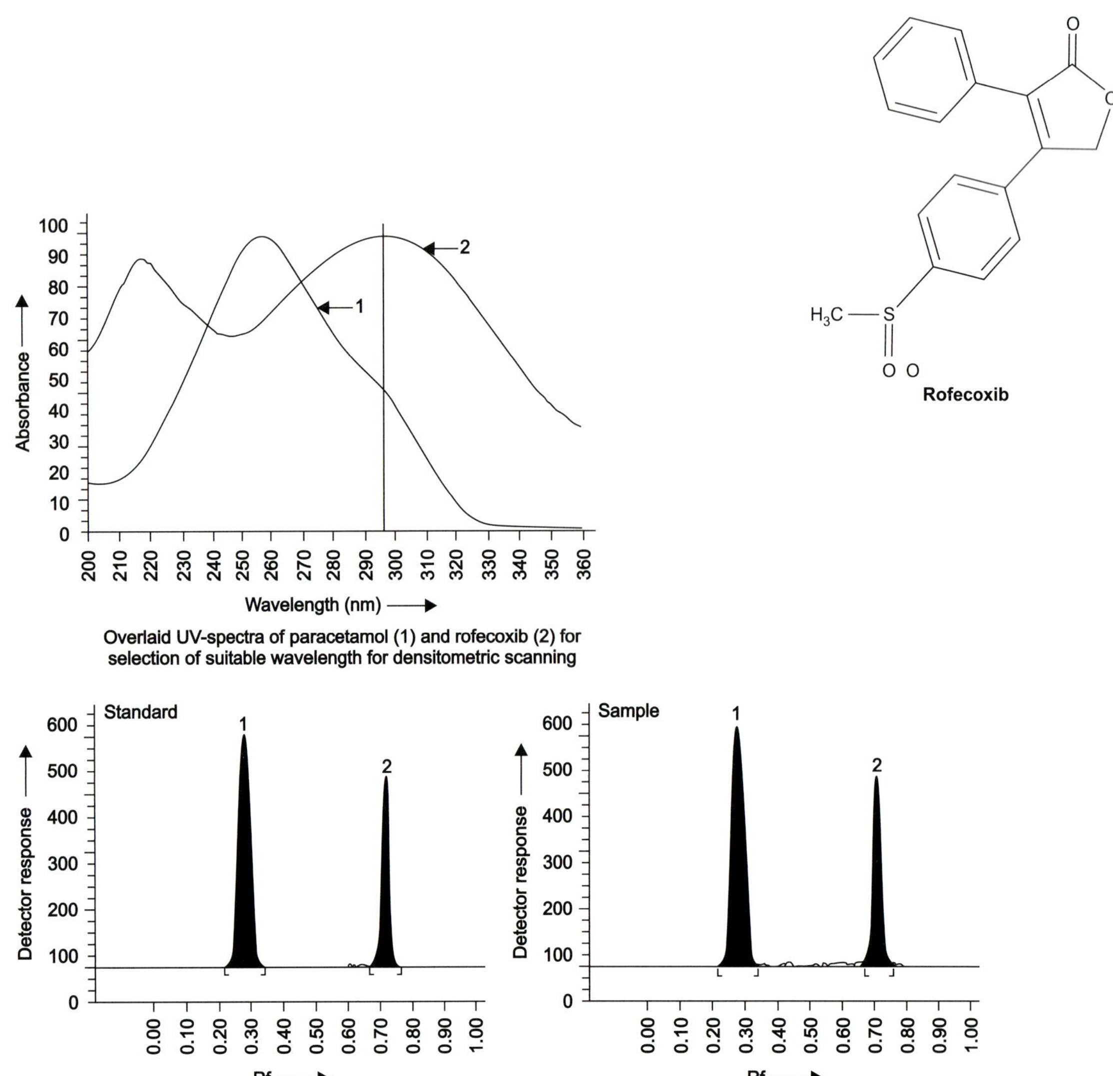

Typical densitogram of the standard and sample containing paracetamol and rofecoxib. For detailed experimental and chromatographic conditions, refer to Protocol No. 161. Peaks identification: 1. Rofecoxib; 2. Paracetamol.

PROTOCOL FOR HPTLC ANALYSIS OF PHARMACEUTICAL FORMULATION

Protocol No. 161

Formulation: **Paracetamol, Rofecoxib**

Classification: Musculoskeletal Disorders **Dosage form:** Tablets

Standard preparation: Prepare mixed standard solution in methanol to contain 200 μg/ml rofecoxib and 4000 μg/ml of paracetamol. Further serial dilutions made with methanol. Apply 4 μl of each solution for linearity profile.

Sample preparation: Powdered sample equivalent to 5 mg of rofecoxib suspended in 20 ml of methanol, sonicated for 15 min, diluted to 25 ml, filtered through Whatman No. 1 filter paper and filtrate used as sample solution. Apply 4 μl for chromatographic separation and evaluation.

Chromatographic equipments:

Sample applicator: Camag Linomat–IV automatic sample applicator

Development chamber: Camag twin–trough glass chamber

Densitometric scanner: Camag TLC Scanner–III

Chromatographic conditions:

1. Stationary phase: Silica gel $60F_{254}$ TLC pre-coated plates, 10 × 10 cm (200 μm) – Merck
2. Mobile phase (MP): Methanol–toluene–chloroform–triethylamine (10 : 6 : 3 : 0.5 v/v)
3. Standard/Sample application:
   Band length: 4 mm Volume applied: 4 μl Spacing: 8 mm
4. Chamber saturation: 10 min (MP)
5. RH (%): 55 ± 5
6. Temperature °C: 20 ± 2
7. Separation technique: Ascending
8. Quantity of mobile phase: 19 ml
9. Migration distance: 70 mm
10. Migration time: 20 min

Densitometric evaluation:

Wavelength: UV–297 nm Scanning mode: Reflectance/Absorbance

HRF: Rofecoxib—29; Paracetamol—72

Linearity (μg/band): Rofecoxib—0.7–1.5; 9.6–21.3

Recovery (%): 98.06–99.31 for both the compounds

References: Anonymous.

Comments: The method validated for accuracy, precision, linearity, LOD, LOQ, specificity, robustness and ruggedness.

HPTLC : High Performance Thin Layer Chromatography
HPTLC Densitogram

No. 162

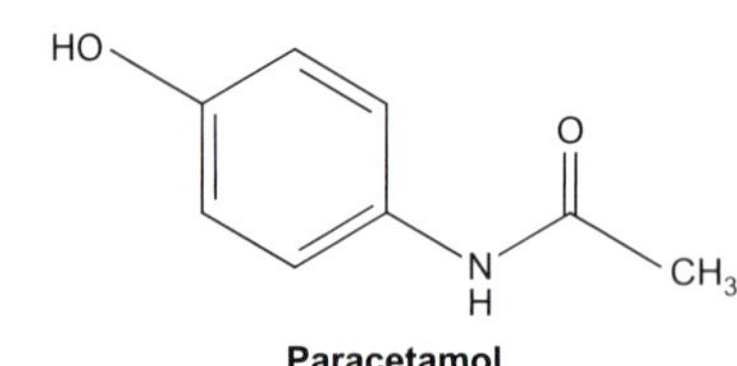

Paracetamol

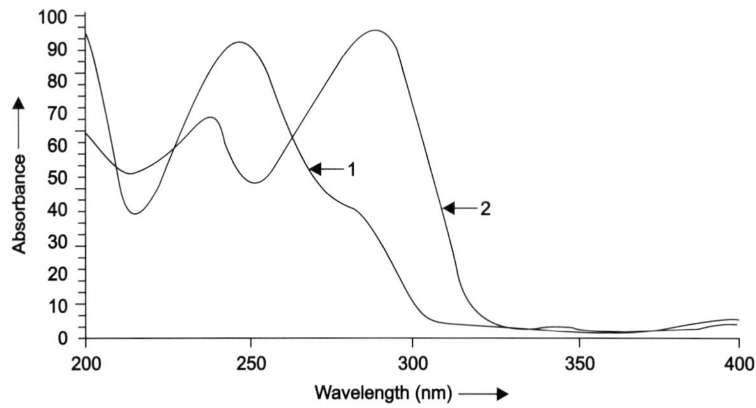

Overlaid UV-spectra of paracetamol (1) and etoricoxib (2) for selection of suitable wavelength for densitometric scanning

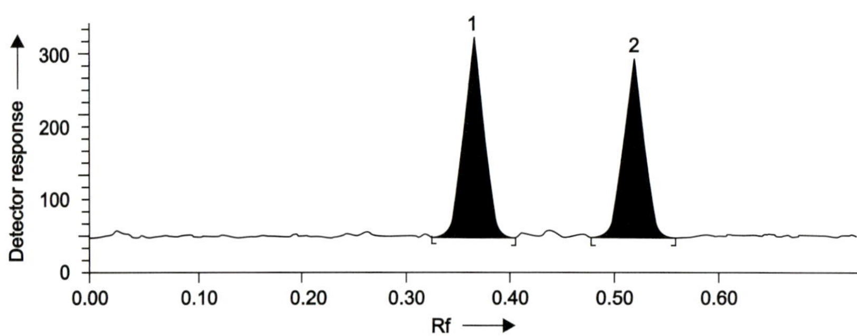

Typical densitogram of the standard containing paracetamol and etoricoxib. For detailed experimental and chromatographic conditions, refer to Protocol No. 162. Peaks identification: 1. Paracetamol; 2. Etoricoxib.

PROTOCOL FOR HPTLC ANALYSIS OF PHARMACEUTICAL FORMULATION

Protocol No. 162

Formulation: Paracetamol, Etoricoxib

Classification: Musculoskeletal Disorders **Dosage form:** Tablets

Standard preparation: Prepare 1 mg/ml solution of each compound in methanol. Further dilute 1 ml to 100 ml with methanol. Apply varying volumes for linearity profile.

Sample preparation: Powdered sample equivalent to 10 mg of etoricoxib suspended in 7 ml of methanol, sonicated for 5 min, diluted to 10 ml with methanol. Filter and further dilute suitably for assay. Apply volume equivalent to 200 ng and carry out chromatographic evaluation.

Chromatographic equipments:

Sample applicator: Camag Linomat–V

Development chamber: Camag twin–trough glass chamber, 10 × 10 cm

Densitometric scanner: Camag TLC Scanner–III

Chromatographic conditions:

1. Stationary phase: Silica gel 60F_{254} pre-coated HPTLC plates, 10 × 10 cm (200 μm) – Merck, pre-washed with methanol, activated at 110°C for 5 min prior to use
2. Mobile phase (MP): Toluene–methanol–chloroform (5 : 2 : 3 v/v)
3. Standard/Sample application:
   Band length: 5 mm Volume applied: 1–5 μl Spacing: 10 mm
4. Chamber saturation: 10 min (MP)
5. RH (%): 55 ± 5
6. Temperature °C: 22 ± 2
7. Separation technique: Ascending
8. Quantity of mobile phase: 10 ml
9. Migration distance: 80 mm
10. Migration time: 20 min

Densitometric evaluation:

Wavelength: UV–240 nm Scanning mode: Reflectance/Absorbance

HRF: Paracetamol—38; Etoricoxib—53

Linearity: 100–500 ng/band for both the drugs

Recovery (%): Paracetamol—99.15–99.99; Etoricoxib—99.75–100.10

References: P.B. Deshpande, Santosh V. Gandhi, Yogeshwari S. Bhangale and Vasudha B. Pisal, *J. Pharm. Biomed. Sci.*, **3(3)**, 1–4, 2010.

Comments: The method validated for accuracy, precision, linearity, LOD, LOQ, specificity, robustness and ruggedness.

HPTLC : High Performance Thin Layer Chromatography
HPTLC Densitogram

No. 163

HO, O, N, H, CH_3

Paracetamol

H_2NO_2S, CH_3, O, N

Valdecoxib

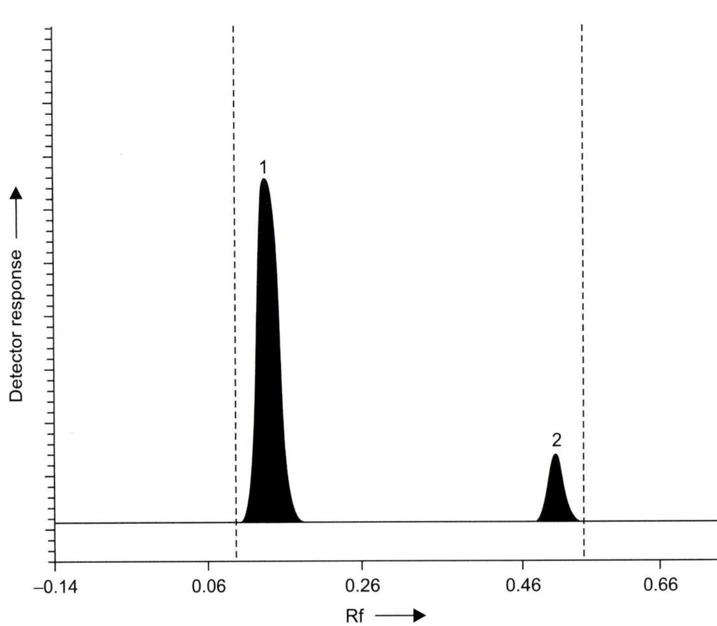

Typical densitogram of the sample containing paracetamol and valdecoxib. For detailed experimental and chromatographic conditions, refer to Protocol No. 163. Peaks identification: 1. Paracetamol; 2. Valdecoxib.

PROTOCOL FOR HPTLC ANALYSIS OF PHARMACEUTICAL FORMULATION

Protocol No. 163

Formulation: Paracetamol, Valdecoxib

Classification: Musculoskeletal Disorders **Dosage form:** Tablets

Standard preparation: Prepare solution of both the compounds separately in ethanol to get 2.5 mg/ml of paracetamol and 100 μg/ml valdecoxib. Further dilutions made to study linearity profile. Apply 5 μl of each solution.

Sample preparation: Powdered sample equivalent to 10 mg of valdecoxib suspended in ethanol, sonicated, diluted to 100 ml, filtered and filtrate suitably diluted. Apply 5 μl of resulting solution for chromatographic evaluation.

Chromatographic equipments:

Sample applicator: Camag Linomat–V

Development chamber: Camag twin–trough glass chamber, 20 × 10 cm

Densitometric scanner: Camag TLC Scanner–III

Chromatographic conditions:

1. Stationary phase: Silica gel $60F_{254}$ pre-coated TLC plates, 10 × 10 cm (250 μm) – Merck
2. Mobile phase (MP): Chloroform–isopropyl alcohol–glacial acetic acid (9.5 : 1 : 0.2 v/v)
3. Standard/Sample application:
   Band length: 10 mm Volume applied: 5 μl Spacing: 10 mm
4. Chamber saturation: 15 min (FP)
5. RH (%): 55 ± 2
6. Temperature °C: 22 ± 2
7. Separation technique: Ascending
8. Quantity of mobile phase: 20 ml
9. Migration distance: 82 mm
10. Migration time: 20 min

Densitometric evaluation:

Wavelength: UV–250 nm Scanning mode: Reflectance/Absorbance

HRF: Paracetamol—14; Valdecoxib—51

Linearity (μg/band): Paracetamol—25–12.5; Valdecoxib—0.1–0.5

Recovery (%): 98.60–99.20 for both the compounds

References: M. Gandhimathi, T.K. Ravi, Nilima Shukla and B. Sowmiya, *Ind. J. Pharm. Sci.*, **69(1)**, 145–146, 2007.

Comments: The method validated for accuracy, precision, linearity, LOD, LOQ, specificity, robustness and ruggedness.

HPTLC : High Performance Thin Layer Chromatography
HPTLC Densitogram

No. 164

Paracetamol

Oxyphenbutazone

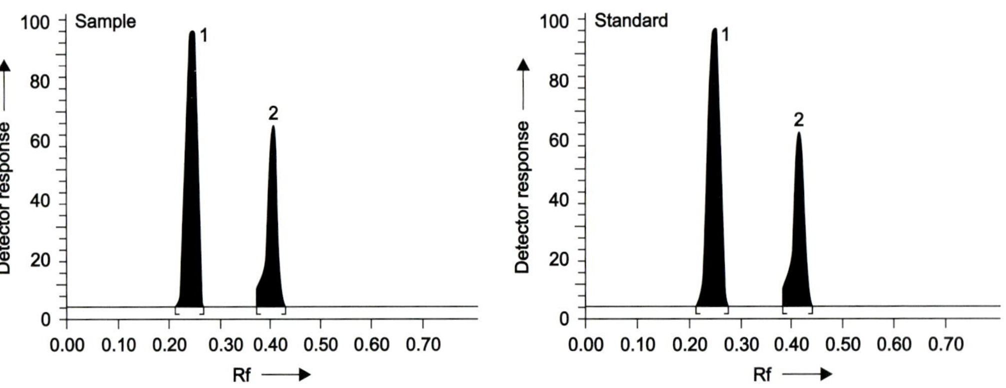

Typical densitogram of the sample and the standard containing paracetamol and oxyphenbutazone. For detailed experimental and chromatographic conditions, refer to Protocol No.164. Peaks identification: 1. Paracetamol; 2. Oxyphenbutazone.

PROTOCOL FOR HPTLC ANALYSIS OF PHARMACEUTICAL FORMULATION

Protocol No. 164

Formulation: Paracetamol, Oxyphenbutazone

Classification: Musculoskeletal Disorders **Dosage form:** Tablets

Standard preparation: (1) Prepare 4 mg/ml solution of paracetamol in methanol; (2) Prepare 1 mg/ml solution of oxyphenbutazone in methanol. Mix 0.25 ml of solutions (1) and (2) and dilute to 10 ml with methanol and use the resulting solution for chromatographic evaluation.

Sample preparation: Weigh powdered sample accurately equivalent to 40 mg of paracetamol, suspend in 50–60 ml methanol, sonicate for 5 min, and dilute to 100 ml. Filer and dilute 2.5 ml to 10 ml. Apply 4 μl of the resulting solution for chromatographic separation and analysis.

Chromatographic equipments:

Sample applicator: Camag Linomat–IV

Development chamber: Camag twin–trough glass chamber, 10 × 10 cm

Densitometric scanner: Camag TLC Scanner–II

Chromatographic conditions:

1. Stationary phase: Silica gel $60F_{254}$ pre-coated HPTLC plates, 5 × 10 cm (200 μm) – Merck
2. Mobile phase (MP): Toluene–acetone (6.5 : 3.5 v/v)
3. Standard/Sample application:
   Band length: 5 mm Volume applied: 4 μl Spacing: 5 mm
4. Chamber saturation: 10 min (MP)
5. RH (%): 55 ± 5
6. Temperature °C: 22 ± 2
7. Separation technique: Ascending
8. Quantity of mobile phase: 10 ml
9. Migration distance: 50 mm
10. Migration time: 13 min

Densitometric evaluation:

Wavelength: UV–244 nm Scanning mode: Reflectance/Absorbance

HRF: Paracetamol—25; Oxyphenbutazone—40

Linearity (ng/band): Paracetamol—100–1000; Oxyphenbutazone—50–250

Recovery (%): 99.54–101.97 for both the compounds

References: —

Comments:

- The method was optimized and analytical work carried out at **Anchrom's HPTLC Application Laboratory**, Mumbai, India.
- Several market samples of similar composition were analysed by the proposed method with reproducible results.
- The method is not suitably for estimation of p-aminophenol as it does not get resolved.

HPTLC : High Performance Thin Layer Chromatography
HPTLC Densitogram

No. 165

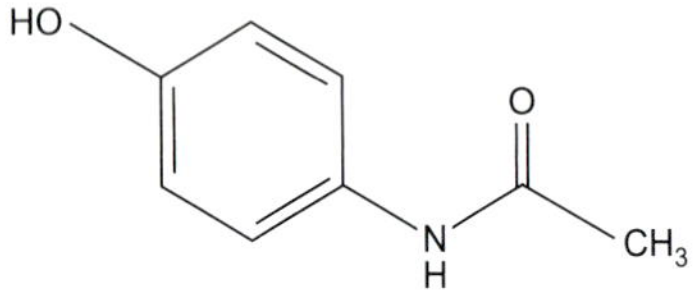

Paracetamol

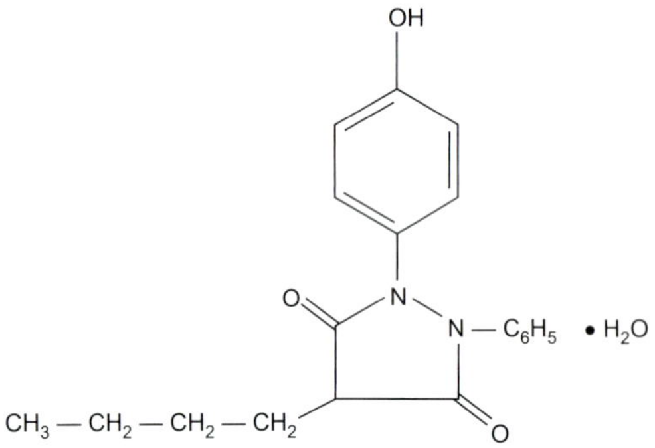

Oxyphenbutazone

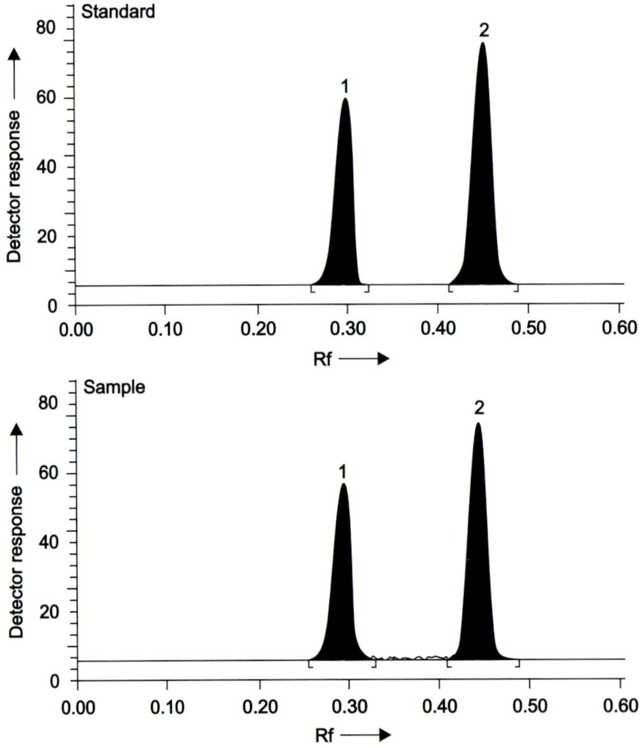

Typical densitogram of the sample and the standard containing paracetamol and oxyphenbutazone. For detailed experimental and chromatographic conditions, refer to Protocol No. 165. Peaks identification: 1. Oxyphenbutazone; 2. Paracetamol.

PROTOCOL FOR HPTLC ANALYSIS OF PHARMACEUTICAL FORMULATION

Protocol No. 165

Formulation: **Paracetamol, Oxyphenbutazone**
Classification: Musculoskeletal Disorders **Dosage form:** Tablets
Standard preparation: (1) Prepare 4 mg/ml solution of paracetamol in methanol; (2) Prepare 1 mg/ml solution of oxyphenbutazone in methanol. Mix 0.25 ml of solutions (1) and (2) and dilute to 10 ml with methanol and use the resulting solution for chromatographic evaluation.
Sample preparation: Weigh powdered sample accurately equivalent to 40 mg of paracetamol, suspend in 50–60 ml methanol, sonicate for 5 min, and dilute to 100 ml. Filter and dilute 2.5 ml to 10 ml. Apply 4 µl of the resulting solution for chromatographic separation and analysis.
Chromatographic equipments:
Sample applicator: Camag Linomat–IV
Development chamber: Camag twin–trough glass chamber, 10 × 10 cm
Densitometric scanner: Camag TLC Scanner–II
Chromatographic conditions:
1. Stationary phase: Silica gel 60 RP-18F_{254s} pre-coated HPTLC plates, 10 × 10 cm (200 µm) – Merck
2. Mobile phase (MP): 0.5 M sodium chloride–methanol–glacial acetic acid (12 : 8 : 0.01 v/v)
3. Standard/Sample application:
   Band length: 5 mm Volume applied: 4 µl Spacing: 5 mm
4. Chamber saturation: 30 min (MP)
5. RH (%): 55 ± 5
6. Temperature °C: 22 ± 2
7. Separation technique: Ascending
8. Quantity of mobile phase: 20 ml
9. Migration distance: 50 mm
10. Migration time: 40 min

Densitometric evaluation:
Wavelength: UV–244 nm Scanning mode: Reflectance/Absorbance
HRF: Oxyphenbutazone—30; Paracetamol—45
Linearity (ng/band): Paracetamol—100–1000; Oxyphenbutazone—50–250
Recovery (%): 100.25–101.75 for both the compounds
References: —
Comments:
- The method was optimized and analytical work carried out at **Anchrom's HPTLC Application Laboratory**, Mumbai, India.
- Several market samples of similar composition were analysed by the proposed method with reproducible results.
- Reversed-phase chromatography resulted in reversal of retention order as compared to NP-chromatography.

HPTLC : High Performance Thin Layer Chromatography
HPTLC Densitogram

No. 167

Paracetamol

Ketoprofen

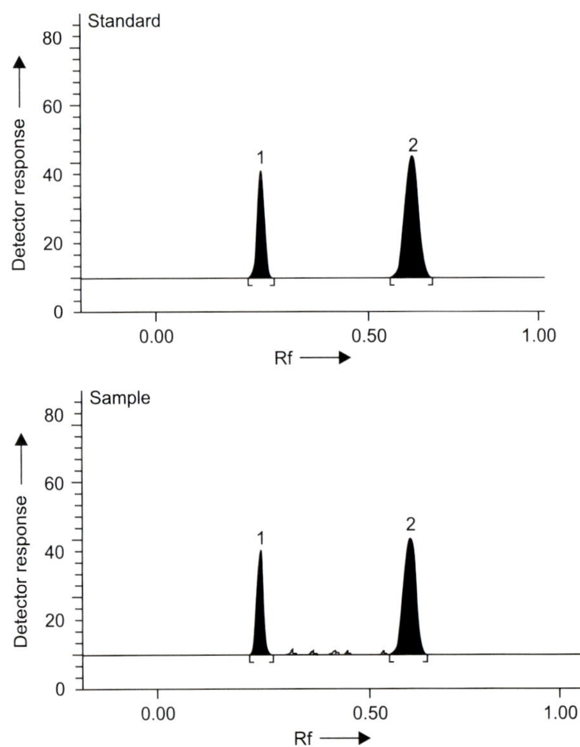

Typical densitogram of the sample and the standard containing paracetamol and ketoprofen. For detailed experimental and chromatographic conditions, refer to Protocol No. 167. Peaks identification: 1. Ketoprofen; 2. Paracetamol.

PROTOCOL FOR HPTLC ANALYSIS OF PHARMACEUTICAL FORMULATION

Protocol No. 167

Formulation: Paracetamol, Ketoprofen

Classification: Musculoskeletal Disorders **Dosage form:** Tablets

Standard preparation: (1) Prepare 0.5 mg/ml solution of ketoprofen in methanol; (2) 1 mg/ml solution of paracetamol in methanol. Mix 0.2 ml of solution (1) and 0.9 ml of solution (2) and dilute to 10 ml with methanol. Apply 5 μl for chromatographic analysis.

Sample preparation: Weigh powdered sample accurately equivalent to 25 mg of ketoprofen, suspend in 30–40 ml methanol, sonicate for 5 min, dilute to 50 ml, filter and dilute 0.2 ml to 10 ml with methanol. Apply 5 μl for chromatographic evaluation.

Chromatographic equipments:

Sample applicator: Camag Linomat–IV

Development chamber: Camag twin–trough glass chamber, 10 × 10 cm

Densitometric scanner: Camag TLC Scanner–II

Chromatographic conditions:

1. Stationary phase: Silica gel 60 RP-18F_{254s} pre-coated HPTLC plates, 10 × 10 cm (200 μm) – Merck
2. Mobile phase (MP): 0.5 M sodium chloride–methanol–glacial acetic acid (12 : 8 : 0.01 v/v)
3. Standard/Sample application:
   Band length: 10 mm Volume applied: 5 μl Spacing: 10 mm
4. Chamber saturation: 30 min (MP)
5. RH (%): 55 ± 5
6. Temperature °C: 22 ± 2
7. Separation technique: Ascending
8. Quantity of mobile phase: 20 ml
9. Migration distance: 50 mm
10. Migration time: 40 min

Densitometric evaluation:

Wavelength: UV–267 nm Scanning mode: Reflectance/Absorbance

HRF: Ketoprofen—24; Paracetamol—60

Linearity (ng/band): Paracetamol—100–1000; Oxyphenbutazone—25–100

Recovery (%): 100.20–102.75 for both the compounds

References: —

Comments:

- The method was optimized and analytical work carried out at **Anchrom's HPTLC Application Laboratory**, Mumbai, India.
- Reversed-phase chromatography resulted in reversal of retention order as compared to NP-chromatography.

HPTLC : High Performance Thin Layer Chromatography
HPTLC Densitogram

No. 168

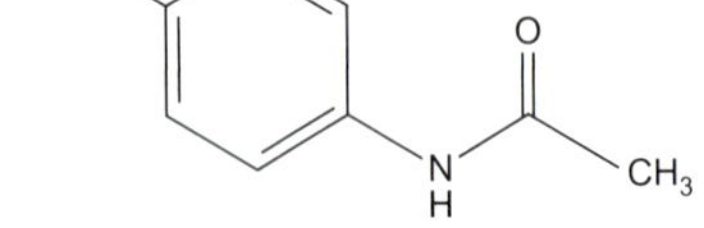

Paracetamol

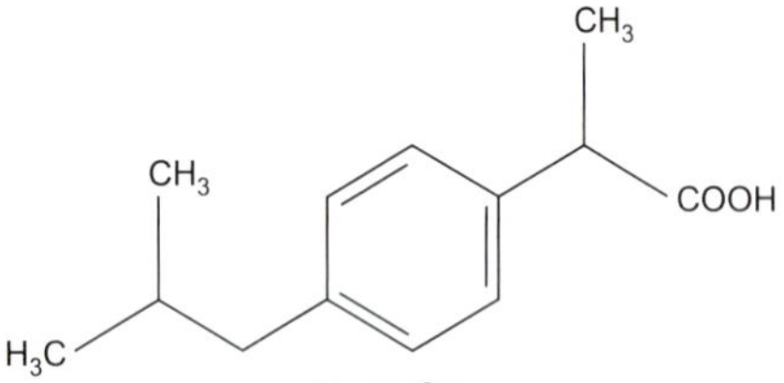

Ibuprofen

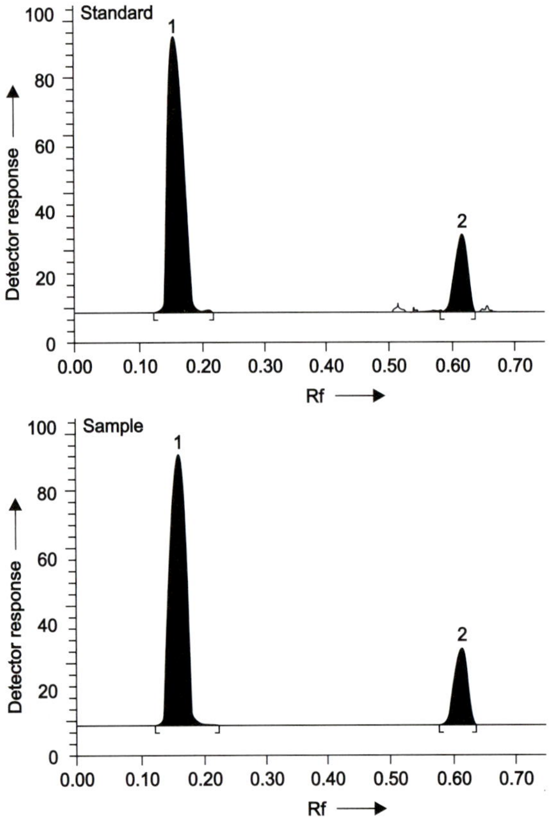

Typical densitogram of the sample and the standard containing paracetamol and ibuprofen. For detailed experimental and chromatographic conditions, refer to Protocol No. 168. Peaks identification: 1. Paracetamol; 2. Ibuprofen.

PROTOCOL FOR HPTLC ANALYSIS OF PHARMACEUTICAL FORMULATION

Protocol No. 168

Formulation: Paracetamol, Ibuprofen

Classification: Musculoskeletal Disorders **Dosage form:**

Standard preparation: Weigh accurately about 25 mg of paracetamol (P) and about 30 mg of ibuprofen (I), dissolve in methanol to make 25 ml. Dilute further 1 ml to 10 ml with methanol and use for chromatographic analysis.

Sample preparation: Weigh accurately powdered sample equivalent to 50 mg of paracetamol, suspend in 30–40 ml methanol, sonicate for 5 min, dilute to 50 ml, filter and dilute 1 ml to 10 ml for chromatographic application.

Chromatographic equipments:

Sample applicator: Camag Linomat–IV

Development chamber: Camag twin–trough glass chamber, 10 × 10 cm

Densitometric scanner: Camag TLC Scanner–II

Chromatographic conditions:

1. Stationary phase: Silica gel 60F_{254} pre-coated HPTLC plates, 10 × 10 cm (200 μm) – Merck
2. Mobile phase (MP): (i) n-hexane–ethyl acetate–glacial acetic acid (9 : 2.5 : 1 v/v); (ii) Ethyl acetate–acetone–n-butanol–25% ammonia (3 : 4 : 3 : 1 v/v)
3. Standard/Sample application:
   Band length: 5 mm   Volume applied: 5 μl   Spacing: 5 mm
4. Chamber saturation: 10 min (MP)
5. RH (%): 55 ± 5
6. Temperature °C: 22 ± 2
7. Separation technique: Ascending
8. Quantity of mobile phase: 12 ml
9. Migration distance: 60 mm
10. Migration time: 18 min

Densitometric evaluation:

Wavelength: UV–235 nm or 265 nm   Scanning mode: Reflectance/Absorbance

HRF: Paracetamol—16, 86; Ibuprofen—62, 32

Linearity (ng/band): Paracetamol—100–1000, 130–650; Ibuprofen—200–2000, 120–600

Recovery (%): 99.75–101.5 for both the compounds

References: (i) P.P. Shirke, M.K. Patel, V.M. Tamhane, V.B. Tirodkar, *Indian Drugs*, **30(12)**, 653–654, 1993; (ii) R. Rele and S. Sawant, *Analytical Chemistry – An Indian Journal*, 2010.

Comments: As ibuprofen is a poor UV absorbing compound, the scanning should preferably be done at 235 nm.

HPTLC : High Performance Thin Layer Chromatography
HPTLC Densitogram

No. 170

Paracetamol

Chlormezanone

Typical densitogram of the sample and the standard containing paracetamol and chlorzoxazone. For detailed experimental and chromatographic conditions, refer to Protocol No. 170. Peaks identification: 1. Paracetamol; 2. Chlormezanone.

PROTOCOL FOR HPTLC ANALYSIS OF PHARMACEUTICAL FORMULATION

Protocol No. 170

Formulation: Paracetamol, Chlormezanone

Classification: Musculoskeletal Disorders **Dosage form:** Tablets

Standard preparation: Weigh accurately about 45 mg of paracetamol (P) and 10 mg of chlormezanone (C), dissolve in methanol to make 50 ml, dilute 1 ml to 10 ml with methanol and use for chromatographic analysis.

Sample preparation: Weigh powdered sample equivalent to 45 mg of paracetamol, suspend in 30–40 ml methanol, sonicate for 5 min, dilute to 50 ml, filter and dilute 1 ml to 10 ml with methanol for chromatographic application.

Chromatographic equipments:

Sample applicator: Camag Linomat–IV

Development chamber: Camag twin–trough glass chamber, 10 × 10 cm

Densitometric scanner: Camag TLC Scanner–II

Chromatographic conditions:

1. Stationary phase: Silica gel $60F_{254}$ pre-coated HPTLC plates, 10 × 10 cm (200 μm) – Merck
2. Mobile phase (MP): n-hexane–ethyl acetate–glacial acetic acid (7 : 5 : 1 v/v)
3. Standard/Sample application:
   Band length: 5 mm Volume applied: 5 μl Spacing: 5 mm
4. Chamber saturation: 10 min (MP)
5. RH (%): 55 ± 5
6. Temperature °C: 22 ± 2
7. Separation technique: Ascending
8. Quantity of mobile phase: 13 ml
9. Migration distance: 50 mm
10. Migration time: 14 min

Densitometric evaluation:

Wavelength: UV–225 nm Scanning mode: Reflectance/Absorbance

HRF: Paracetamol—25; Chlormezanone—32

Linearity (ng/band): Paracetamol—100–1000; Chlormezanone—50–200

Recovery (%): 99.0–102.70 for both the compounds

References: —

Comments:

- The method was optimized and analytical work carried out at **Anchrom's HPTLC Application Laboratory**, Mumbai, India.
- Several market samples of similar composition were analysed by the proposed method with reproducible results.

HPTLC : High Performance Thin Layer Chromatography
HPTLC Densitogram

No. 171

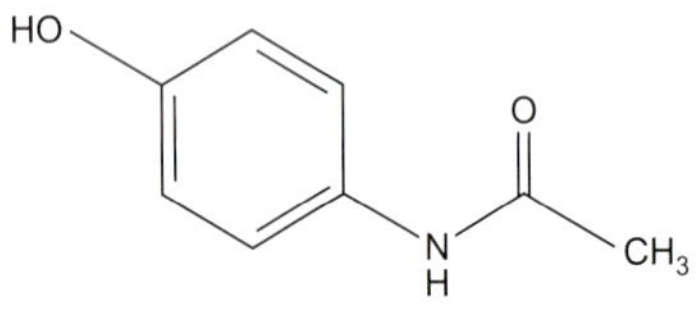

HO
O
N
H
CH_3
Paracetamol

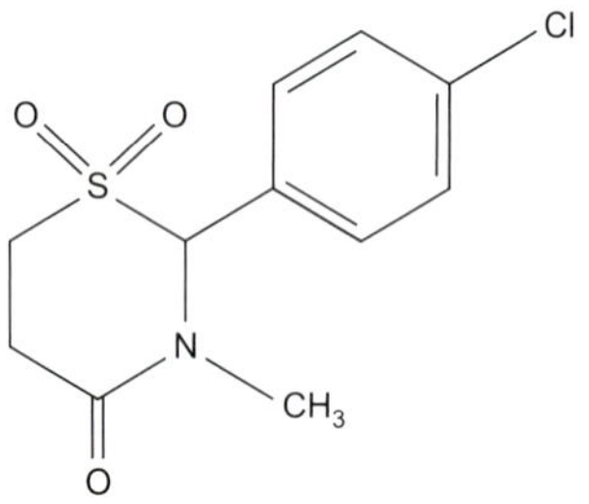

Cl
O
O
S
N
CH_3
O
Chlormezanone

Standard
Detector response
80
60
40
20
0
1
2
0.00 0.10 0.20 0.30 0.40 0.50
Rf

Sample
Detector response
80
60
40
20
0
1
2
0.00 0.10 0.20 0.30 0.40 0.50
Rf

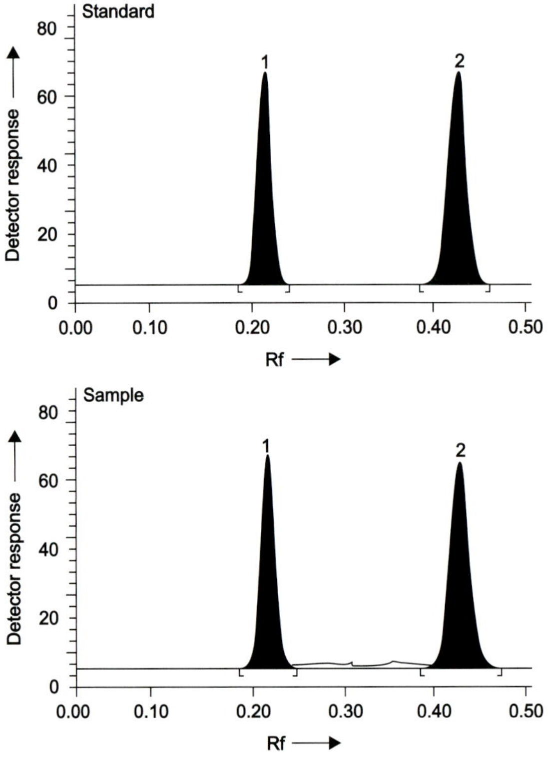

Typical densitogram of the sample and the standard containing paracetamol and chlormezanone. For detailed experimental and chromatographic conditions, refer to Protocol No. 171. Peaks identification: 1. Chlormezanone; 2. Paracetamol.

PROTOCOL FOR HPTLC ANALYSIS OF PHARMACEUTICAL FORMULATION

Protocol No. 171

Formulation: **Paracetamol, Chlormezanone**
Classification: Musculoskeletal Disorders **Dosage form:** Tablets
Standard preparation: Weigh accurately about 45 mg of paracetamol (P) and 10 mg of chlormezanone (C), dissolve in methanol to make 50 ml, dilute 1 ml to 10 ml with methanol and use for chromatographic analysis.
Sample preparation: Weigh powdered sample equivalent to 45 mg of paracetamol, suspend in 30–40 ml methanol, sonicate for 5 min, dilute to 50 ml, filter and dilute 1 ml to 10 ml with methanol for chromatographic application.
Chromatographic equipments:
Sample applicator: Camag Linomat–IV
Development chamber: Camag twin–trough glass chamber, 10 × 10 cm
Densitometric scanner: Camag TLC Scanner–II
Chromatographic conditions:
1. Stationary phase: Silica gel 60 RP-18F_{254s} pre-coated HPTLC plates, 10 × 10 cm (200 μm) – Merck
2. Mobile phase (MP): 0.5 M sodium chloride–methanol–glacial acetic acid (12 : 8 : 0.01 v/v)
3. Standard/Sample application:
   Band length: 5 mm Volume applied: 5 μl Spacing: 5 mm
4. Chamber saturation: 30 min (MP)
5. RH (%): 55 ± 5
6. Temperature °C: 22 ± 2
7. Separation technique: Ascending
8. Quantity of mobile phase: 20 ml
9. Migration distance: 50 mm
10. Migration time: 40 min

Densitometric evaluation:
Wavelength: UV–225 nm Scanning mode: Reflectance/Absorbance
HRF: Chlormezanone—22; Paracetamol—43
Linearity (ng/band): Paracetamol—100–1000; Chlormezanone—50–200
Recovery (%): 100.45–101.35 for both the compounds
References: —
Comments:
- The method was optimized and analytical work carried out at **Anchrom's HPTLC Application Laboratory**, Mumbai, India.
- Reversed-phase chromatography resulted in reversal of retention order as compared to NP-chromatography.
- Resolution of two compounds is superior with RP-chromatography.

HPTLC : High Performance Thin Layer Chromatography
HPTLC Densitogram

No. 172

Paracetamol

Chlorzoxazone

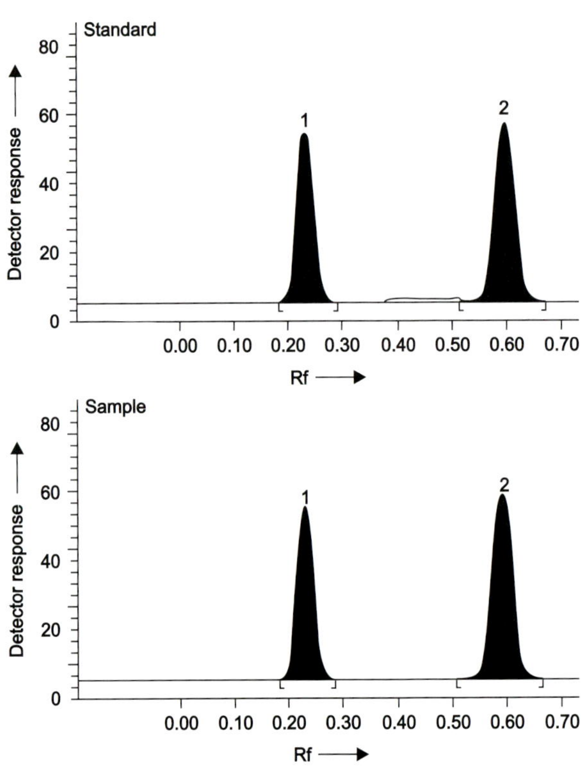

Typical densitogram of the sample and the standard containing paracetamol and chlorzoxazone. For detailed experimental and chromatographic conditions, refer to Protocol No. 172. Peaks identification: 1. Paracetamol; 2. Chlorzoxazone.

PROTOCOL FOR HPTLC ANALYSIS OF PHARMACEUTICAL FORMULATION

Protocol No. 172

Formulation: Paracetamol, Chlorzoxazone

Classification: Musculoskeletal Disorders **Dosage form:** Tablets

Standard preparation: Weigh accurately about 30 mg of paracetamol and 25 mg of chlorzoxazone, dissolve in methanol to make 100 ml, further dilute 2 ml to 10 ml with methanol for chromatographic analysis.

Sample preparation: Weigh powdered sample equivalent to 30 mg of paracetamol, suspend in 60–70 ml methanol, sonicate and dilute to 100 ml. Filter and dilute 2 ml to 10 ml with methanol for chromatographic analysis.

Chromatographic equipments:

Sample applicator: Camag Linomat–IV

Development chamber: Camag twin–trough glass chamber, 10 × 10 cm

Densitometric scanner: Camag TLC Scanner–II

Chromatographic conditions:

1. Stationary phase: Silica gel $60F_{254}$ pre-coated TLC plates, 10 × 10 cm (250 μm) – Merck
2. Mobile phase (MP): Toluene–acetone (7 : 3 v/v)
3. Standard/Sample application:
   Band length: 5 mm Volume applied: 5 μl Spacing: 5 mm
4. Chamber saturation: 10 min (MP)
5. RH (%): 55 ± 5
6. Temperature °C: 22 ± 2
7. Separation technique: Ascending
8. Quantity of mobile phase: 10 ml
9. Migration distance: 50 mm
10. Migration time: 14 min

Densitometric evaluation:

Wavelength: UV–278 nm Scanning mode: Reflectance/Absorbance

HRF: Paracetamol—23; Chlorzoxazone—60

Linearity: Paracetamol and chlorzoxazone—100–1000 ng/band

Recovery (%): 99.75–102.25 for both the compounds

References: —

Comments:

- The method was optimized and analytical work carried out at **Anchrom's HPTLC Application Laboratory**, Mumbai, India.
- Several market samples of similar composition were analysed by the proposed method with reproducible results.

HPTLC : High Performance Thin Layer Chromatography
HPTLC Densitogram

No. 173

HO, O, N, H, CH_3

Paracetamol

O, OH, N, Cl

Chlorzoxazone

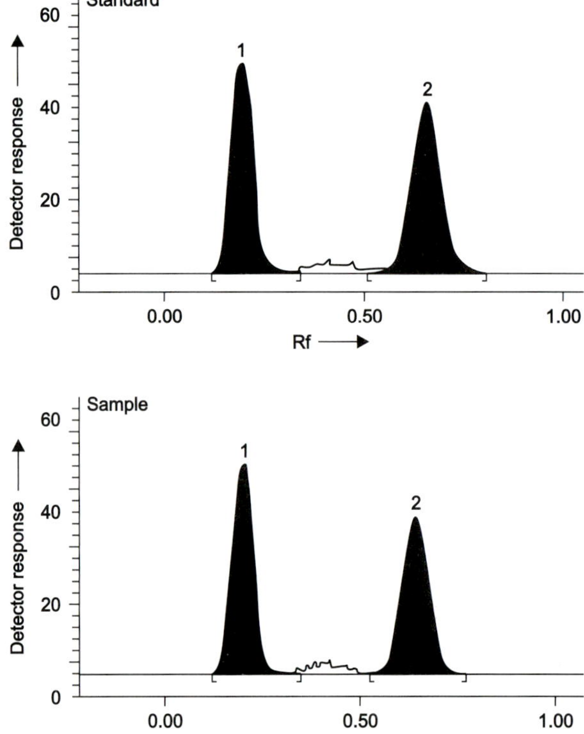

Typical densitogram of the sample and the standard containing paracetamol and chlorzoxazone. For detailed experimental and chromatographic conditions, refer to Protocol No. 173. Peaks identification: 1. Chlorzoxazone; 2. Paracetamol.

PROTOCOL FOR HPTLC ANALYSIS OF PHARMACEUTICAL FORMULATION

Protocol No. 173

Formulation: Paracetamol, Chlorzoxazone
Classification: Musculoskeletal Disorders **Dosage form:** Tablets
Standard preparation: Weigh accurately about 30 mg of paracetamol and 25 mg of chlorzoxazone, dissolve in methanol to make 100 ml, further dilute 2 ml to 10 ml with methanol for chromatographic analysis.
Sample preparation: Weigh powdered sample equivalent to 30 mg of paracetamol, suspend in 60–70 ml methanol, sonicate and dilute to 100 ml. Filter and dilute 2 ml to 10 ml with methanol for chromatographic analysis.
Chromatographic equipments:
Sample applicator: Camag Linomat–IV
Development chamber: Camag twin–trough glass chamber, 10 × 10 cm
Densitometric scanner: Camag TLC Scanner–II
Chromatographic conditions:

1. Stationary phase: Silica gel 60 RP-18F_{254s} pre-coated HPTLC plates, 10 × 10 cm (200 μm) – Merck
2. Mobile phase (MP): 0.5 M sodium chloride–methanol–glacial acetic acid (12 : 8 : 0.01 v/v)
3. Standard/Sample application:
   Band length: 5 mm Volume applied: 5 μl Spacing: 5 mm
4. Chamber saturation: 10 min (MP)
5. RH (%): 55 ± 5
6. Temperature °C: 22 ± 2
7. Separation technique: Ascending
8. Quantity of mobile phase: 20 ml
9. Migration distance: 50 mm
10. Migration time: 40 min

Densitometric evaluation:
Wavelength: UV–278 nm Scanning mode: Reflectance/Absorbance
HRF: Chlorzoxazone—19; Paracetamol—64
Linearity: Paracetamol and chlorzoxazone—100–1000 ng/band
Recovery (%): 99.85–101.25 for both the compounds
References: —
Comments:

- The method was optimized and analytical work carried out at **Anchrom's HPTLC Application Laboratory**, Mumbai, India.
- Reversed-phase chromatography resulted in reversal of retention order as compared to NP-chromatography.
- Several market samples of similar composition were analysed by the proposed method with reproducible results.

HPTLC : High Performance Thin Layer Chromatography
HPTLC Densitogram

No. 174

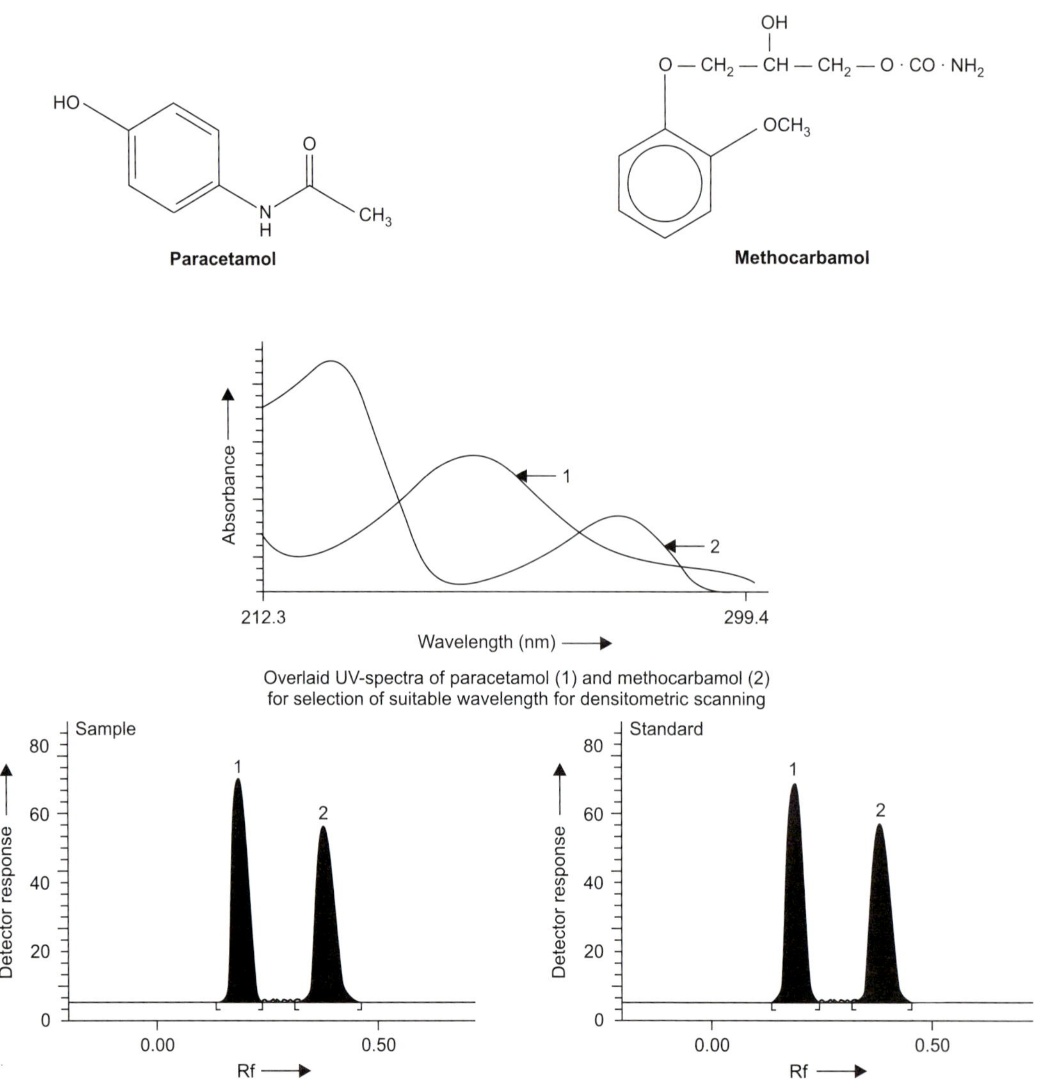

Typical densitogram of the sample and the standard containing paracetamol and methocarbamol. For detailed experimental and chromatographic conditions, refer to Protocol No. 174. Peaks identification: 1. Paracetamol; 2. Methocarbamol.

PROTOCOL FOR HPTLC ANALYSIS OF PHARMACEUTICAL FORMULATION

Protocol No. 174

Formulation: Paracetamol, Methocarbamol

Classification: Musculoskeletal Disorders **Dosage form:** Tablets

Standard preparation: Weigh accurately about 40 mg of methocarbamol (M) and 32.5 mg of paracetamol (P) and dissolve in methanol to make 100 ml, further dilute 1 ml of the solution to 10 ml with methanol. Apply 6 μl for chromatographic evaluation.

Sample preparation: Weigh accurately powdered sample equivalent to about 40 mg of methocarbamol, add about 80 ml of methanol, vortex for 10 min, and dilute to 100 ml. Further dilute 1 ml to 10 ml with methanol and use for chromatographic separation.

Chromatographic equipments:

Sample applicator: Camag Linomat–IV
Development chamber: Camag twin–trough glass chamber, 10 × 10 cm
Densitometric scanner: Camag TLC Scanner–II

Chromatographic conditions:

1. Stationary phase: Silica gel $60F_{254}$ pre-coated HPTLC plates, 10 × 10 cm (200 μm) – Merck
2. Mobile phase (MP): Chloroform–methanol–glacial acetic acid (9.5 : 0.5 : 0.2 v/v)
3. Standard/Sample application:
   Band length: 10 mm Volume applied: 6 μl Spacing: 10 mm
4. Chamber saturation: 20 min (MP)
5. RH (%): 55 ± 5
6. Temperature °C: 22 ± 2
7. Separation technique: Ascending
8. Quantity of mobile phase: 10 ml
9. Migration distance: 50 mm
10. Migration time: 20 min

Densitometric evaluation:

Wavelength: UV–275 nm Scanning mode: Reflectance/Absorbance
HRF: Paracetamol—19; Methocarbamol—38
Linearity (ng/band): Paracetamol—50–500; Methocarbamol—100–500
Recovery (%): 98.20–99.57 for both the compounds

References: —

Comments:

- The method was optimized and analytical work carried out at **Anchrom's HPTLC Application Laboratory**, Mumbai, India.
- Several market samples of similar composition were analysed by the proposed method with reproducible results.
- p-Aminophenol, the decomposition product of paracetamol, did not interfere.

HPTLC : High Performance Thin Layer Chromatography
HPTLC Densitogram

No. 175

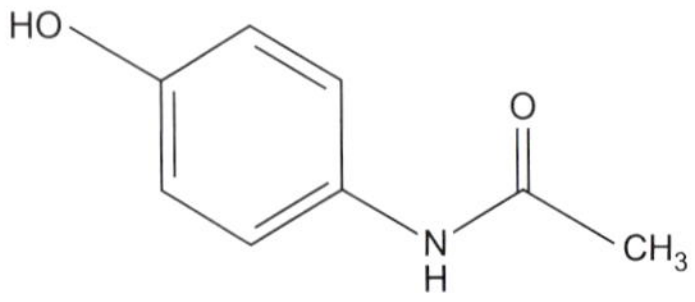
HO
O
N
H
CH3

Paracetamol

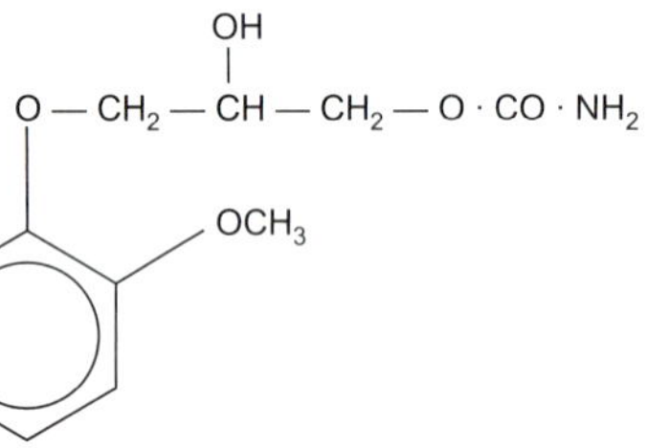
OH
O — CH2 — CH — CH2 — O · CO · NH2
OCH3

Methocarbamol

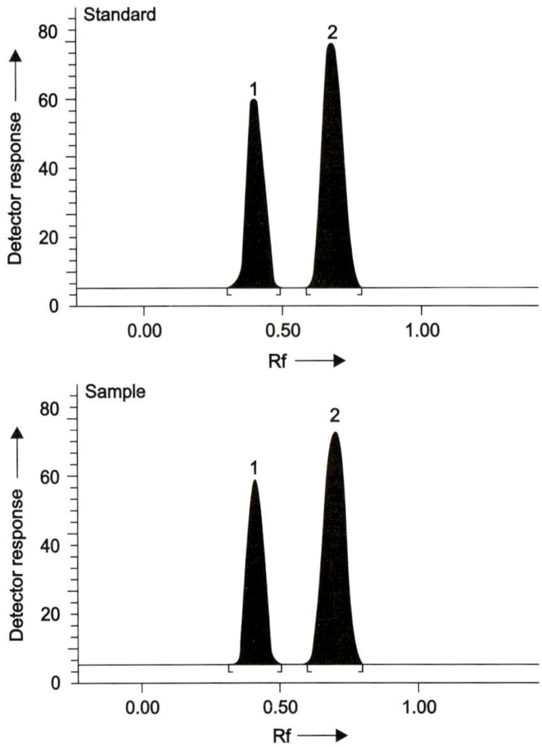
Standard
Detector response
80
60
40
20
0
1
2
0.00
0.50
1.00
Rf
Sample
Detector response
80
60
40
20
0
1
2
0.00
0.50
1.00
Rf

Typical densitogram of the sample and the standard containing paracetamol and methocarbamol. For detailed experimental and chromatographic conditions, refer to Protocol No. 175. Peaks identification: 1. Methocarbamol; 2. Paracetamol.

PROTOCOL FOR HPTLC ANALYSIS OF PHARMACEUTICAL FORMULATION

Protocol No. 175

Formulation: **Paracetamol, Methocarbamol**

Classification: Musculoskeletal Disorders **Dosage form:** Tablets

Standard preparation: Weigh accurately about 40 mg of methocarbamol (M) and 32.5 mg of paracetamol (P) and dissolve in methanol to make 100 ml, further dilute 1 ml of the solution to 10 ml with methanol. Apply 6 μl for chromatographic evaluation.

Sample preparation: Weigh accurately powdered sample equivalent to about 40 mg of methocarbamol, add about 80 ml of methanol, vortex for 10 min, and dilute to 100 ml. Further dilute 1 ml to 10 ml with methanol and use for chromatographic separation.

Chromatographic equipments:

Sample applicator: Camag Linomat–IV
Development chamber: Camag twin–trough glass chamber, 10 × 10 cm
Densitometric scanner: Camag TLC Scanner–II

Chromatographic conditions:

1. Stationary phase: Silica gel 60 RP-18F_{254s} pre-coated HPTLC plates, 10 × 10 cm (200 μm) – Merck
2. Mobile phase (MP): 0.5 M sodium chloride–methanol–glacial acetic acid (12 : 8 : 0.01 v/v)
3. Standard/Sample application:
   Band length: 10 mm Volume applied: 6 μl Spacing: 10 mm
4. Chamber saturation: 30 min (MP)
5. RH (%): 55 ± 5
6. Temperature °C: 22 ± 2
7. Separation technique: Ascending
8. Quantity of mobile phase: 20 ml
9. Migration distance: 50 mm
10. Migration time: 40 min

Densitometric evaluation:

Wavelength: UV–275 nm Scanning mode: Reflectance/Absorbance
HRF: Methocarbamol—40; Paracetamol—60
Linearity (ng/band): Paracetamol—50–500; Methocarbamol—100–500
Recovery (%): 102.14–103.50 for both the compounds

References: —

Comments:

- The method was optimized and analytical work carried out at **Anchrom's HPTLC Application Laboratory**, Mumbai, India.
- Reversed-phase chromatography resulted in reversal of retention order as compared to NP-chromatography.

HPTLC : High Performance Thin Layer Chromatography
HPTLC Densitogram

No. 176

HO

O

N
H

CH_3

Paracetamol

H_3C CH_3
N
H
H_3CO
OH

Tramadol

Standard
2
1
Detector response
0.20 0.40 0.60 0.80 1.00
Rf

Sample
2
1
Detector response
0.20 0.40 0.60 0.80 1.00
Rf

Typical densitogram of the sample and the standard containing paracetamol and tramadol HCl For detailed experimental and chromatographic conditions, refer to Protocol No. 176. Peaks identification: 1. Tramadol HCl; 2. Paracetamol.

PROTOCOL FOR HPTLC ANALYSIS OF PHARMACEUTICAL FORMULATION

Protocol No. 176

Formulation: Paracetamol, Tramadol hydrochloride

Classification: Musculoskeletal Disorders **Dosage form:** Tablets

Standard preparation: Prepare solution of each compound separately in methanol to get 1 mg/ml of tramadol HCl and 9 mg/ml of paracetamol. Further dilutions made suitably with methanol and used for linearity studies.

Sample preparation: Powdered sample equivalent to 10 mg of tramadol suspended in methanol, sonicated, diluted to 10 ml, filtered and the filtrate suitable diluted for chromatographic application and assay.

Chromatographic equipments:

Sample applicator: Camag Linomat–V

Development chamber: Camag twin–trough glass chamber, 10 × 10 cm

Densitometric scanner: Camag TLC Scanner–III

Chromatographic conditions:

1. Stationary phase: Silica gel $60F_{254}$ pre-coated HPTLC plates, 10 × 10 cm (200 μm) – Merck
2. Mobile phase (MP): Ethyl acetate–toluene–25% ammonia (6 : 4 : 0.1 v/v)
3. Standard/Sample application:
   Band length: 10 mm Volume applied: 1–5 μl Spacing: 10 mm
4. Chamber saturation: 15 min (MP)
5. RH (%): 55 ± 5
6. Temperature °C: 22 ± 2
7. Separation technique: Ascending
8. Quantity of mobile phase: 10 ml
9. Migration distance: 75 mm
10. Migration time: 18 min

Densitometric evaluation:

Wavelength: UV–254 nm Scanning mode: Reflectance/Absorbance

HRF: Tramadol HCl—28; Paracetamol—57

Linearity (ng/band): Tramadol HCl—100–500; Paracetamol—900–4500

Recovery (%): 99.66–99.84 for both the compounds

References: M. Gandhimathi and T.K. Ravi, *Asian J. Chem.*, **20(6)**, 4940–4942, 2008.

Comments: The method validated for accuracy, precision, linearity, LOD, LOQ, specificity, robustness and ruggedness.

HPTLC : High Performance Thin Layer Chromatography
HPTLC Densitogram

No. 177

HO

O

N
H

CH_3

Paracetamol

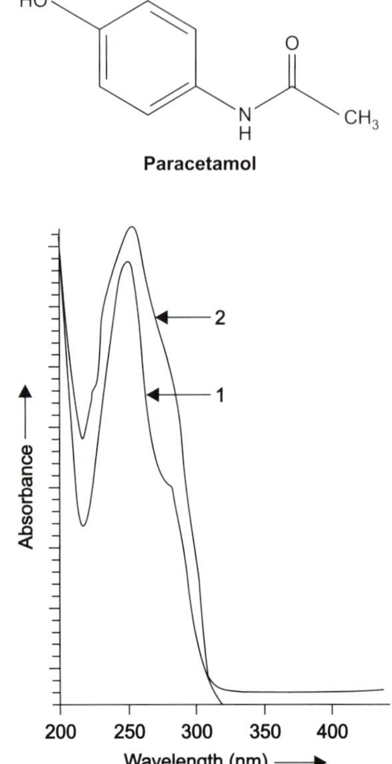

Overlaid UV-spectra of paracetamol (1) and tramadol HCl (2) for selection of suitable wavelength for densitometric scanning

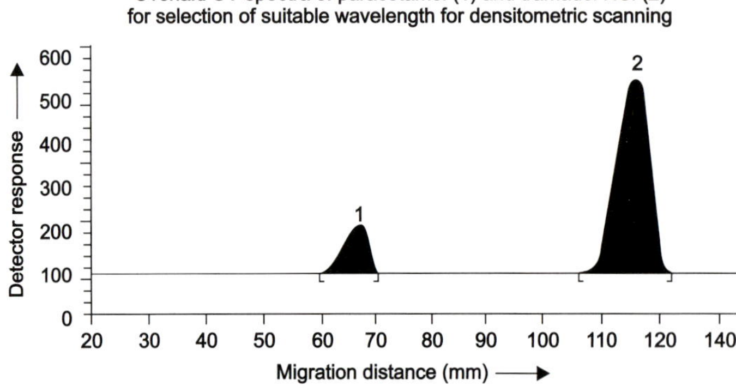

Typical densitogram of the standard containing paracetamol and tramadol HCl. For detailed experimental and chromatographic conditions, refer to Protocol No. 177. Peaks identification: 1. Tramadol HCl; 2. Paracetamol.

PROTOCOL FOR HPTLC ANALYSIS OF PHARMACEUTICAL FORMULATION

Protocol No. 177

Formulation: **Paracetamol, Tramadol hydrochloride**

Classification: Musculoskeletal Disorders **Dosage form:** Tablets

Standard preparation: Prepare solution of each compound separately in methanol to get 1 mg/ml of tramadol HCl and 9 mg/ml of paracetamol. Further dilutions made suitably with methanol and used for linearity studies.

Sample preparation: Powdered sample equivalent to 10 mg of tramadol suspended in methanol, sonicated, diluted to 10 ml, filtered and the filtrate suitably diluted for chromatographic application and assay.

Chromatographic equipments:

Sample applicator: Camag Linomat–IV

Development chamber: Camag twin–trough glass chamber, 10 × 10 cm

Densitometric scanner: Camag TLC Scanner–III

Chromatographic conditions:

1. Stationary phase: Silica gel $60F_{254}$ pre-coated HPTLC plates, 10 × 10 cm (200 μm) – Merck
2. Mobile phase (MP): Chloroform–methanol–glacial acetic acid (9 : 2 : 0.1 v/v)
3. Standard/Sample application:
   Band length: 16 mm Volume applied: 1 μl Spacing: 10 mm
4. Chamber saturation: 10 min (MP)
5. RH (%): 55 ± 5
6. Temperature °C: 22 ± 2
7. Separation technique: Ascending
8. Quantity of mobile phase: 11 ml
9. Migration distance: 80 mm
10. Migration time: 20 min

Densitometric evaluation:

Wavelength: UV–270 nm Scanning mode: Reflectance/Absorbance

HRF: See densitogram

Linearity (ng/band): Paracetamol—1950–4550; Tramadol HCl—225–525

Recovery (%): 99.70–99.90 for both the compounds

References: C. Roosewelt et al., *Asian J. Chem.*, **22(2)**, 850–854, 2010.

Comments: The method validated for accuracy, precision, linearity, LOD, LOQ, specificity, robustness and ruggedness.

HPTLC : High Performance Thin Layer Chromatography
HPTLC Densitogram

No. 178

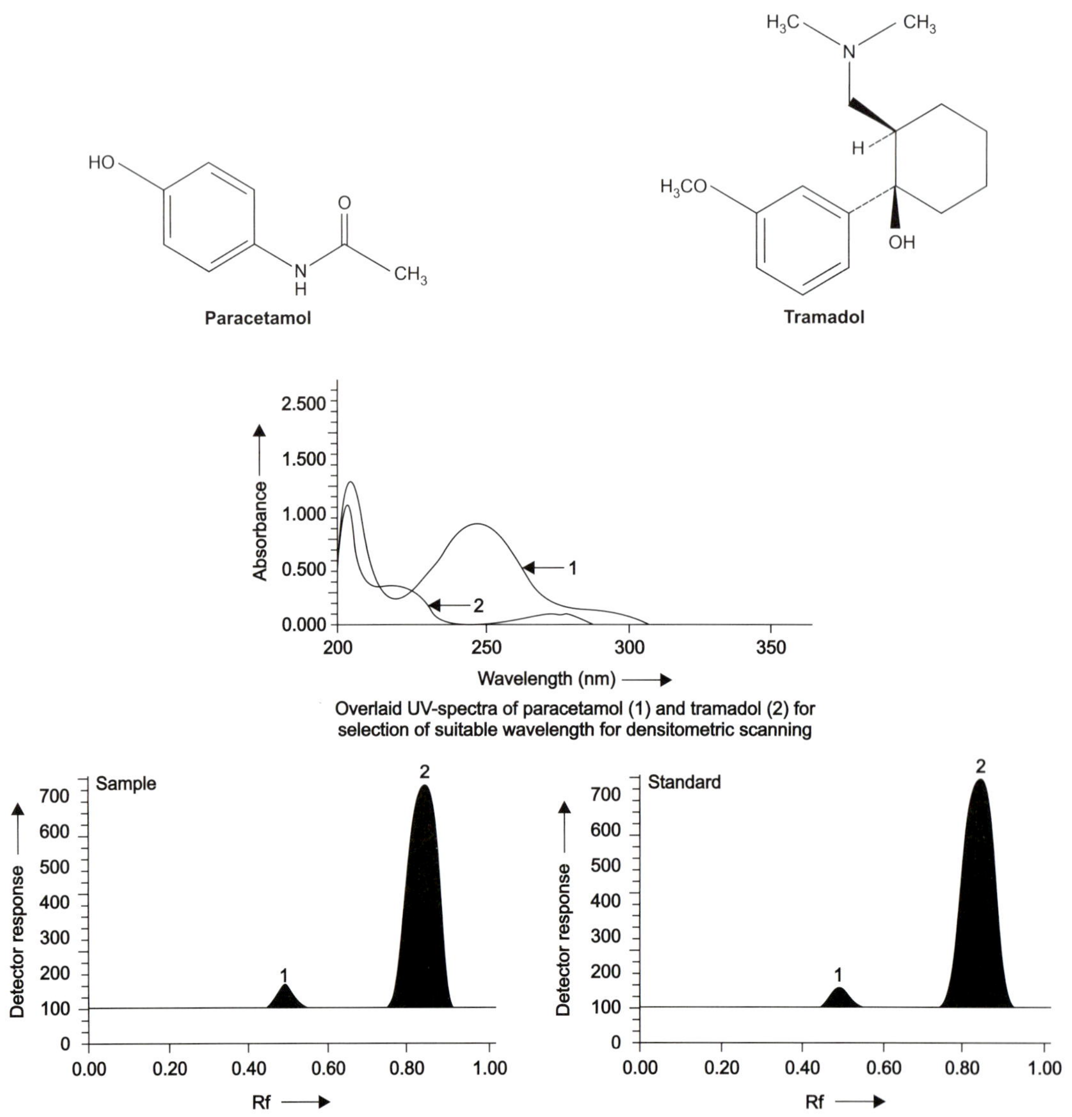

Overlaid UV-spectra of paracetamol (1) and tramadol (2) for selection of suitable wavelength for densitometric scanning

Typical densitogram of the sample and standard containing paracetamol and tramadol HCl. For detailed experimental and chromatographic conditions, refer to Protocol No. 178. Peaks identification: 1. Tramadol HCl; 2. Paracetamol.

PROTOCOL FOR HPTLC ANALYSIS OF PHARMACEUTICAL FORMULATION

Protocol No. 178

Formulation: Paracetamol, Tramadol hydrochloride

Classification: Musculoskeletal Disorders **Dosage form:** Tablets

Standard preparation: Prepare 5 mg/ml solution of tramadol HCl and 10 mg/ml solution of paracetamol, both in methanol, and use for analysis.

Sample preparation: Powdered sample equivalent to 100 mg of paracetamol suspended in methanol, sonicated, centrifuged and supernatant liquid diluted to 10 ml with methanol. Apply 5 µl for chromatographic analysis.

Chromatographic equipments:

Sample applicator: Camag Linomat–V

Development chamber: Camag twin–trough glass chamber, 20 × 10 cm

Densitometric scanner: Camag TLC Scanner–III

Chromatographic conditions:

1. Stationary phase: Silica gel 60F_{254} pre-coated HPTLC plates, 10 × 10 cm (200 µm) – Merck, pre-washed with methanol and activated at 115°C for 30 min prior to use
2. Mobile phase (MP): Chloroform–ethanol (7 : 3 v/v)
3. Standard/Sample application:
   Band length: 5 mm Volume applied: 0.5–5 µl Spacing: 5 mm
4. Chamber saturation: 15 min (MP)
5. RH (%): 55 ± 5
6. Temperature °C: 22 ± 2
7. Separation technique: Ascending
8. Quantity of mobile phase: 20 ml
9. Migration distance: 90 mm
10. Migration time: 25 min

Densitometric evaluation:

Wavelength: UV–254 nm Scanning mode: Reflectance/Absorbance

HRF: Tramadol HCl—48; Paracetamol—83

Linearity (µg/band): Paracetamol—10–50; Tramadol HCl—2.5–32.5

Recovery (%): Paracetamol—100.67–100.97; Tramadol HCl—101.4–102

References: W.D. Sam Solomon, P.R. Vijai Anand, Rajesh Shukla, R. Sivakumar and R. Venkatnarayanan, *Int. J. Chem. Tech. Research*, **2(2)**, 1188–1193, 2010.

Comments: The method validated for accuracy, precision, linearity, LOD, LOQ, specificity, robustness and ruggedness.

HPTLC : High Performance Thin Layer Chromatography
HPTLC Densitogram

No. 179

HO, O, N, H, CH_3

Paracetamol

HO, HCCH$_3$, N — CH_2 CH=C$(CH_3)_2$, CH_3, • HCl

Pentazocine hydrochloride

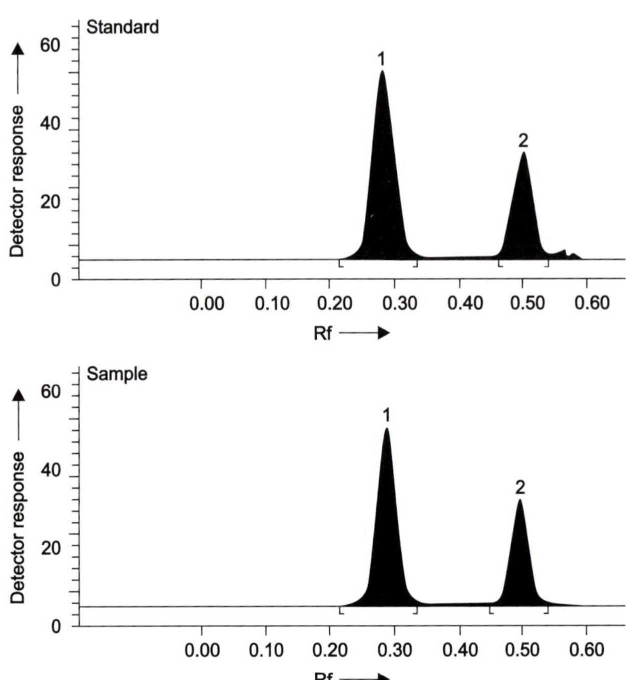

Typical densitogram of the sample and standard containing paracetamol and pentazocine HCl. For detailed experimental and chromatographic conditions, refer to Protocol No. 179. Peaks identification: 1. Paracetamol; 2. Pentazocine HCl.

PROTOCOL FOR HPTLC ANALYSIS OF PHARMACEUTICAL FORMULATION

Protocol No. 179

Formulation: **Paracetamol, Pentazocine hydrochloride**

Classification: Musculoskeletal Disorders **Dosage form:** Tablets

Standard preparation: Prepare 100 μg/ml solution of paracetamol and 150 μg/ml solution of pentazocine hydrochloride, both in methanol, and use for chromatographic evaluation.

Sample preparation: Weigh sample accurately equivalent to about 50 mg of paracetamol, dissolve in methanol to make 10 ml, dilute 0.2 ml of solution to 10 ml and use for chromatographic analysis.

Chromatographic equipments:

Sample applicator: Camag Linomat–IV
Development chamber: Camag twin–trough glass chamber, 10 × 10 cm
Densitometric scanner: Camag TLC Scanner–II

Chromatographic conditions:

1. Stationary phase: Silica gel $60F_{254}$ pre-coated TLC plate, 10 × 10 cm (250 μm) – Merck
2. Mobile phase (MP): Toluene–acetone–25% ammonia (6 : 4 : 0.1 v/v)
3. Standard/Sample application:
   Band length: 10 mm Volume applied: 10 μl Spacing: 10 mm
4. Chamber saturation: 20 min (MP)
5. RH (%): 55 ± 5
6. Temperature °C: 22 ± 2
7. Separation technique: Ascending
8. Quantity of mobile phase: 10 ml
9. Migration distance: 50 mm
10. Migration time: 12 min

Densitometric evaluation:

Wavelength: UV–245 nm (paracetamol); 280 nm (pentazocine HCl)
Scanning mode: Reflectance/Absorbance
HRF: Paracetamol—30; Pentazocine HCl—50
Linearity (ng/band): Paracetamol—100–1000; Pentazocine HCl—500–2000
Recovery (%): 98.10–102.10 for both the compounds

References: —

Comments:

- The method was optimized and analytical work carried out at **Anchrom's HPTLC Application Laboratory**, Mumbai, India.
- Several market samples of similar composition were analysed by the proposed method with reproducible results.
- The densitogram may preferably to scanned at 280 nm for both the compounds.

HPTLC : High Performance Thin Layer Chromatography
HPTLC Densitogram

No. 180

HO, O, N, H, CH_3

Paracetamol

$COOCH_2CH_2N(C_2H5)_2$ • HCl

Dicyclomine hydrochloride

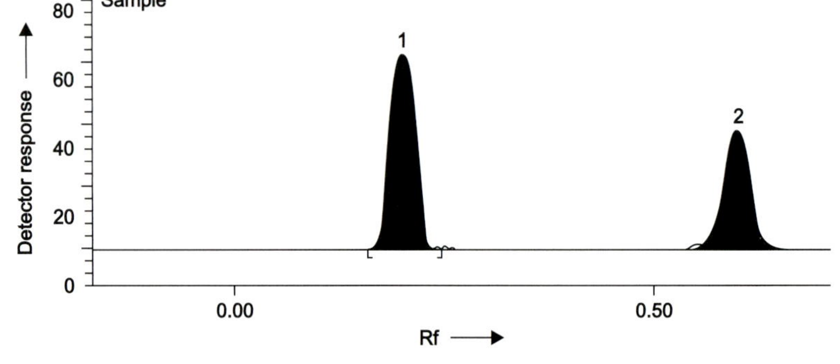

Typical densitogram of the sample and standard containing paracetamol and dicyclomine HCl. For detailed experimental and chromatographic conditions, refer to Protocol No. 180. Peaks identification: 1. Paracetamol; 2. Dicyclomine HCl.

PROTOCOL FOR HPTLC ANALYSIS OF PHARMACEUTICAL FORMULATION

Protocol No. 180

Formulation: **Paracetamol, Dicyclomine hydrochloride**
Classification: Musculoskeletal Disorders **Dosage form:** Tablets
Standard preparation: (a) Prepare 1 mg and 0.4 mg/ml solution of dicyclomine HCl in methanol. (b) Prepare 1 mg and 0.5 mg/ml solution of paracetamol in methanol and use for chromatographic analysis.
Sample preparation: Weigh powdered sample accurately equivalent to 20 mg of dicyclomine hydrochloride, suspend in 30–40 methanol, sonicate for 10 min, make up to 50 ml, filter (stock solution). Further dilute with methanol to get 100 μg/ml solution in respect of paracetamol (dilute solution) and use for application.
Chromatographic equipments:
Sample applicator: Camag Linomat–IV
Development chamber: Camag twin–trough glass chamber, 10 × 10 cm
Densitometric scanner: Camag TLC Scanner–II
Chromatographic conditions:
1. Stationary phase: Silica gel $60F_{254}$ pre-coated HPTLC plates, 10 × 10 cm (200 μm) – Merck
2. Mobile phase (MP): Toluene–acetone–25% ammonia (7 : 3 : 0.5 v/v)
3. Standard/Sample application:
   Band length: 10 mm Volume applied: 5 and 20 μl Spacing: 10 mm
4. Chamber saturation: 10 min (MP)
5. RH (%): 55 ± 5
6. Temperature °C: 22 ± 2
7. Separation technique: Ascending
8. Quantity of mobile phase: 10 ml
9. Migration distance: 50 mm
10. Migration time: 14 min

Densitometric evaluation:
Wavelength: UV–244 nm and 623 nm (dicyclomine HCl)
Scanning mode: Reflectance/Absorbance
HRF: Paracetamol—21; Dicyclomine HCl—64
Linearity (ng/band): Paracetamol—100–2000; Dicyclomine HCl—1000–10000
Recovery (%): 100.75–101.89 for both the compounds
References: —
Comments:
- The method was optimized and analytical work carried out at **Anchrom's HPTLC Application Laboratory**, Mumbai, India.
- After scanning chromatoplate at 244 nm for paracetamol, the plate was treated with cobalt thiocyanate reagent and then scanned at 623 nm. For details and preparation of dipping reagent, (refer to Protocol No. 232).
- Several market samples of similar composition were analysed by the proposed method with reproducible results.

HPTLC : High Performance Thin Layer Chromatography
HPTLC Densitogram

No. 181

HO, N H, O, CH_3

Paracetamol

COOH, H N, CH_3, CH_3

Mefenamic acid

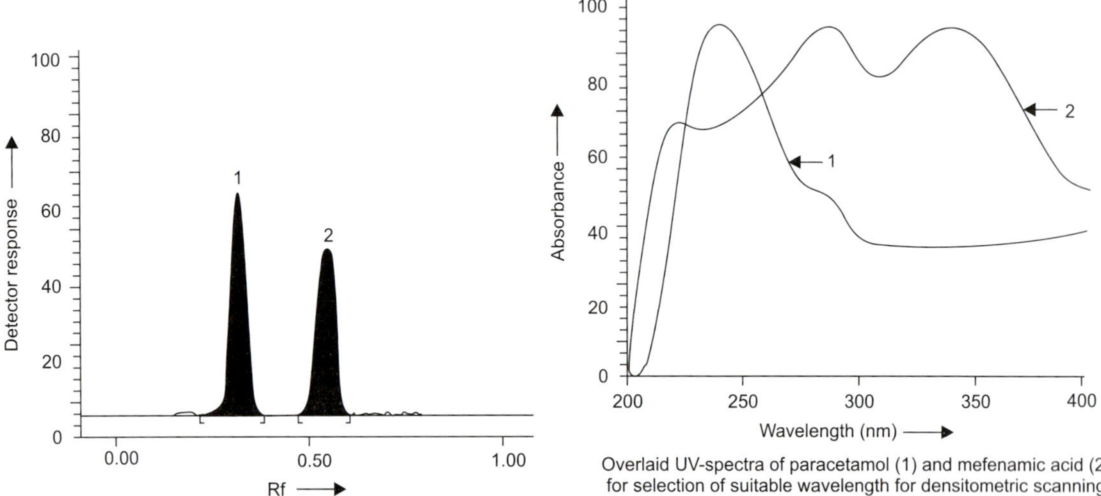

Overlaid UV-spectra of paracetamol (1) and mefenamic acid (2) for selection of suitable wavelength for densitometric scanning

Typical densitogram of the standard containing paracetamol and mefenamic acid. For detailed experimental and chromatographic conditions, refer to Protocol No. 181. Peaks identification: 1. Paracetamol; 2. Mefenamic acid.

PROTOCOL FOR HPTLC ANALYSIS OF PHARMACEUTICAL FORMULATION

Protocol No. 181

Formulation: Paracetamol, Mefenamic acid
Classification: Musculoskeletal Disorders **Dosage form:** Tablets
Standard preparation: Prepare 200 μg/ml solution of each compound in methanol. Prepare serial dilutions of each for linearity studies by applying 5 μl of each solution.
Sample preparation: Powdered sample equivalent to 50 mg of paracetamol suspended in 40 ml of methanol. Sonicate for 15 min, dilute to 50 ml with methanol, filter through Whatman No. 42 filter paper, dilute 2 ml of the filtrate to 10 ml with methanol and use for chromatographic analysis.
Chromatographic equipments:
Sample applicator: Camag Linomat–IV
Development chamber: Camag twin–trough glass chamber, 20 × 10 cm
Densitometric scanner: Camag TLC Scanner–II
Chromatographic conditions:

1. Stationary phase: Silica gel $60F_{254}$ pre-coated HPTLC plates, 20 × 10 cm (200 μm) – Merck
2. Mobile phase (MP): Toluene–acetone–methanol (8 : 1 : 1 v/v)
3. Standard/Sample application:
   Band length: 6 mm Volume applied: 5 μl Spacing: 10 mm
4. Chamber saturation: 20 min (MP)
5. RH (%): 55 ± 5
6. Temperature °C: 25 ± 1
7. Separation technique: Ascending
8. Quantity of mobile phase: 20 ml
9. Migration distance: 50 mm
10. Migration time: 14 min

Densitometric evaluation:
Wavelength: UV–263 nm Scanning mode: Reflectance/Absorbance
HRF: Paracetamol—29; Mefenamic acid—58
Linearity: 600–1800 ng/band for both the drugs
Recovery (%): Paracetamol—95.80–102.70; Mefenamic acid—99.40–100.50
References: A.P. Argekar and J.G. Sawant, *J. Planar Chromatogr.*, **12(5)**, 361–364, 1999.
Comments:

- The method validated for accuracy, precision, linearity, LOD, LOQ and specificity.
- The method is stability indicating (acid, base, oxidative, thermal, photolytic). The degradation products were separated from main compounds.

HPTLC : High Performance Thin Layer Chromatography
HPTLC Densitogram

No. 182

Paracetamol

Lornoxicam

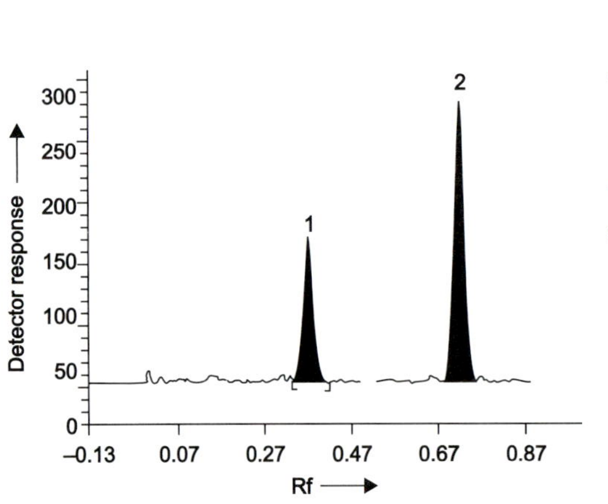

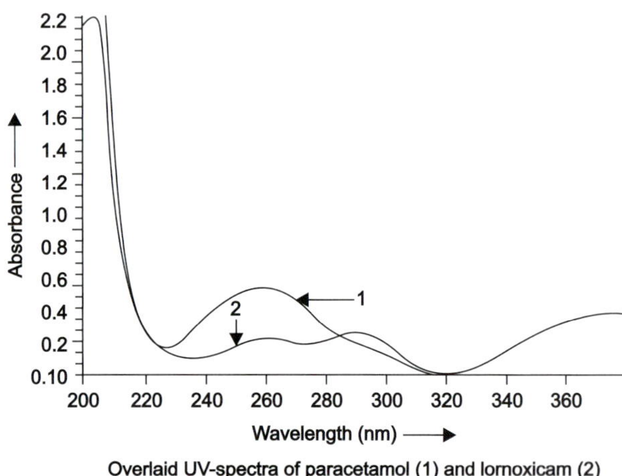

Overlaid UV-spectra of paracetamol (1) and lornoxicam (2) for selection of suitable wavelength for densitometric scanning

Typical densitogram of the standard containing paracetamol and lornoxicam. For detailed experimental and chromatographic conditions, refer to Protocol No. 182. Peaks identification: 1. Lornoxicam; 2. Paracetamol.

PROTOCOL FOR HPTLC ANALYSIS OF PHARMACEUTICAL FORMULATION

Protocol No. 182

Formulation: Paracetamol, Lornoxicam

Classification: Musculoskeletal Disorders **Dosage form:** Tablets

Standard preparation: Prepare solution of both the drugs in methanol to get 200 μg/ml of paracetamol and 100 μg/ml of lornoxicam. Apply 1–6 μl of each solution for linearity profile of both the drugs.

Sample preparation: Powdered sample equivalent to 2 mg of lornoxicam suspended in 80 ml of methanol, sonicated for 30 min, and diluted to 100 ml with methanol, filtered through 0.45 μm filter. Apply 2 μl of resulting solution for chromatographic analysis.

Chromatographic equipments:

Sample applicator: Camag Linomat–V

Development chamber: Camag twin–trough glass chamber, 20 × 10 cm

Densitometric scanner: Camag TLC Scanner–II

Chromatographic conditions:

1. Stationary phase: Silica gel $60F_{254}$ pre-coated TLC plates, 10 × 10 cm (250 μm) – Merck, pre-washed with methanol, activated at 110°C for 5 min prior to use
2. Mobile phase (MP): Ethyl acetate–methanol–toluene–glacial acetic acid (7 : 2.5 : 10 : 0.5 v/v)
3. Standard/Sample application:
   Band length: 6 mm Volume applied: 1–6 μl Spacing: 11.6 mm
4. Chamber saturation: 35 min (MP)
5. RH (%): 55 ± 5
6. Temperature °C: 25 ± 2
7. Separation technique: Ascending
8. Quantity of mobile phase: 20 ml
9. Migration distance: 80 mm
10. Migration time: 18 min

Densitometric evaluation:

Wavelength: UV–270 nm Scanning mode: Reflectance/Absorbance

HRF: Lornoxicam—39; Paracetamol—72

Linearity (ng/band): Paracetamol—200–1200; Lornoxicam—100–600

Recovery (%): Paracetamol—99.0–99.79; Lornoxicam—99.77–100.98

References: Dhara J. Patel and Vivek P. Patel, *Int. J. Chem. Tech. Research*, **2(4)**, 1929–1932, 2010.

Comments: The method validated for accuracy, precision, linearity, LOD, LOQ, specificity, robustness and ruggedness.

HPTLC : High Performance Thin Layer Chromatography
HPTLC Densitogram

No. 184

HO, N, H, O, CH_3

Paracetamol

O, O, S, N, CH_3, Cl, S, H, N, N, OH, O

Lornoxicam

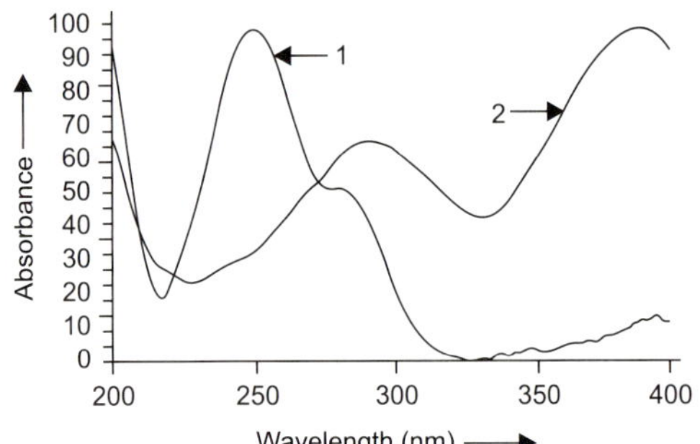

Overlaid UV-spectra of paracetamol (1) and lornoxicam (2) for selection of suitable wavelength for densitometric scanning

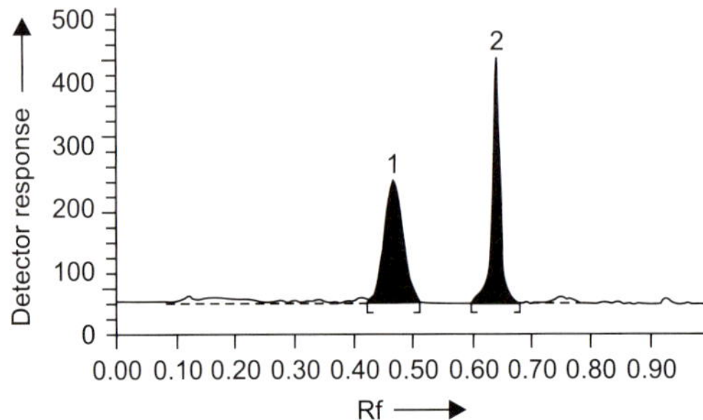

Typical densitogram of the standard containing paracetamol and lornoxicam. For detailed experimental and chromatographic conditions, refer to Protocol No. 184. Peaks identification: 1. Paracetamol; 2. Lornoxicam.

PROTOCOL FOR HPTLC ANALYSIS OF PHARMACEUTICAL FORMULATION

Protocol No. 184

Formulation: Paracetamol, Lornoxicam

Classification: Musculoskeletal Disorders **Dosage form:** Tablets

Standard preparation: Prepare 100 μg/ml solution of each compound in methanol. Apply 1–6 μl for linearity studies.

Sample preparation: Powdered sample equivalent to 10 mg of paracetamol and 10 mg of lornoxicam suspended in 60 ml of methanol, sonicated for 10 min, diluted to 100 ml, filtered and applied 2 μl of final solution for assay.

Chromatographic equipments:

Sample applicator: Camag Linomat–V

Development chamber: Camag twin–trough glass chamber, 10 × 10 cm

Densitometric scanner: Camag TLC Scanner–III

Chromatographic conditions:

1. Stationary phase: Silica gel $60F_{254}$ pre-coated TLC plate, 10 × 10 cm (250 μm) – Merck
2. Mobile phase (MP): Toluene–methanolic sodium hydroxide–glacial acetic acid (7 : 2 : 1.5 v/v)
3. Standard/Sample application:
   Band length: 6 mm Volume applied: 1–6 μl Spacing: 10 mm
4. Chamber saturation: 20 min (MP)
5. RH (%): 55 ± 5
6. Temperature °C: Ambient
7. Separation technique: Ascending
8. Quantity of mobile phase: 10 ml
9. Migration distance: 90 mm
10. Migration time: 30 min

Densitometric evaluation:

Wavelength: UV–265 nm Scanning mode: Reflectance/Absorbance

HRF: Paracetamol—47; Lornoxicam—65

Linearity (ng/band): 100–600 for both the compounds

Recovery (%): 99.93–100.04 for both the compounds

References: Veena G. Kulkarni, Santosh V. Gandhi, Padmanabh B. Deshpande and Poonam H. Chaube, *Pelagia Res. Library (Der Chemica Sinica)*, **2(1)**, 182–188, 2011.

Comments: The method validated for accuracy, precision, linearity, LOD, LOQ, specificity, robustness and ruggedness.

HPTLC : High Performance Thin Layer Chromatography
HPTLC Densitogram

No. 186

Paracetamol **Caffeine** **Ascorbic acid**

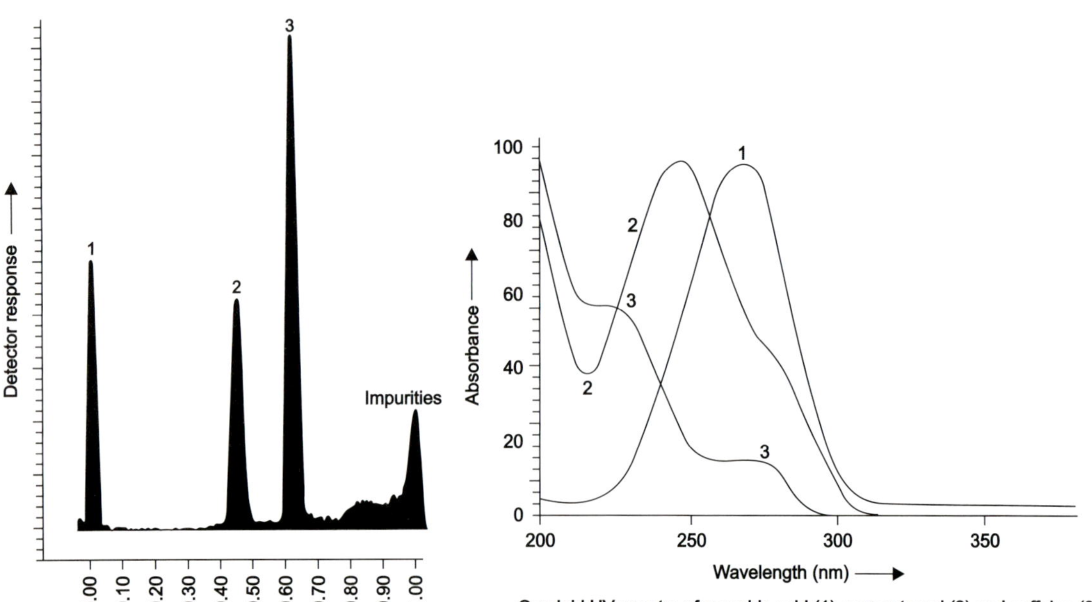

Overlaid UV-spectra of ascorbic acid (1), paracetamol (2) and caffeine (3) for selection of suitable wavelength for densitometric scanning

Typical densitogram of the sample containing paracetamol, caffeine and ascorbic acid. For detailed experimental and chromatographic conditions, refer to Protocol No. 186. Peaks identification: 1. Ascorbic acid; 2. Caffeine; 3. Paracetamol.

PROTOCOL FOR HPTLC ANALYSIS OF PHARMACEUTICAL FORMULATION

Protocol No. 186

Formulation: Paracetamol, Caffeine citrate, Ascorbic acid

Classification: Musculoskeletal Disorders **Dosage form:** Tablets/Capsules

Standard preparation: Weigh 400 mg of paracetamol, 30 mg of caffeine, 60 mg of ascorbic acid, dilute to 25 ml with methanol for estimation of ascorbic acid or to 100 ml for estimation of paracetamol and caffeine. Apply 5 μl for chromatographic separation.

Sample preparation: Take powdered sample equivalent to 60 mg of ascorbic acid, dilute to 25 ml with methanol and use for analysis of ascorbic acid. Further dilute 2.5 ml of the solution to 25 ml with methanol and use for estimation of paracetamol and caffeine.

Chromatographic equipments:

Sample applicator: Camag Linomat–IV

Development chamber: Rectangular flat bottom glass chamber, 20 × 20 cm

Densitometric scanner: Camag TLC Scanner–II

Chromatographic conditions:

1. Stationary phase: Silica gel $60F_{254}$ pre-coated HPTLC plates, 10 × 10 cm (200 μm) – Merck
2. Mobile phase (MP): Dichloromethane–ethyl acetate–ethanol (5 : 5 : 1 v/v)
3. Standard/Sample application:
   Band length: 5 mm Volume applied: 5 μl Spacing: 5 mm
4. Chamber saturation: 20 min (MP)
5. RH (%): 55 ± 5
6. Temperature °C: 22 ± 2
7. Separation technique: Ascending
8. Quantity of mobile phase: 22 ml
9. Migration distance: 100 mm
10. Migration time: 27 min

Densitometric evaluation:

Wavelength: UV–254 nm Scanning mode: Reflectance/Absorbance

HRF: Ascorbic acid—05; Caffeine citrate—45; Paracetamol—65

Linearity (ng/band): Paracetamol—50–500; Caffeine citrate—50–300; Ascorbic acid—100–1000

Recovery (%): 98.5–102.5 for all the three compounds

References: M. El Sadek et al., *Analyst*, **115**, 1181–1184, 1990.

Comments: The method validated for accuracy, precision, linearity, LOD, LOQ and specificity.

HPTLC : High Performance Thin Layer Chromatography
HPTLC Densitogram

No. 189

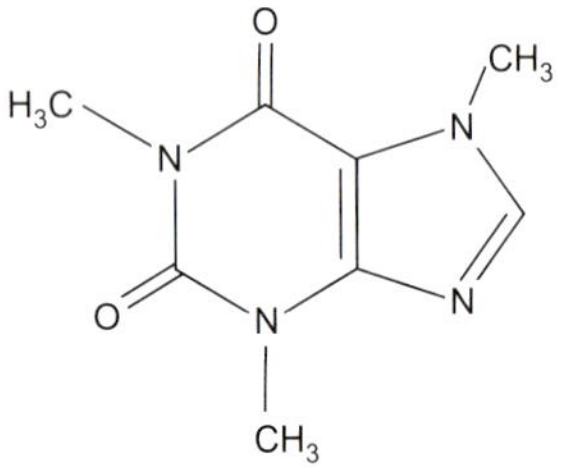

Caffeine

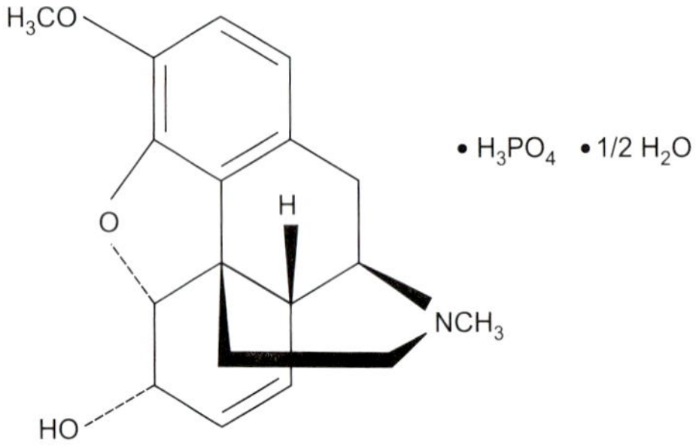

Codeine phosphate • H_3PO_4 • 1/2 H_2O

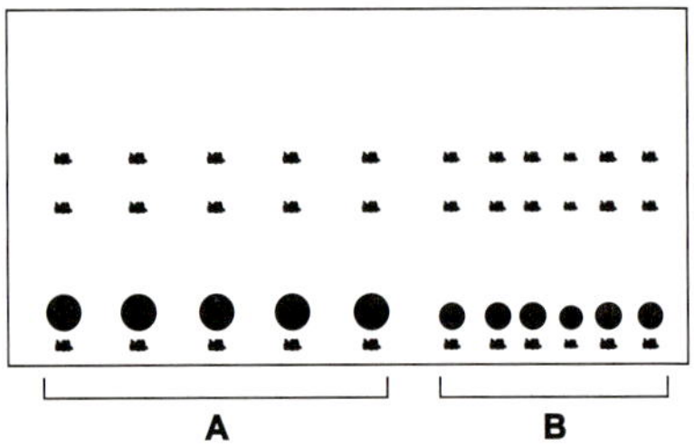

TLC finger-print profile of tablets containing
A, Paracetamol—325 mg; Codeine phosphate—30 mg and Caffeine—30 mg
B. Paracetamol—150 mg; Codeine phosphate—30 mg and Caffeine—15 mg using MP–1

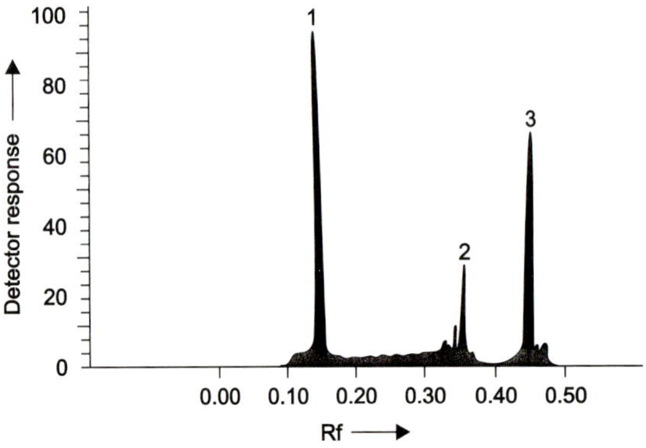

Typical densitogram of the sample containing paracetamol, caffeine citrate and codeine phosphate. For detailed experimental and chromatographic conditions, refer to Protocol No. 189. Peaks identification: 1. Paracetamol; 2. Codeine phosphate; 3. Caffeine citrate.

PROTOCOL FOR HPTLC ANALYSIS OF PHARMACEUTICAL FORMULATION

Protocol No. 189

Formulation: Paracetamol, Caffeine citrate, Codeine phosphate

Classification: Musculoskeletal Disorders **Dosage form:** Tablets/Drugs

Standard preparation: Paracetamol (P) 60 mcg/ml; codeine phosphate (CP) 200 mcg/ml; Caffeine (C) 120 mcg/ml in methanol–water (9 + 1) mixture.

Sample preparation: Sample equivalent to 10 mg of codeine phosphate extracted with methanol–water (9 + 1) by sonication, made up to 50 ml. Use as such for codeine phosphate. Further dilute 2 ml to 10 ml for caffeine and 2 ml to 20 ml for paracetamol.

Chromatographic equipments:

Sample applicator: Camag Linomat–IV

Development chamber: Camag twin–trough glass chamber, 10 × 10 cm

Densitometric scanner: Camag TLC Scanner–II

Chromatographic conditions:

1. Stationary phase: Silica gel 60F_{254} pre-coated HPTLC plates, 10 × 10 cm (200 μm) – Merck
2. Mobile phase (MP): (i) Chloroform–cyclohexane–acetone–diethylamine (6 : 2 : 1 : 1 v/v); (ii) n-butanol–methanol–toluene–water–glacial acetic acid (3 : 4 : 1 : 2 : 0.1 v/v)
3. Standard/Sample application:
   Band length: 10 mm Volume applied: 10 μl Spacing: 10 mm
4. Chamber saturation: 20 min (MP)
5. RH (%): 50 ± 5
6. Temperature °C: 22 ± 2
7. Separation technique: Ascending
8. Quantity of mobile phase: 10 ml
9. Migration distance: 60 mm
10. Migration time: 30 min

Densitometric evaluation:

Wavelength: UV–254 nm (paracetamol and caffeine); 285 nm (codeine)

Scanning mode: Reflectance/Absorbance

HRF: Paracetamol—15; Codeine phosphate—35; Caffeine citrate—45

Linearity (ng/band): Paracetamol—200–800; Caffeine citrate—600–1600; Codeine phosphate—900–3000

Recovery (%): 98.05–99.50 for all the three compounds

References: (i) N. Rusu, V. Tamas and M.S. Ionescu, *Rev. Chem.*, **43**, 730–733, 1993 through AA 55(12) G 17, 1993; (ii) Camag Application Notes A–16.2, p. 1–8, 1987, Courtesy: Camag, Switzerland; (iii) H.N. al-Kaysi, *Anal. Lett.*, **19**, 915, 1986.

Comments: It is preferable to scan the densitogram at 265 nm for evaluation of all the three compounds.

HPTLC : High Performance Thin Layer Chromatography
HPTLC Densitogram

No. 190

Caffeine

Analgin

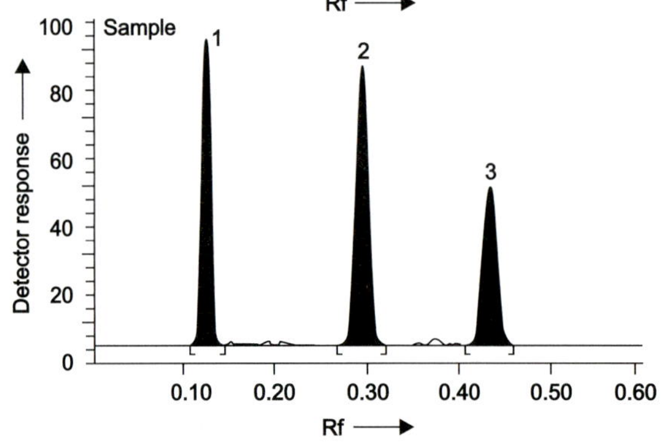

Typical densitogram of the sample and standard containing paracetamol, analgin and caffeine citrate. For detailed experimental and chromatographic conditions, refer to Protocol No. 190. Peaks identification: 1. Analgin; 2. Paracetamol; 3. Caffeine citrate.

PROTOCOL FOR HPTLC ANALYSIS OF PHARMACEUTICAL FORMULATION

Protocol No. 190

Formulation: Paracetamol, Caffeine citrate, Analgin

Classification: Musculoskeletal Disorders **Dosage form:** Tablets

Standard preparation: Prepare 1.5 mg/ml solution of caffeine citrate in methanol (CC); weigh 25 mg each of paracetamol and analgin, add 1 ml of solution (CC), dilute to 10 ml with methanol. Further dilute 2 ml to 10 ml with methanol and use for chromatographic analysis.

Sample preparation: Weight accurately powdered sample equivalent to 250 mg of paracetamol, suspend in 50–60 ml of methanol, sonicate for 5 min, make up to 100 ml, filter and dilute 2 ml and 10 ml with methanol and use for chromatographic analysis.

Chromatographic equipments:

Sample applicator: Camag Linomat–IV

Development chamber: Camag twin–trough glass chamber, 10 × 10 cm

Densitometric scanner: Camag TLC Scanner–II

Chromatographic conditions:

1. Stationary phase: Silica gel $60F_{254}$ pre-coated HPTLC plates, 10 × 10 cm (200 μm) – Merck
2. Mobile phase (MP): Chloroform–methanol–toluene (9 : 1 : 1 v/v)
3. Standard/Sample application:
   Band length: 10 mm Volume applied: 5 μl Spacing: 10 mm
4. Chamber saturation: 20 min (MP)
5. RH (%): 55 ± 5
6. Temperature °C: 22 ± 2
7. Separation technique: Ascending
8. Quantity of mobile phase: 11 ml
9. Migration distance: 60 mm
10. Migration time: 16 min

Densitometric evaluation:

Wavelength: UV–278 nm Scanning mode: Reflectance/Absorbance

HRF: Analgin—12; Paracetamol—30; Caffeine citrate—44

Linearity (ng/band): Analgin and paracetamol—200–2000; Caffeine citrate—10–50

Recovery (%): Analgin—99.90; Paracetamol—98.90; Caffeine citrate—97.0

References: —

Comments:

- The method was optimized and analytical work carried out at **Anchrom's HPTLC Application Laboratory**, Mumbai, India.
- Several market samples of similar composition were analysed by the proposed method with reproducible results.

HPTLC : High Performance Thin Layer Chromatography
HPTLC Densitogram

No. 192

HO N H O CH3 **Paracetamol**

Cl O N OH **Chlorzoxazone**

O COOH O NH Cl Cl **Aceclofenac**

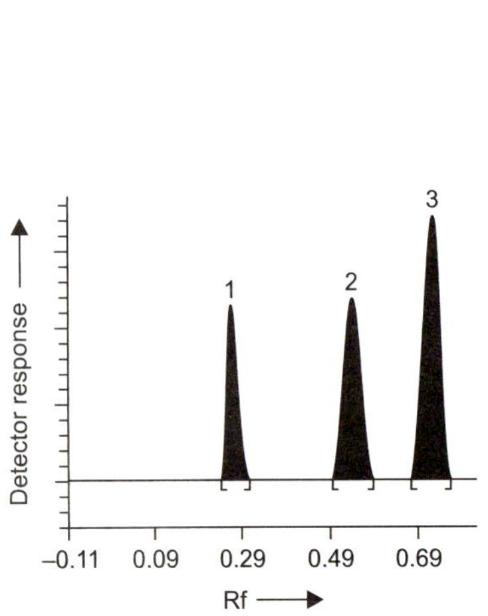

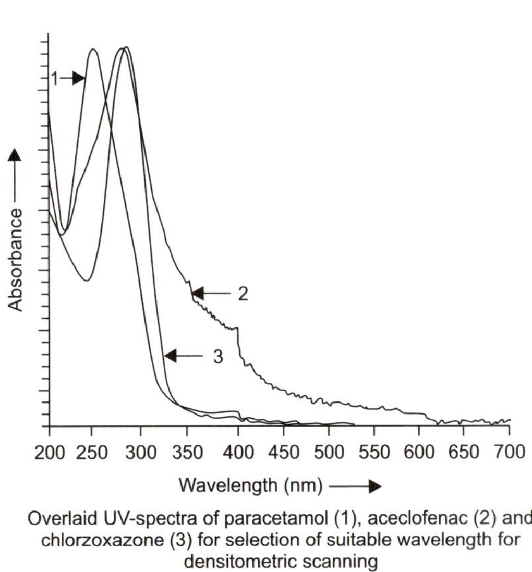

Overlaid UV-spectra of paracetamol (1), aceclofenac (2) and chlorzoxazone (3) for selection of suitable wavelength for densitometric scanning

Typical densitogram of the sample containing paracetamol, aceclofenac and chlorzoxazone. For detailed experimental and chromatographic conditions, refer to Protocol No. 192. Peaks identification: 1. Aceclofenac; 2. Chlorzoxazone; 3. Paracetamol.

PROTOCOL FOR HPTLC ANALYSIS OF PHARMACEUTICAL FORMULATION

Protocol No. 192

Formulation: Paracetamol, Aceclofenac, Chlorzoxazone

Classification: Musculoskeletal Disorders **Dosage form:** Tablets

Standard preparation: Prepare solution of each compound separately in methanol to get 1 mg/ml (aceclofenac), 5 mg/ml (paracetamol) and 2.5 mg/ml (chlorzoxazone). Apply varying volumes of each solution for linearity profile.

Sample preparation: Powdered sample equivalent to 100 mg of aceclofenac suspended in methanol, sonicated for 10 min, adjusted to 100 ml with methanol (1 mg/ml), filtered and 1 ml of the filtrate diluted to 10 ml with methanol. Apply 5 μl of the resulting solution for chromatographic analysis.

Chromatographic equipments:

Sample applicator: Camag Linomat–V

Development chamber: Camag twin–trough glass chamber, 10 × 10 cm

Densitometric scanner: Camag TLC Scanner–III

Chromatographic conditions:

1. Stationary phase: Silica gel $60F_{254}$ pre-coated HPTLC plates, 10 × 10 cm (200 μm) – Merck, pre-washed with methanol, dried at 110°C for 5 min prior to use
2. Mobile phase (MP): Toluene–isopropanol–25% ammonia (4 : 4 : 0.4 v/v)
3. Standard/Sample application:
   Band length: 6 mm Volume applied: 5 μl Spacing: 10 mm
4. Chamber saturation: 30 min (MP)
5. RH (%): 55 ± 5
6. Temperature °C: 25 ± 2
7. Separation technique: Ascending
8. Quantity of mobile phase: 16 ml
9. Migration distance: 80 mm
10. Migration time: 20 min

Densitometric evaluation:

Wavelength: UV–274 nm Scanning mode: Reflectance/Absorbance

HRF: Aceclofenac—28; Chlorzoxazone—51; Paracetamol—72

Linearity (ng/band): Paracetamol—2000–7000; Aceclofenac—400–1400; Chlorzoxazone—1000–3500

Recovery (%): Paracetamol—100.02–100.47; Aceclofenac—98.97–100.44; Chlorzoxazone—99.25–99.84

References: V.K. Mahajan, S.B. Bari, A.A. Shirkhedkar and S.J. Surana, *Acta Chromatographica*, **20(4)**, 625–636, 2008.

Comments: The method validated for accuracy, precision, linearity, LOD, LOQ, specificity, robustness and ruggedness.

HPTLC : High Performance Thin Layer Chromatography
HPTLC Densitogram

No. 193

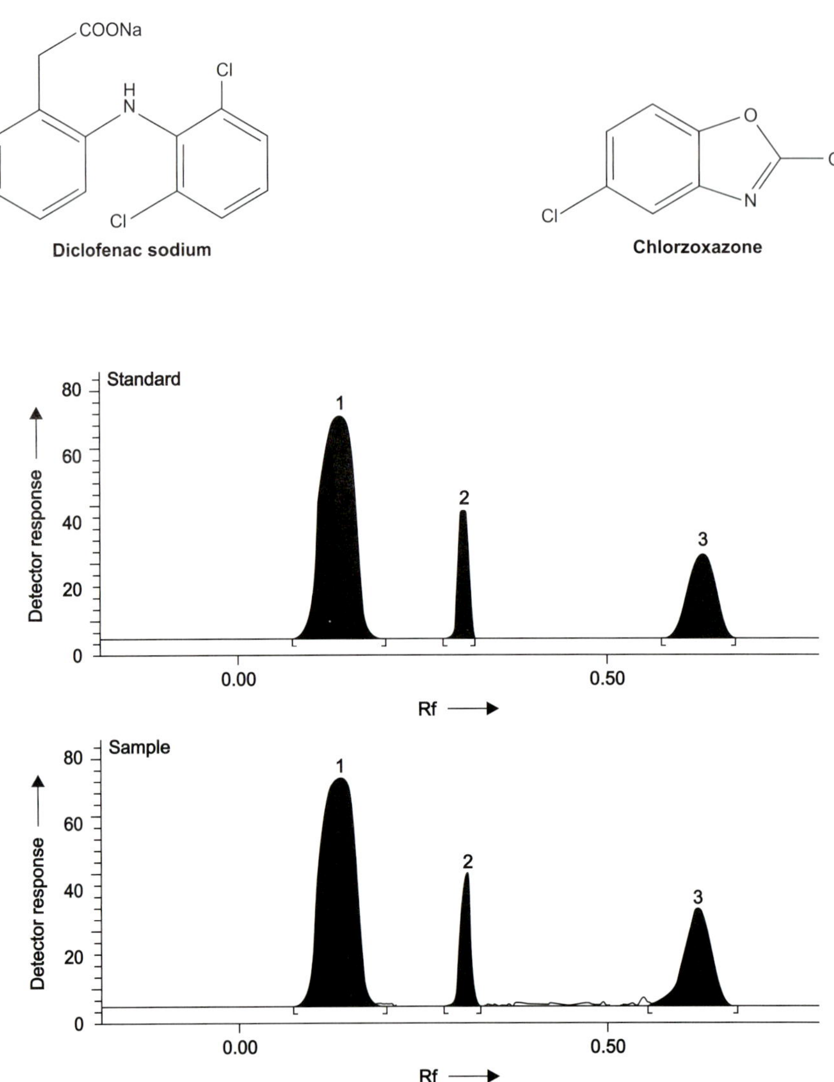

Typical densitogram of the sample and standard containing paracetamol, chlorzoxazone and diclofenac sodium. For detailed experimental and chromatographic conditions, refer to Protocol No. 193. Peaks identification: 1. Paracetamol; 2. Diclofenac sodium; 3. Chlorzoxazone.

PROTOCOL FOR HPTLC ANALYSIS OF PHARMACEUTICAL FORMULATION

Protocol No. 193

Formulation: Paracetamol, Diclofenac sodium, Chlorzoxazone

Classification: Musculoskeletal Disorders **Dosage form:** Tablets

Standard preparation: (a) Weigh accurately 10 mg of diclofenac sodium and dissolve in methanol to make 10 ml; (b) Dissolve 10 mg each of paracetamol and chlorzoxazone accurately weighed in methanol, add 1 ml of solution (a) to it and make up to 100 ml. Use the resulting solution for chromatographic analysis.

Sample preparation: Weigh powdered sample equivalent to 50 mg of paracetamol, add about 70 ml of methanol, vortex for 10 to 15 min, dilute to 100 ml. Filter and dilute 2 ml of filtrate to 10 ml with methanol for chromatographic analysis.

Chromatographic equipments:

Sample applicator: Camag Linomat–IV

Development chamber: Camag twin–trough glass chamber, 10 × 10 cm

Densitometric scanner: Camag TLC Scanner–II

Chromatographic conditions:

1. Stationary phase: Silica gel $60F_{254}$ pre-coated HPTLC plates, 10 × 10 cm (200 μm) – Merck
2. Mobile phase (MP): Toluene–ethyl acetate–glacial acetic acid (6 : 4 : 0.2 v/v)
3. Standard/Sample application:
   Band length: 5 mm Volume applied: 5 μl Spacing: 5 mm
4. Chamber saturation: 10 min (MP)
5. RH (%): 55 ± 5
6. Temperature °C: 22 ± 2
7. Separation technique: Ascending
8. Quantity of mobile phase: 10 ml
9. Migration distance: 50 mm
10. Migration time: 14 min

Densitometric evaluation:

Wavelength: UV–286 nm Scanning mode: Reflectance/Absorbance

HRF: Paracetamol—13; Diclofenac sodium—30; Chlorzoxazone—62

Linearity (ng/band): Paracetamol and chlorzoxazone—100–1000; Diclofenac sodium—10–100

Recovery (%): 99.66–100.65 for all the three compounds

References: —

Comments:

- The method was optimized and analytical work carried out at **Anchrom's HPTLC Application Laboratory**, Mumbai, India.
- Several market samples of similar composition were analysed by the proposed method with reproducible results.

HPTLC : High Performance Thin Layer Chromatography
HPTLC Densitogram

No. 194

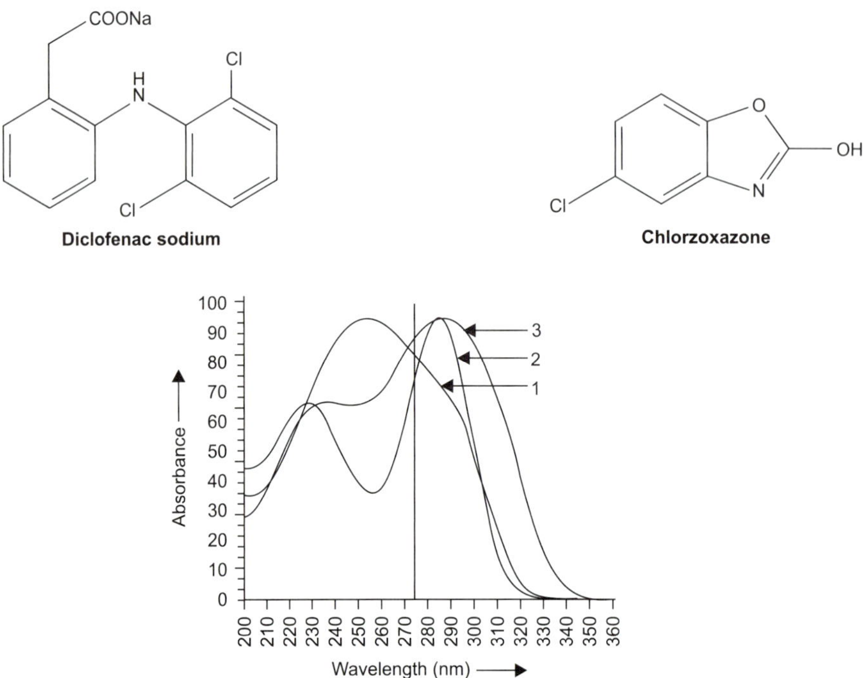

Overlaid UV-spectra of paracetamol (1), diclofenac sodium (2) and chlorzoxazone (3) for selection of suitable wavelength for densitometric scanning

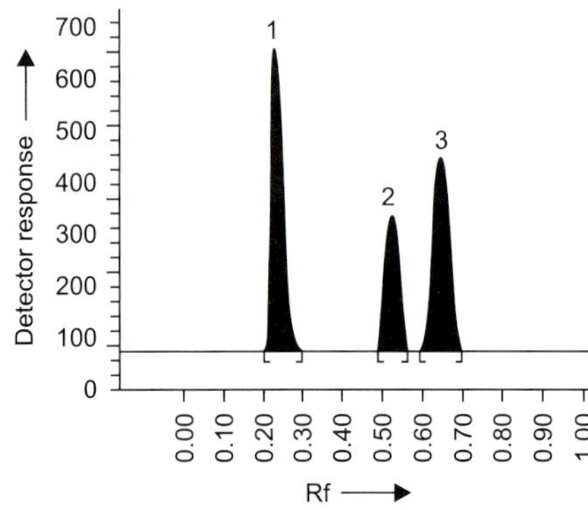

Typical densitogram of the standard containing paracetamol, diclofenac sodium and chlorzoxazone. For detailed experimental and chromatographic conditions, refer to Protocol No. 194. Peaks identification: 1. Chlorzoxazone; 2. Diclofenac sodium; 3. Paracetamol.

PROTOCOL FOR HPTLC ANALYSIS OF PHARMACEUTICAL FORMULATION

Protocol No. 194

Formulation: Paracetamol, Diclofenac sodium, Chlorzoxazone

Classification: Musculoskeletal Disorders **Dosage form:** Tablets

Standard preparation: Prepare solution of each drug in methanol to get 350 μg/ml of paracetamol, 50 μg/ml of diclofenac sodium and 250 μg/ml of chlorzoxazone. Dilute 2–8 ml of each solution to 10 ml with methanol and apply 4 μl of each solution for linearity profile.

Sample preparation: Powdered sample equivalent to 10 mg of diclofenac sodium suspended in 5 ml of methanol, sonicated for 10 min, diluted to 10 ml, centrifuged (2000 rpm) for 5 min. Apply 2 μl of a supernatant solution for chromatographic separation and assay.

Chromatographic equipments:

Sample applicator: Camag Linomat–IV
Development chamber: Camag twin–trough glass chamber, 20 × 10 cm
Densitometric scanner: Camag TLC Scanner–III

Chromatographic conditions:

1. Stationary phase: Silica gel $60F_{254}$ pre-coated HPTLC plates, 20 × 10 cm (200 μm) – Merck, pre-washed with methanol and activated at 110°C for 5 min prior to use
2. Mobile phase (MP): Toluene–ethyl acetate–glacial acetic acid (6.5 : 3.5 : 0.02 v/v)
3. Standard/Sample application:
   Band length: 5 mm Volume applied: 4 μl Spacing: 4 mm
4. Chamber saturation: 10 min (MP)
5. RH (%): 60 ± 5
6. Temperature °C: 20 ± 2
7. Separation technique: Ascending
8. Quantity of mobile phase: 20 ml
9. Migration distance: 80 mm
10. Migration time: 20 min

Densitometric evaluation:

Wavelength: UV–274 nm Scanning mode: Reflectance/Absorbance
HRF: Chlorzoxazone—23; Diclofenac sodium—51; Paracetamol—62
Linearity (ng/band): Paracetamol—260–1040; Diclofenac sodium—40–160; Chlorzoxazone—200–800
Recovery (%): Paracetamol—100.15–101.24; Diclofenac sodium—99.54–100.26; Chlorzoxazone—99.81–101.01

References: M.R. Tajne, A.V. Kasture and S.G. Wadekar, *J. Planar Chromatogr. – Modern TLC* (under press).

Comments:

- The method validated for accuracy, precision, linearity, LOD, LOQ, specificity, robustness and ruggedness.
- The method is stability indicating (acid, base, oxidative, thermal, photolytic). The degradation products were separated from main compounds.

HPTLC : High Performance Thin Layer Chromatography
HPTLC Densitogram

No. 195

Chlorzoxazone **Paracetamol** **Diclofenac sodium**

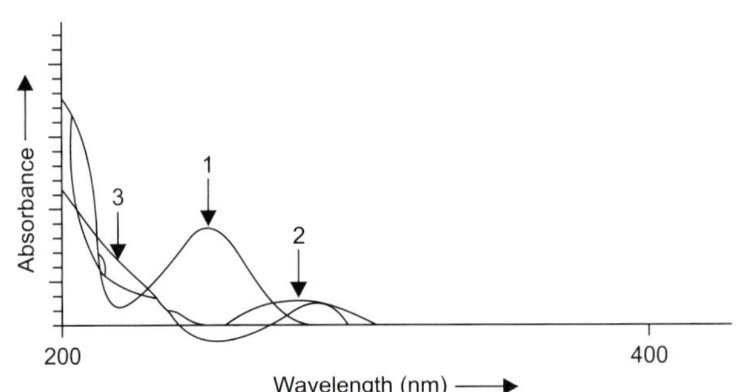

Overlaid UV-spectra of paracetamol (1), diclofenac (2) and chlorzoxazone (3) for selection of suitable wavelength for densitometric scanning

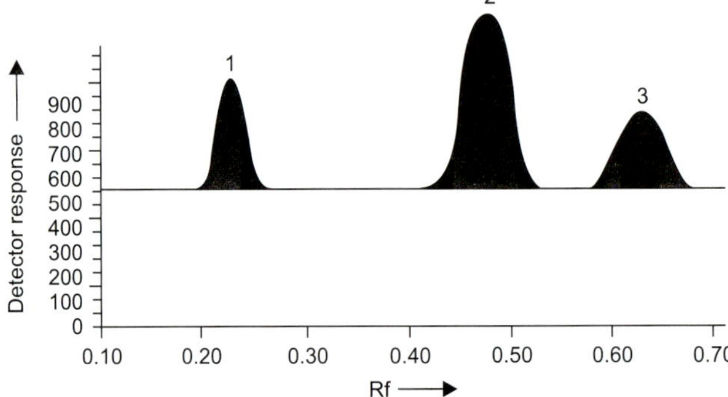

Typical densitogram of the standard containing paracetamol, diclofenac sodium and chlorzoxazone. For detailed experimental and chromatographic conditions, refer to Protocol No. 195. Peaks identification: 1. Diclofenac sodium; 2. Paracetamol; 3. Chlorzoxazone.

PROTOCOL FOR HPTLC ANALYSIS OF PHARMACEUTICAL FORMULATION

Protocol No. 195

Formulation: Paracetamol, Diclofenac sodium, Chlorzoxazone

Classification: Musculoskeletal Disorders **Dosage form:** Tablets

Standard preparation: Prepare 500 μg/ml solution of each compound separately in methanol. Apply varying volumes of each solution for linearity profile.

Sample preparation: Powdered sample equivalent to 500 mg of paracetamol suspended in 20 ml of methanol, sonicated for 15 min, diluted to 250 ml with methanol. Filter and dilute 1 ml of filtrate to 10 ml with methanol. Apply 6 μl for chromatographic analysis.

Chromatographic equipments:

Sample applicator: Camag Linomat–V

Development chamber: Camag twin-trough glass chamber, 20 × 10 cm

Densitometric scanner: Camag TLC Scanner–II

Chromatographic conditions:

1. Stationary phase (MP): Silica gel $60F_{254}$ pre-coated HPTLC plates, 20 × 10 cm (200 μm), pre-washed with methanol, dried at 50°C for 5 min prior to use
2. Mobile phase (MP): Chloroform–methanol–25% ammonia (20 : 5 : 0.2 v/v)
3. Standard/Sample application:

   Band length: 6 mm Volume applied: 2–10 μl Spacing: 10 mm
4. Chamber saturation: 20 min (MP)
5. RH (%): 55 ± 5
6. Temperature °C: 25 ± 2
7. Separation technique: Ascending
8. Quantity of mobile phase: 25 ml
9. Migration distance: 80 mm
10. Migration time: 20 min

Densitometric evaluation:

Wavelength: UV–254 nm Scanning mode: Reflectance/Absorbance

HRF: Diclofenac—23; Paracetamol—48; Chlorzoxazone—64

Linearity (ng/band): 1000–5000 ng/band for all the three drugs

Recovery (%): Paracetamol—99.73–100.04; Diclofenac sodium—99.13–99.98; Chlorzoxazone—99.96–100.08

References: Smita J. Pawar, Amol P. Kale, A. Manoj, P. Amrutkar, Jyotsna J. Jagade, Nikhil S. Pore and Ashok V. Bhosle, *Asian J. Research Chem.*, **2(3)**, 306–309, 2009.

Comments: The method validated for accuracy, precision, linearity, LOD, LOQ and specificity.

HPTLC : High Performance Thin Layer Chromatography
HPTLC Densitogram

No. 196

Paracetamol

Famotidine

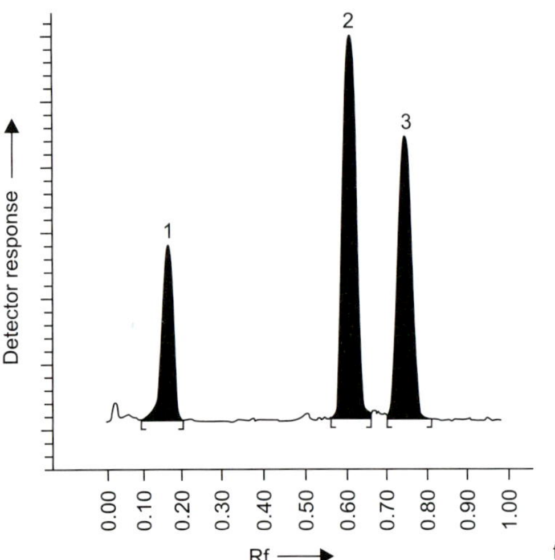

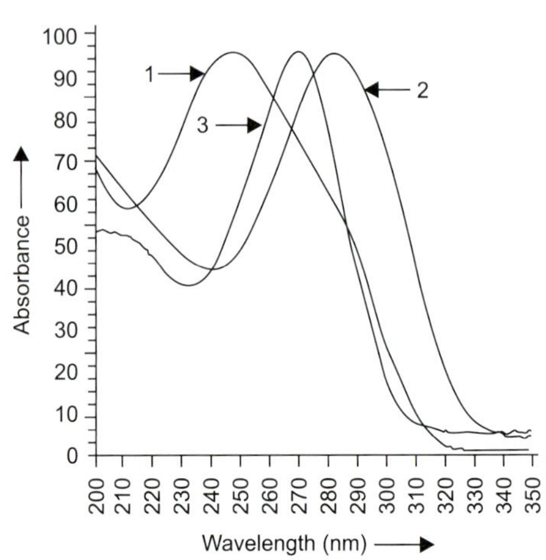

Overlaid UV-spectra of paracetamol (1), diclofenac K^+ (2) and famotidine (3) for selection of suitable wavelength for densitometric scanning

Typical densitogram of the sample containing paracetamol, diclofenac potassium and famotidine. For detailed experimental and chromatographic conditions, refer to Protocol No. 196. Peaks identification: 1. Famotidine; 2. Paracetamol; 3. Diclofenac K^+.

PROTOCOL FOR HPTLC ANALYSIS OF PHARMACEUTICAL FORMULATION

Protocol No. 196

Formulation: **Paracetamol, Diclofenac potassium, Famotidine**

Classification: Musculoskeletal Disorders **Dosage form:** Tablets

Standard preparation: Prepare solution of each compound separately in methanol to get 3.25 mg/ml of paracetamol; 0.5 mg/ml of diclofenac and 0.2 mg/ml of famotidine. Apply 1–6 μl of each solution for linearity profile.

Sample preparation: Powdered sample equivalent to 50 mg of diclofenac suspended in methanol, sonicated for 30 min, diluted and filtered. The filtrate suitably diluted for assay. Apply 2 μl of the resulting solution for chromatographic analysis.

Chromatographic equipments:

Sample applicator: Camag Linomat–IV

Development chamber: Camag twin–trough glass chamber, 10 × 10 cm

Densitometric scanner: Camag TLC Scanner–II

Chromatographic conditions:

1. Stationary phase: Silica gel $60F_{254}$ pre-coated TLC plates, 10 × 10 cm (250 μm) – Merck, pre-washed with methanol and dried at 110°C for 5 min prior to use
2. Mobile phase (MP): Toluene–acetone–methanol–formic acid (5 : 2 : 2 : 0.01 v/v)
3. Standard/Sample application:
   Band length: 5 mm Volume applied: 1–6 μl Spacing: 5 mm
4. Chamber saturation: 30 min (MP)
5. RH (%): 60 ± 5
6. Temperature °C: 25 ± 2
7. Separation technique: Ascending
8. Quantity of mobile phase: 9 ml
9. Migration distance: 80 mm
10. Migration time: 18 min

Densitometric evaluation:

Wavelength: UV–274 nm Scanning mode: Reflectance/Absorbance

HRF: Famotidine—17; Paracetamol—62; Diclofenac potassium—75

Linearity (ng/band): Paracetamol—1625–9750; Diclofenac potassium—250–1500; Famotidine—100–600

Recovery (%): 95.65–98.15 for all the three compounds

References: Laxman D. Khatel, Asmita Y. Kamble, M.V. Mahadik and S.R. Dhaneshwar, *J. AOAC Int.*, **93(3)**, 765–770, 2010.

Comments: The method validated for accuracy, precision, linearity, LOD, LOQ, specificity, robustness and ruggedness.

HPTLC : High Performance Thin Layer Chromatography
HPTLC Densitogram

No. 197

Ibuprofen

Paracetamol

Famotidine

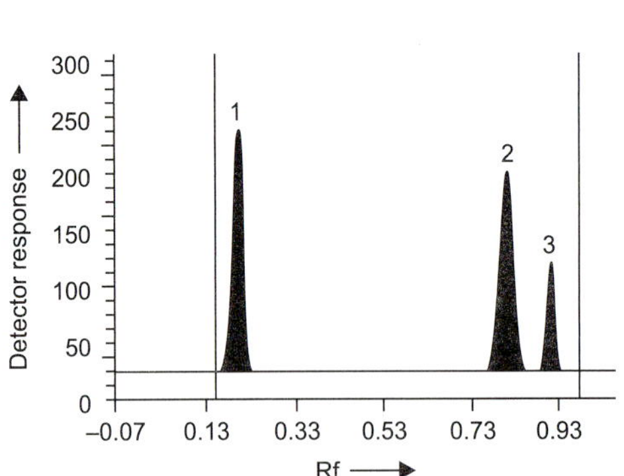

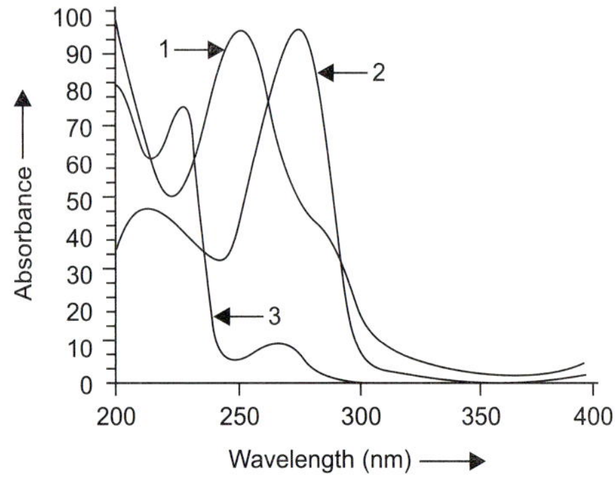

Overlaid UV-spectra of paracetamol (1), famotidine (2) and ibuprofen (3) for selection of suitable wavelength for densitometric scanning

Typical densitogram of the sample containing paracetamol, famotidine and ibuprofen. For detailed experimental and chromatographic conditions, refer to Protocol No. 197. Peaks identification: 1. Famotidine; 2. Paracetamol; 3. Ibuprofen.

PROTOCOL FOR HPTLC ANALYSIS OF PHARMACEUTICAL FORMULATION

Protocol No. 197

Formulation: Paracetamol, Famotidine, Ibuprofen

Classification: Musculoskeletal Disorders **Dosage form:** Tablets

Standard preparation: Prepare solution of each compound separately in methanol to get 80 μg/ml of paracetamol, 32 μg/ml of famotidine and 120 μg/ml of ibuprofen. Apply 5–30 μl of each solution for linearity profile.

Sample preparation: Powdered sample equivalent to 10 mg of famotidine suspended in 50 ml of methanol, sonicated for 20 min, diluted to 100 ml, filtered and 2 ml of filtrate diluted to 10 ml with methanol. Apply 10 μl for assay.

Chromatographic equipments:

Sample applicator: Camag Linomat–V

Development chamber: Camag twin-trough glass chamber, 10 × 10 cm

Densitometric scanner: Camag TLC Scanner–III

Chromatographic conditions:

1. Stationary phase: Silica gel $60F_{254}$ pre-coated HPTLC plates, 10 × 10 cm (200 μm) – Merck
2. Mobile phase (MP): Chloroform–methanol–ethyl acetate–acetic acid (21.5 : 16.1 : 59.1 : 3.2 v/v)
3. Standard/Sample application:
   Band length: 6 mm Volume applied: 10 μl Spacing: 10 mm
4. Chamber saturation: 20 min (MP)
5. RH (%): 55 ± 5
6. Temperature °C: 25 ± 2
7. Separation technique: Ascending
8. Quantity of mobile phase: 10 ml
9. Migration distance: 85 mm
10. Migration time: 20 min

Densitometric evaluation:

Wavelength: UV–256 nm

Scanning mode: Reflectance/Absorbance

HRF: Famotidine—21; Paracetamol—80; Ibuprofen—89

Linearity (ng/band): Paracetamol—400–2400; Famotidine—160–960, Ibuprofen—600–3600

Recovery (%): 98.21–100.35 for all the three compounds

References: Nitin Dubey, Dinesh K. Jain and Subash Jadhawani, *J. Planar Chromatogr.* 25(2), 162–167, 2012.

Comments:

- The method validated for accuracy, precision, linearity, LOD, LOQ, specificity and robustness as per ICH guidelines.
- The method is stability (acid, base, oxidative, thermal, photolytic) indicating.

HPTLC : High Performance Thin Layer Chromatography
HPTLC Densitogram

No. 198

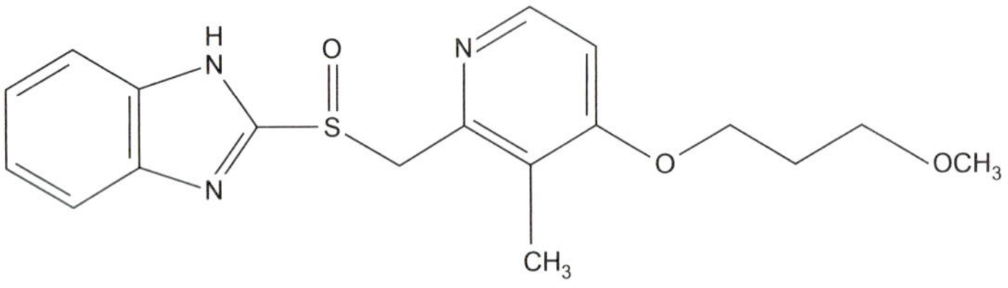

Rabeprazole

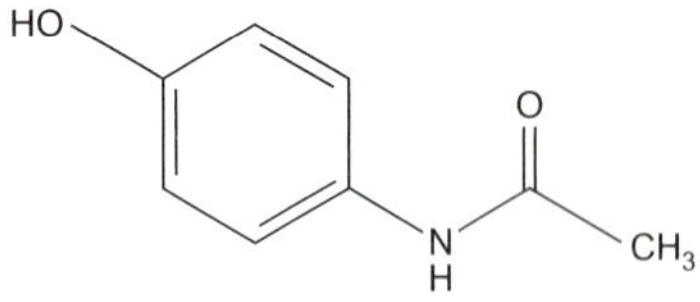

Paracetamol

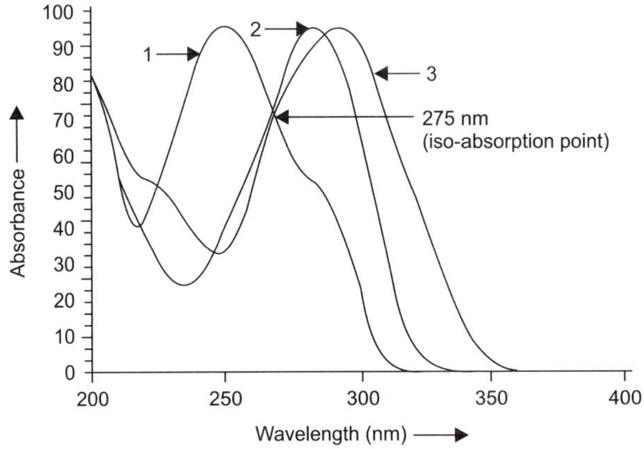

Overlaid UV-spectra of paracetamol (1), aceclofenac (2) and rabeprazole (3) for selection of suitable wavelength for densitometric scanning

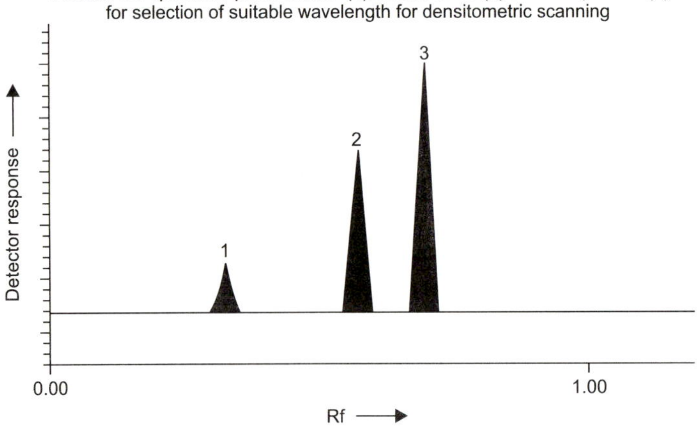

Typical densitogram of the standard containing paracetamol, aceclofenac and rabeprazole sodium. For detailed experimental and chromatographic conditions, refer to Protocol No. 198. Peaks identification: 1. Rabeprazole sodium; 2. Aceclofenac; 3. Paracetamol.

PROTOCOL FOR HPTLC ANALYSIS OF PHARMACEUTICAL FORMULATION

Protocol No. 198

Formulation: **Paracetamol, Aceclofenac, Rabeprazole sodium**

Classification: Musculoskeletal Disorders **Dosage form:** Tablets

Standard preparation: Prepare solution of each compound separately in methanol to get 50 mg/ml of paracetamol, 10 mg/ml of aceclofenac and 1 mg/ml of rabeprazole. These solutions further diluted to get 100–500 μg/ml of paracetamol, 20–100 μg/ml of aceclofenac and 2–10 μg/ml of rabeprazole. Apply 0.2–1 μl of each solution for linearity profile.

Sample preparation: Powdered sample equivalent to 50 mg of aceclofenac suspended in 40 ml of methanol, sonicated for 5 min, diluted to 50 ml with methanol, filtered and used for chromatographic evaluation.

Chromatographic equipments:

Sample applicator: Camag Linomat–V

Development chamber: Camag twin-trough glass chamber, 20 × 10 cm

Densitometric scanner: Camag TLC Scanner–III

Chromatographic conditions:

1. Stationary phase: Silica gel $60F_{254}$ pre-coated HPTLC plates, 20 × 10 cm (200 μm)
2. Mobile phase (MP): Ethyl acetate–methanol–glacial acetic acid (9 : 1 : 0.1 v/v)
3. Standard/Sample application:
   Band length: 6 mm Volume applied: 0.2–1 μl Spacing: 10 mm
4. Chamber saturation: 10 min (MP)
5. RH (%): 55 ± 5
6. Temperature °C: 25 ± 2
7. Separation technique: Ascending
8. Quantity of mobile phase: 20 ml
9. Migration distance: 80 mm
10. Migration time: 20 min

Densitometric evaluation:

Wavelength: UV–275 nm Scanning mode: Reflectance/Absorbance

HRF: Rabeprazole sodium—42; Aceclofenac—63; Paracetamol—79

Linearity (ng/band): Paracetamol—100–500; Aceclofenac—20–100; Rabeprazole sodium—2–10

Recovery (%): Paracetamol—98.89–101.04; Aceclofenac—99.88–100.08; Rabeprazole sodium—98.98–99.22

References: Mallikarjuna Rao N. and Gowri Sankar D., *Int. J. Pharm. Tech. Res.*, **3(2)**, 909–918, 2011.

Comments: The method validated for accuracy, precision, linearity, LOD, LOQ, specificity, robustness and ruggedness.

HPTLC : High Performance Thin Layer Chromatography
HPTLC Densitogram

No. 199

CH_3 CH_3 COOH H_3C

Ibuprofen

O OH N Cl

Chlorzoxazone

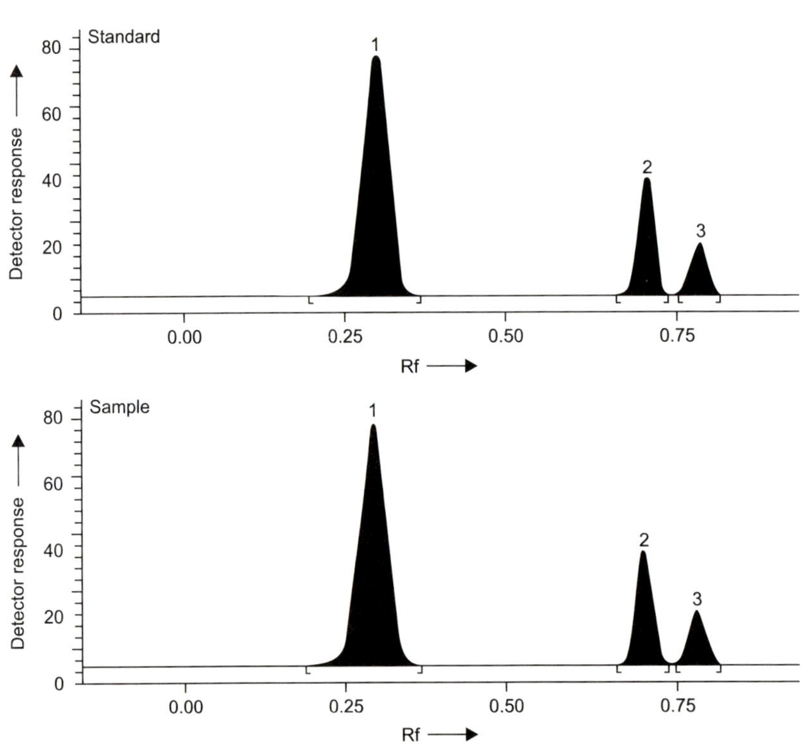

Typical densitogram of the sample and standard containing paracetamol, ibuprofen and chlorzoxazone. For detailed experimental and chromatographic conditions, refer to Protocol No. 199. Peaks identification: 1. Paracetamol; 2. Chlorzoxazone; 3. Ibuprofen.

PROTOCOL FOR HPTLC ANALYSIS OF PHARMACEUTICAL FORMULATION

Protocol No. 199

Formulation: Paracetamol, Ibuprofen, Chlorzoxazone

Classification: Musculoskeletal Disorders **Dosage form:** Tablets

Standard preparation: Weigh accurately about 30 mg of paracetamol (P), 25 mg of chlorzoxazone (C) and 40 mg of ibuprofen (I), dissolve in methanol to make 100 ml. Dilute 2 ml to 10 with methanol for chromatographic analysis.

Sample preparation: Weigh powdered sample equivalent to 30 mg of paracetamol, add 80 ml of methanol, vortex for 15 min and dilute to 100 ml, filter and dilute 2 ml to 10 ml with methanol for chromatographic analysis.

Chromatographic equipments:

Sample applicator: Camag Linomat–IV

Development chamber: Camag twin–trough glass chamber, 10 × 10 cm

Densitometric scanner: Camag TLC Scanner–II

Chromatographic conditions:

1. Stationary phase: Silica gel 60F_{254} pre-coated HPTLC plates, 10 × 10 cm (200 μm) – Merck
2. Mobile phase (MP): (i) Toluene–ethyl acetate–glacial acetic acid (6 : 3 : 0.5 v/v); (ii) Chloroform–toluene–dioxane (7 : 2 : 2 v/v)
3. Standard/Sample application:
   Band length: 10 mm Volume applied: 5 μl Spacing: 10 mm
4. Chamber saturation: —
5. RH (%): 55 ± 5
6. Temperature °C: 22 ± 2
7. Separation technique: Ascending
8. Quantity of mobile phase: 9.5 ml
9. Migration distance: 60 mm
10. Migration time: 15 min

Densitometric evaluation:

Wavelength: UV–210 nm or 254 nm Scanning mode: Reflectance/Absorbance

HRF: Paracetamol—29; Chlorzoxazone—72; Ibuprofen—80

Linearity (ng/band): Paracetamol—100–500; Ibuprofen—100–900; Chlorzoxazone—75–500

Recovery (%): 98.82–99.97 for all the three compounds

References: Renu A. Sodhi, Jyoti L. Chawla and Ramesh T. Sane, *Indian Drugs*, **33(6)**, 280–285, 1996.

Comments: —

HPTLC : High Performance Thin Layer Chromatography
HPTLC Densitogram

No. 200

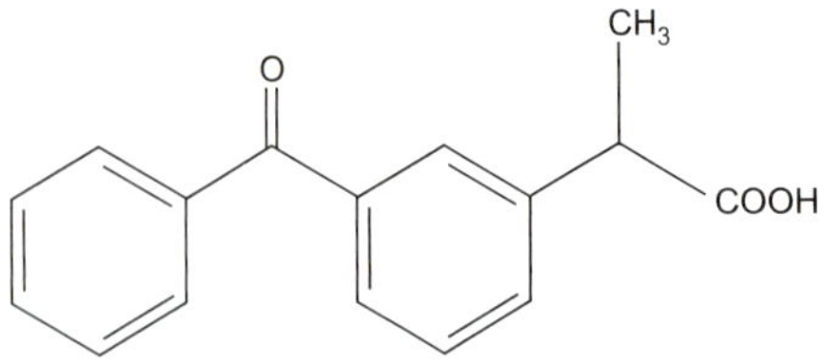

Ketoprofen

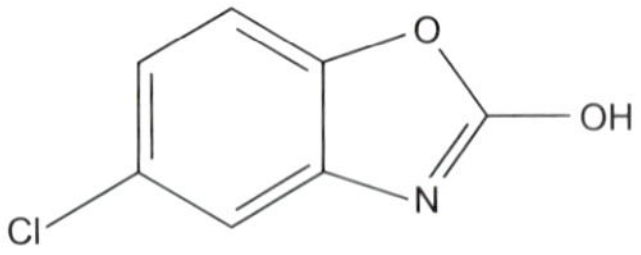

Chlorzoxazone

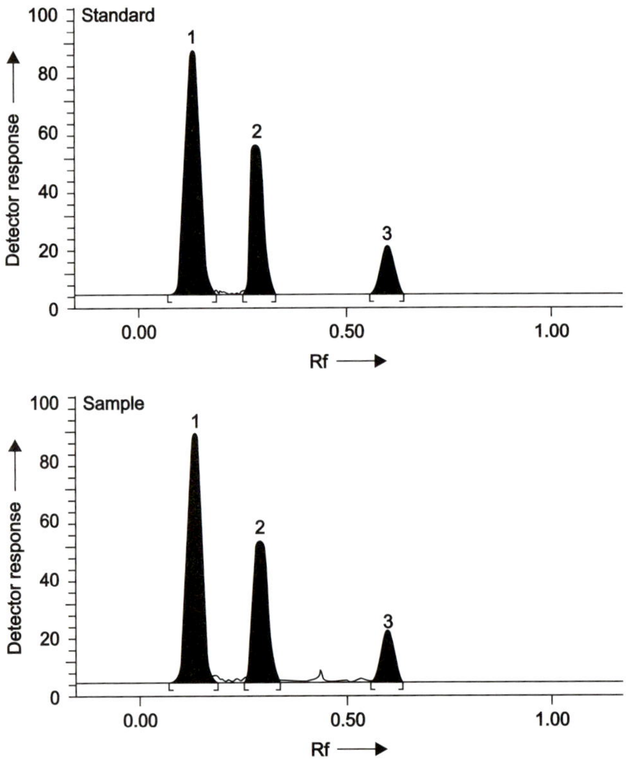

Typical densitogram of the sample and standard containing paracetamol, chlorzoxazone and ketoprofen. For detailed experimental and chromatographic conditions, refer to Protocol No. 200. Peaks identification: 1. Paracetamol; 2. Ketoprofen; 3. Chlorzoxazone.

PROTOCOL FOR HPTLC ANALYSIS OF PHARMACEUTICAL FORMULATION

Protocol No. 200

Formulation: Paracetamol, Ketoprofen, Chlorzoxazone

Classification: Musculoskeletal Disorders **Dosage form:** Tablets

Standard preparation: (1) Weigh accurately 30 mg of paracetamol and 25 mg of chlorzoxazone, dissolve in methanol to make 100 ml; (2) Prepare 100 μg/ml solution of ketoprofen in methanol. Mix 4 ml of solution (1) and 2 ml of solution (2) and dilute to make 10 ml with methanol and use for chromatographic analysis.

Sample preparation: Weigh accurately powdered sample equivalent to about 30 mg of paracetamol, suspend in 60–70 ml of methanol, sonicate for 5 min, make up to 100 ml, filter and dilute 4 ml to 10 ml with methanol for chromatographic analysis.

Chromatographic equipments:

Sample applicator: Camag Linomat–IV

Development chamber: Camag twin–trough glass chamber, 10 × 10 cm

Densitometric scanner: Camag TLC Scanner–II

Chromatographic conditions:

1. Stationary phase: Silica gel $60F_{254}$ pre-coated HPTLC plates, 10 × 10 cm (200 μm) – Merck
2. Mobile phase (MP): Toluene–ethyl acetate–glacial acetic acid (6 : 4 : 0.2 v/v)
3. Standard/Sample application:
   Band length: 5 mm Volume applied: 5 μl Spacing: 5 mm
4. Chamber saturation: 10 min (MP)
5. RH (%): 55 ± 5
6. Temperature °C: 22 ± 2
7. Separation technique: Ascending
8. Quantity of mobile phase: 10 ml
9. Migration distance: 50 mm
10. Migration time: 14 min

Densitometric evaluation:

Wavelength: UV–254 nm Scanning mode: Reflectance/Absorbance

HRF: Paracetamol—13; Ketoprofen—28; Chlorzoxazone—61

Linearity (ng/band): Paracetamol—100–1000; Chlorzoxazone—100–1500; Ketoprofen—25–200

Recovery (%): 98.48–101.53 for all the three compounds

References: —

Comments:

- The method was optimized and analytical work carried out at **Anchrom's HPTLC Application Laboratory**, Mumbai, India.
- Several market samples of similar composition were analysed by the proposed method with reproducible results.

HPTLC : High Performance Thin Layer Chromatography
HPTLC Densitogram

No. 201

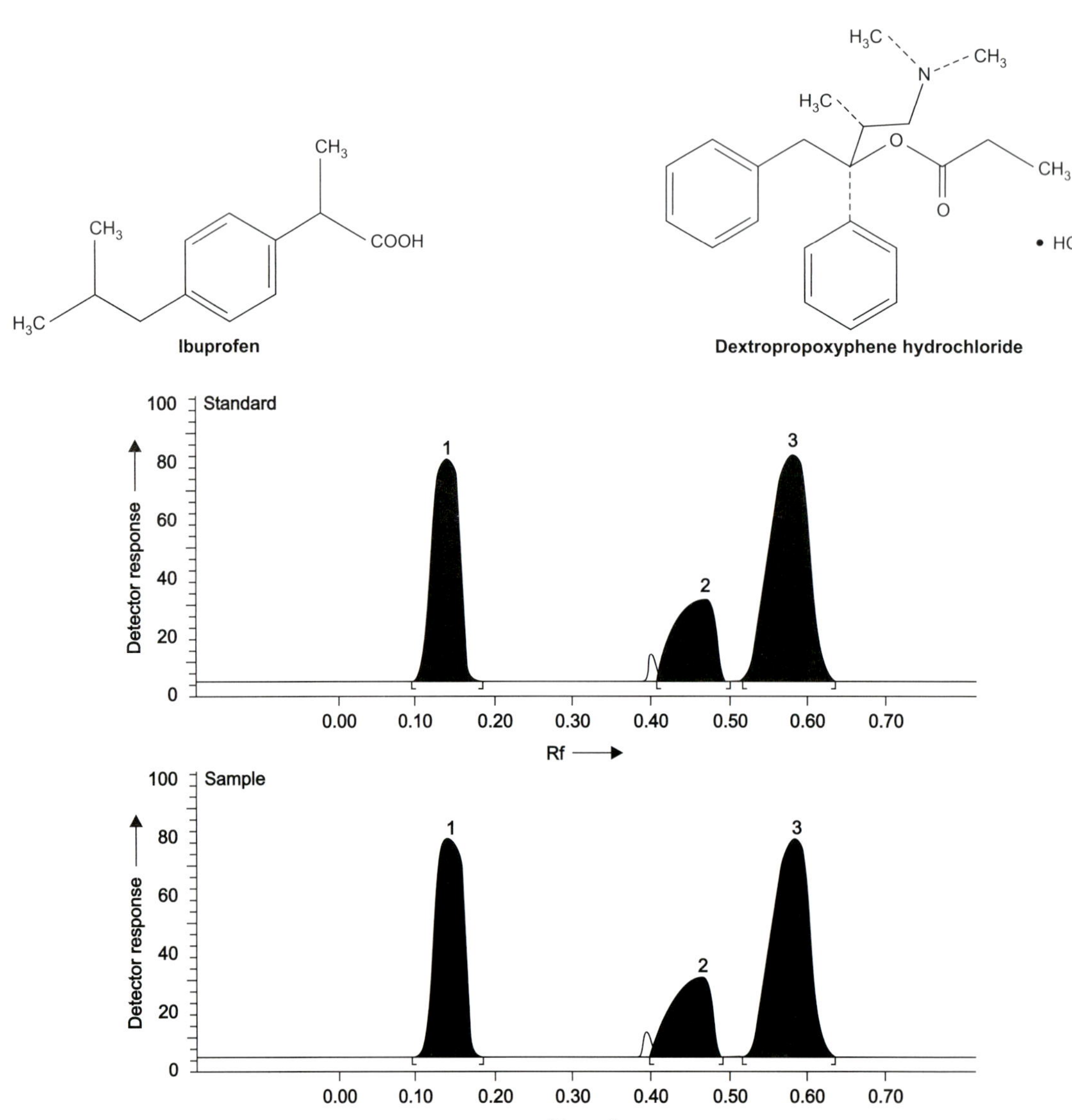

Typical densitogram of the sample and standard containing paracetamol, ibuprofen and dextropropoxyphene HCl. For detailed experimental and chromatographic conditions, refer to Protocol No. 201. Peaks identification: 1. Paracetamol; 2. Ibuprofen; 3. Dextropropoxyphene HCl.

PROTOCOL FOR HPTLC ANALYSIS OF PHARMACEUTICAL FORMULATION

Protocol No. 201

Formulation: **Paracetamol, Ibuprofen, Dextropropoxyphene hydrochloride**
Classification: Musculoskeletal Disorders **Dosage form:** Tablets
Standard preparation: (a) Weigh accurately about 32.5 mg of dextropropoxyphene HCl and dissolve in methanol to make 10 ml. (b) Weigh 40 mg of ibuprofen and 25 mg of paracetamol, add 1 ml of solution (a), dissolve in methanol to make 10 ml, use the resulting solution for chromatographic separation.
Sample preparation: Weigh powdered sample accurately equivalent to 200 mg of ibuprofen, suspend in 30–40 ml methanol, sonicate for 5 min, dilute to 50 ml. Filter and dilute 1 ml to 10 ml with methanol and carry out chromatographic analysis.
Chromatographic equipments:
Sample applicator: Camag Linomat–IV
Development chamber: Camag twin–trough glass chamber, 10 × 10 cm
Densitometric scanner: Camag TLC Scanner–II
Chromatographic conditions:
1. Stationary phase: Silica gel $60F_{254}$ pre-coated HPTLC plates 10 × 10 cm (200 μm) – Merck
2. Mobile phase (MP): (i) Toluene–acetone–25% ammonia (7 : 3 : 0.1 v/v); (ii) Toluene–acetone–glacial acetic acid (7 : 3 : 0.5 v/v)
3. Standard/Sample application:
   Band length: 10 mm Volume applied: 2 and 20 μl Spacing: 10 mm
4. Chamber saturation: 10 min (MP)
5. RH (%): 55 ± 5
6. Temperature °C: 22 ± 2
7. Separation technique: Ascending
8. Quantity of mobile phase: 10 ml
9. Migration distance: 50 (multiple)
10. Migration time: 14 min for each run

Densitometric evaluation:
Wavelength: Paracetamol—245 nm; Ibuprofen—235 nm; Dextropropoxyphene HCl—200 nm/623 nm
Scanning mode: Reflectance/Absorbance
HRF: Paracetamol—13; Ibuprofen—45; Dextropropoxyphene HCl—58
Linearity (ng/band): Paracetamol—100–1000; Ibuprofen—200–2000; Dextropropoxyphene HCl—1000–67500
Recovery (%): 98.53–101.39 for all the three compounds
References: —
Comments:
- The method was optimized and analytical work carried out at **Anchrom's HPTLC Application Laboratory**, Mumbai, India.
- Several market samples of similar composition were analysed by the proposed method with reproducible results.
- After developing the plate in mobile phase (i) scan at 245 nm (paracetamol), and 200 nm (dextropropoxyphene HCl). Redevelop the plate in mobile phase (ii) and then scan at 235 nm (ibuprofen). The plate can be treated with cobalt thiocyanate reagent and scanned at 623 nm for dextropropoxyphene HCl. For preparation of cobalt thiocyanate reagent, see Protocol No. 232.

HPTLC : High Performance Thin Layer Chromatography
HPTLC Densitogram

No. 202

Chlorzoxazone

Nimesulide

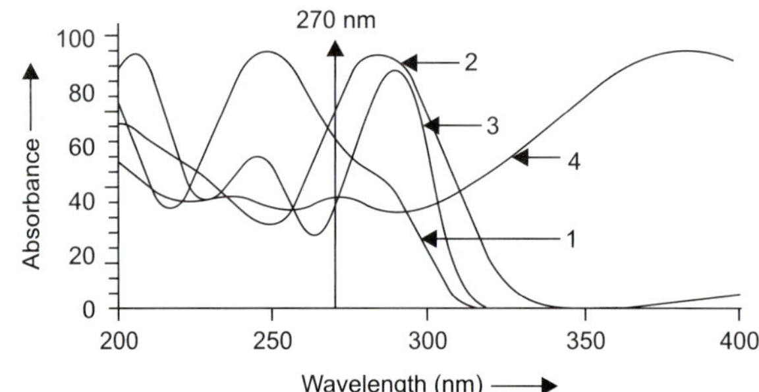

Overlaid UV-spectra of paracetamol (1), diclofenac Na^{+} (2), chlorzoxazone (3) and nimesulide (4) for selection of suitable wavelength for densitometric scanning

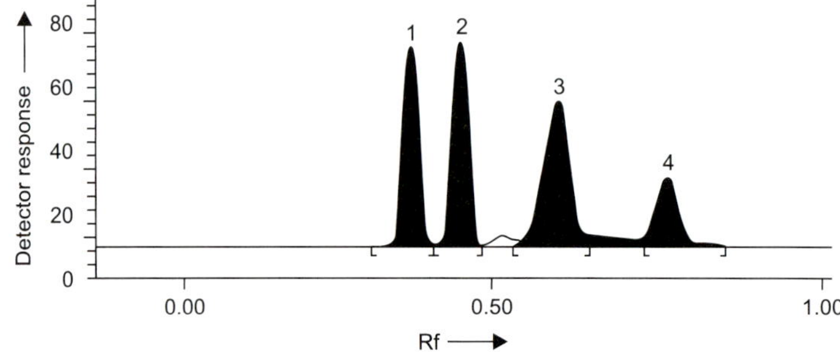

Typical densitogram of the standard containing paracetamol, chlorzoxazone and nimesulide. For detailed experimental and chromatographic conditions, refer to Protocol No. 202. Peaks identification: 1. Paracetamol; 2. Diclofenac sodium (IS); 3. Chlorzoxazone; 4. Nimesulide.

PROTOCOL FOR HPTLC ANALYSIS OF PHARMACEUTICAL FORMULATION

Protocol No. 202

Formulation: Paracetamol, Chlorzoxazone, Nimesulide

Classification: Musculoskeletal Disorders **Dosage form:** Tablets

Standard preparation: Dissolve 163 mg of paracetamol, 188 mg of chlorzoxazone and 50 mg of nimesulide in methanol to produce 50 ml. Add 50 mg diclofenac sodium as (IS). Further dilute with methanol to cover the linearity range. Apply 10 μl of each solution.

Sample preparation: Powdered sample equivalent to 50 mg of nimesulide suspended in methanol, sonicated, diluted and filtered. The filtrate suitably diluted and used. Apply 10 μl for chromatographic separation and analysis.

Chromatographic equipments:

Sample applicator: Camag Linomat–IV

Development chamber: Camag twin–trough glass chamber, 10 × 10 cm

Densitometric scanner: Camag TLC Scanner–II

Chromatographic conditions:

1. Stationary phase: Silica gel $60F_{254}$ pre-coated HPTLC plates 10 × 10 cm (200 μm) – Merck, pre-washed with 10% TEA in methanol, dried at 105°C for 60 min prior to use
2. Mobile phase (MP): Chloroform–methanol–toluene (6 : 0.5 : 1.5 v/v)
3. Standard/Sample application:
   Band length: 10 mm Volume applied: 10 μl Spacing: 10 mm
4. Chamber saturation: 10 min (MP)
5. RH (%): 55 ± 5
6. Temperature °C: 22 ± 2
7. Separation technique: Ascending
8. Quantity of mobile phase: 16 ml
9. Migration distance: 90 mm
10. Migration time: 20 min

Densitometric evaluation:

Wavelength: UV–270 nm Scanning mode: Reflectance/Absorbance

HRF: See densitogram

Linearity (ng/band): Paracetamol—1956–5868; Chlorzoxazone—2251–6754; Nimesulide—60–1822

Recovery (%): 99.30–101.03 for all the compounds

References: Ramesh T. Sane and Manjusha Gadgil, *J. Planar Chromatogr.*, **16(1)**, 76–78, 2002.

Comments: The method validated for accuracy, precision, linearity, LOD, LOQ, specificity, robustness and ruggedness.

HPTLC : High Performance Thin Layer Chromatography
HPTLC Densitogram

No. 203

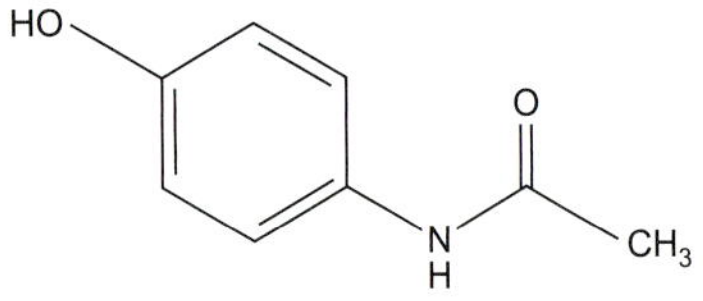

Paracetamol

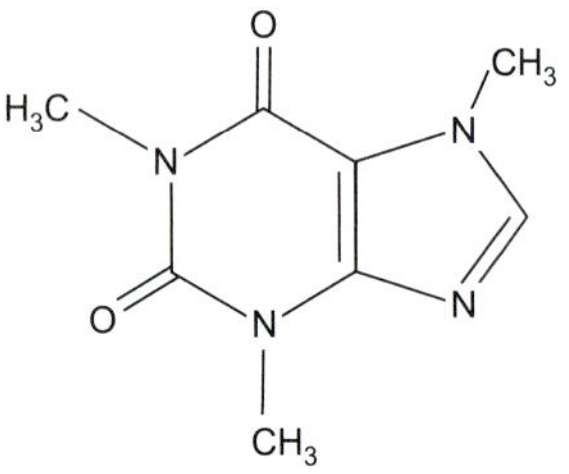

Caffeine

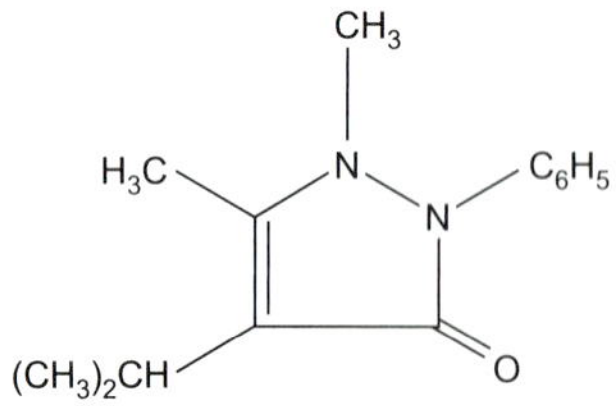

Propyphenazone

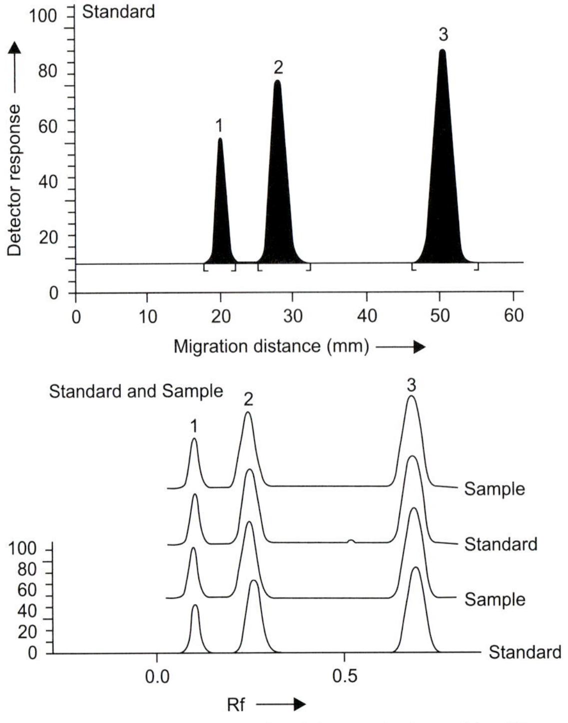

Typical densitogram of sample (tablets) and the standard containing 30 mg of caffeine (1), 250 mg of paracetamol (2) and 150 mg of propyphenazone (3)

Typical densitogram of the standard containing paracetamol, caffeine citrate and propyphenazone. For detailed experimental and chromatographic conditions, refer to Protocol No. 203. Peaks identification: 1. Caffeine citrate; 2. Paracetamol; 3. Propyphenazone.

PROTOCOL FOR HPTLC ANALYSIS OF PHARMACEUTICAL FORMULATION

Protocol No. 203

Formulation: Paracetamol, Caffeine citrate, Propyphenazone

Classification: Musculoskeletal Disorders **Dosage form:** Tablets/Capsules

Standard preparation: Weigh accurately about 15 mg of caffeine (C), 75 mg of propyphenazone (PZ) and 125 mg of paracetamol (P), dissolve in methanol to produce 50 ml, dilute 0.2 ml to 10 ml with methanol and use for analysis.

Sample preparation: Weigh accurately powdered sample equivalent to 30 mg of caffeine, suspend in 60–70 ml of methanol, sonicate for 5 min and dilute to 100 ml, filter and dilute 0.2 ml to 10 ml with methanol for chromatographic analysis.

Chromatographic equipments:

Sample applicator: Camag Linomat–IV

Development chamber: Camag twin–trough glass chamber, 10 × 10 cm

Densitometric scanner: Camag TLC Scanner–II

Chromatographic conditions:

1. Stationary phase: Silica gel $60F_{254}$ pre-coated HPTLC plates 7 × 10 cm (200 μm) – Merck
2. Mobile phase (MP): n-hexane–ethyl acetate–glacial acetic acid (5 : 5 : 0.1 v/v)
3. Standard/Sample application:
   Band length: 5 mm Volume applied: 5 μl Spacing: 5 mm
4. Chamber saturation: 10 min (MP)
5. RH (%): 55 ± 5
6. Temperature °C: 22 ± 2
7. Separation technique: Ascending
8. Quantity of mobile phase: 10 ml
9. Migration distance: 60 mm
10. Migration time: 20 min

Densitometric evaluation:

Wavelength: UV–273 nm Scanning mode: Reflectance/Absorbance

HRF: Caffeine citrate—10; Paracetamol—26; Propyphenazone—71

Linearity (ng/band): Paracetamol—10–1000; Caffeine citrate—10–50; Propyphenazone—100–500

Recovery (%): 99.75–101.25 for all the three compounds

References: —

Comments:

- The method was optimized and analytical work carried out at **Anchrom's HPTLC Application Laboratory**, Mumbai, India.
- Several market samples of similar composition were analysed by the proposed method with reproducible results.
- The densitogram could also be scanned at 280 nm with satisfactory results.

HPTLC : High Performance Thin Layer Chromatography
HPTLC Densitogram

No. 204

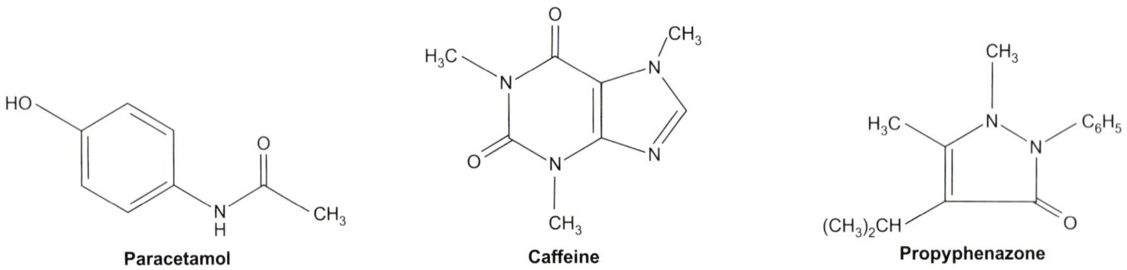

Paracetamol

Caffeine

Propyphenazone

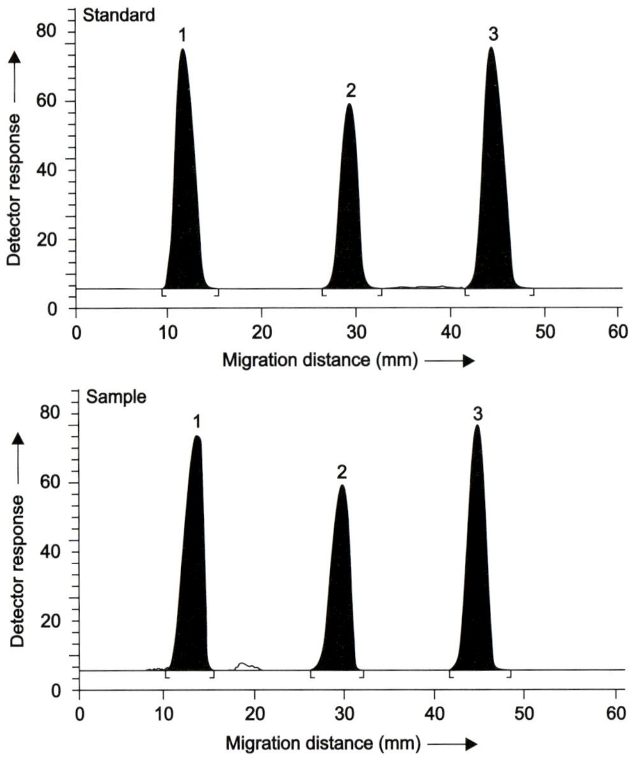

Typical densitogram of the sample and standard containing paracetamol, caffeine citrate and propyphenazone. For detailed experimental and chromatographic conditions, refer to Protocol No. 204. Peaks identification: 1. Propyphenazone; 2. Caffeine citrate; 3. Paracetamol.

PROTOCOL FOR HPTLC ANALYSIS OF PHARMACEUTICAL FORMULATION

Protocol No. 204

Formulation: Paracetamol, Caffeine citrate, Propyphenazone

Classification: Musculoskeletal Disorders **Dosage form:** Tablets

Standard preparation: Weigh accurately about 15 mg of caffeine (C), 75 mg of propyphenazone (PZ) and 125 mg of paracetamol (P), dissolve in methanol to produce 50 ml, dilute 0.2 ml to 10 ml with methanol.

Sample preparation: Weigh accurately powdered sample equivalent to 30 mg of caffeine, suspend in 60–70 ml methanol, sonicate for 5 min, and dilute to 100 ml, filter and dilute 0.2 ml to 10 ml with methanol for chromatographic analysis.

Chromatographic equipments:

Sample applicator: Camag Linomat–IV

Development chamber: Camag twin–trough glass chamber, 10 × 10 cm

Densitometric scanner: Camag TLC Scanner–II

Chromatographic conditions:

1. Stationary phase: Silica gel 60 RP-18F_{254s} pre-coated HPTLC plates 10 × 10 cm (200 μm) – Merck
2. Mobile phase (MP): 0.5 M sodium chloride–methanol–glacial acetic acid (12 : 8 : 0.01 v/v)
3. Standard/Sample application:
   Band length: 5 mm Volume applied: 5 μl Spacing: 10 mm
4. Chamber saturation: 40 min (MP)
5. RH (%): 55 ± 5
6. Temperature °C: 22 ± 2
7. Separation technique: Ascending
8. Quantity of mobile phase: 20 ml
9. Migration distance: 60 mm
10. Migration time: 40 min

Densitometric evaluation:

Wavelength: UV–273 nm Scanning mode: Reflectance/Absorbance

HRF: Propyphenazone—20; Caffeine citrate—55; Paracetamol—80

Linearity (ng/band): Paracetamol—100–1000; Caffeine citrate—10–50; Propyphenazone—100–500

Recovery (%): 99.75–101.65 for all the three compounds

References: —

Comments:

- The method was optimized and analytical work carried out at **Anchrom's HPTLC Application Laboratory**, Mumbai, India.
- Several market samples of similar composition were analysed by the proposed method with reproducible results.
- Reversed-phase chromatography resulted in partial reversal of retention order as compared to normal-phase chromatography.

HPTLC : High Performance Thin Layer Chromatography
HPTLC Densitogram

No. 205

Paracetamol **Caffeine** **Propyphenazone**

Overlaid UV-spectra of paracetamol (1), propyphenazone (2) and caffeine (3) for selection of suitable wavelength for densitometric scanning

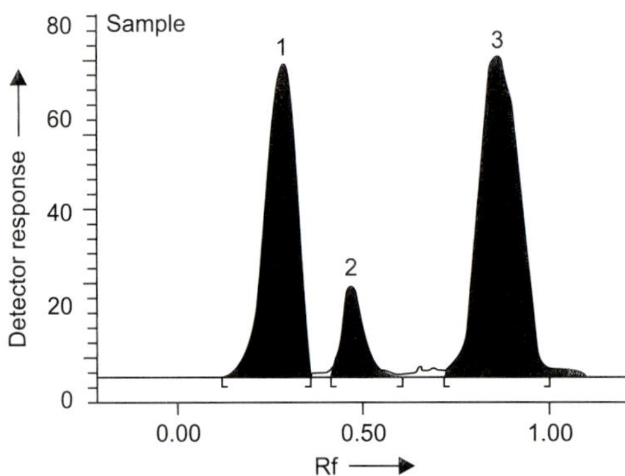

Typical densitogram of the sample containing paracetamol, caffeine citrate and propyphenazone. For detailed experimental and chromatographic conditions, refer to Protocol No. 205. Peaks identification: 1. Paracetamol; 2. Caffeine citrate; 3. Propyphenazone.

PROTOCOL FOR HPTLC ANALYSIS OF PHARMACEUTICAL FORMULATION

Protocol No. 205

Formulation: Paracetamol, Caffeine citrate, Propyphenazone

Classification: Musculoskeletal Disorders **Dosage form:** Tablets

Standard preparation: Dissolve 125 mg of paracetamol, 75 mg of propyphenazone and 15 mg of caffeine in methanol to produce 50 ml. Dilute 0.2 ml to 10 ml with methanol and use for chromatographic analysis.

Sample preparation: Weight accurately powdered sample equivalent to 30 mg of caffeine, suspend in 60–70 ml of methanol, sonicate, dilute to 100 ml with methanol, filter and dilute 0.2 ml to 10 ml with methanol and use for analysis.

Chromatographic equipments:

Sample applicator: Camag Linomat–IV

Development chamber: Camag twin–trough glass chamber, 10 × 10 cm

Densitometric scanner: Camag TLC Scanner–II

Chromatographic conditions:

1. Stationary phase: Silica gel $60F_{254}$ pre-coated TLC plate; 10 × 10 cm (250 μm) – Merck
2. Mobile phase (MP): Dioxane–chloroform (2.5 : 7.5 v/v)
3. Standard/Sample application:
   Band length: 10 mm Volume applied: 5 μl Spacing: 10 mm
4. Chamber saturation: 10 min (MP)
5. RH (%): 55 ± 5
6. Temperature °C: 22 ± 2
7. Separation technique: Ascending
8. Quantity of mobile phase: 10 ml
9. Migration distance: 50 mm
10. Migration time: 12 min

Densitometric evaluation:

Wavelength: UV–273 nm Scanning mode: Reflectance/Absorbance

HRF: Paracetamol—25; Caffeine—50; Propyphenazone—85

Linearity (ng/band): Paracetamol—100–1000; Caffeine citrate—10–50; Propyphenazone—100–500

Recovery (%): 100.15–101.95 for all the three compounds

References: —

Comments:

- The method was optimized and analytical work carried out at **Anchrom's HPTLC Application Laboratory**, Mumbai, India.
- Several market samples of similar composition were analysed by the proposed method with reproducible results.

HPTLC : High Performance Thin Layer Chromatography
HPTLC Densitogram

No. 206

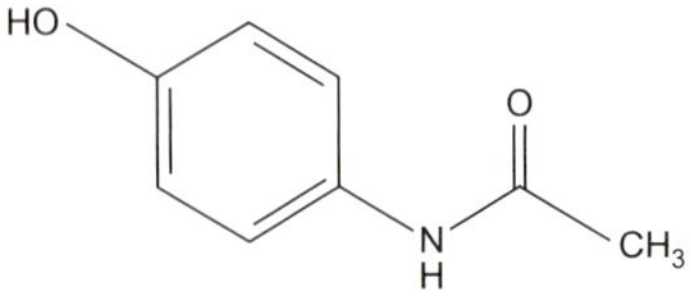

HO, N H, O, CH_3

Paracetamol

$COOCH_2CH_2N(C_2H5)_2$

• HCl

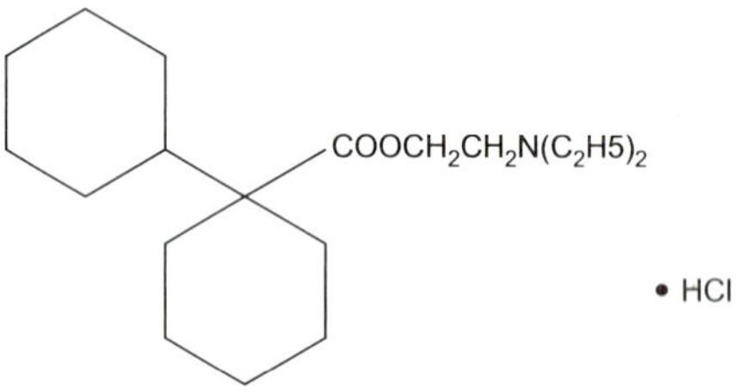

Dicyclomine hydrochloride

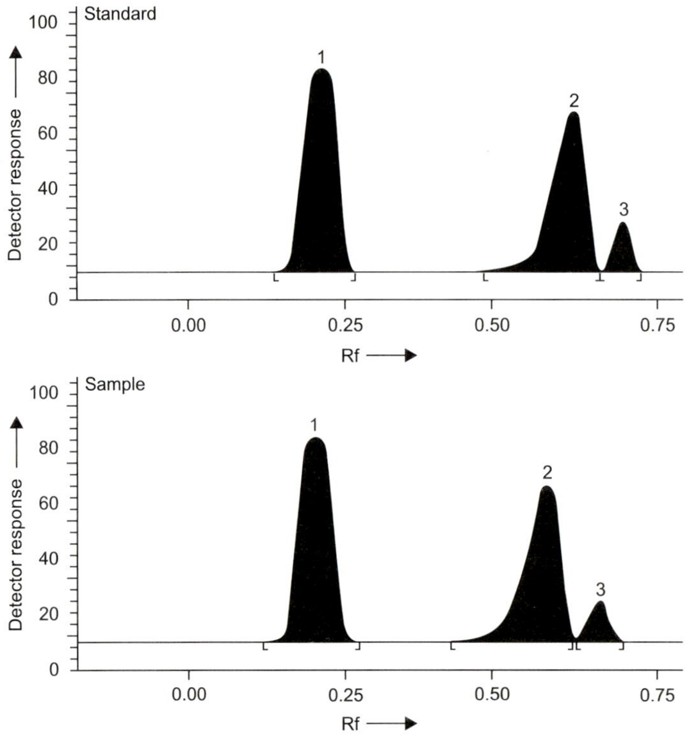

Standard

Detector response; 0, 20, 40, 60, 80, 100; 1, 2, 3; 0.00, 0.25, 0.50, 0.75; Rf

Sample

Detector response; 0, 20, 40, 60, 80, 100; 1, 2, 3; 0.00, 0.25, 0.50, 0.75; Rf

Typical densitogram of the sample and standard containing paracetamol, dextropropoxyphene HCl and dicyclomine HCl. For detailed experimental and chromatographic conditions, refer to Protocol No. 206. Peaks identification: 1. Paracetamol; 2. Dicyclomine HCl; 3. Dextropropoxyphene HCl.

PROTOCOL FOR HPTLC ANALYSIS OF PHARMACEUTICAL FORMULATION

Protocol No. 206

Formulation: **Paracetamol, Dextropropoxyphene hydrochloride, Dicyclomine hydrochloride**

Classification: Musculoskeletal Disorders **Dosage form:** Tablets

Standard preparation: Weigh accurately 32.5 mg of dextropropoxyphene hydrochloride, dissolve in methanol to produce 10 ml (a). Weigh 12.5 mg of paracetamol and 5 mg of dicyclomine HCl, add 1 ml of solution (a), add methanol to produce 10 ml and use for chromatographic analysis.

Sample preparation: (1) Weigh accurately powdered sample equivalent to 10 mg of dicyclomine HCl, suspend in 20 ml methanol, sonicate for 5 min, make up to 25 ml. Dilute 0.25 ml of solution (1) to 100 ml with methanol and use for analysis.

Chromatographic equipments:

Sample applicator: Camag Linomat–IV
Development chamber: Camag twin–trough glass chamber, 10 × 10 cm
Densitometric scanner: Camag TLC Scanner–II

Chromatographic conditions:

1. Stationary phase: Silica gel $60F_{254}$ pre-coated HPTLC plate 10 × 10 cm (200 μm) – Merck
2. Mobile phase (MP): Toluene–acetone–25% ammonia (7 : 3 : 0.05 v/v)
3. Standard/Sample application:
   Band length: 10 mm Volume applied: 2 and 10 μl Spacing: 10 mm
4. Chamber saturation: 10 min (MP)
5. RH (%): 55 ± 5
6. Temperature °C: 22 ± 2
7. Separation technique: Ascending
8. Quantity of mobile phase: 10 ml
9. Migration distance: 50 mm
10. Migration time: 14 min

Densitometric evaluation:

Wavelength: UV–245 nm (paracetamol); UV–200 nm (dextropropoxyphene HCl); 623 nm (dicyclomine HCl) Scanning mode: Reflectance/Absorbance
HRF: Paracetamol—21; Dicyclomine HCl—60; Dextropropoxyphene HCl—70
Linearity (ng/band): Paracetamol—100–1000; Dextropropoxyphene HCl—1000–7500; Dicyclomine HCl—1000–10,000
Recovery (%): 100.61–101.45 for all the three compounds

References: —

Comments:

- The method initially developed and optimized at CDL (CDTL), Bombay. Densitometric evaluation carried out at **Anchrom HPTLC Application Laboratory**, Mulund, Bombay.
- See densitogram No.
- Several market samples of similar composition were analysed by the proposed method with reproducible results.
- After scanning for paracetamol (245 nm), the chromatoplate was treated with cobalt reagent and scanned for dicyclomine HCl and dextropropoxyphene HCl at 623 nm for blue colour formed as a result of post-chromatographic derivatization. For preparation of the reagent, refer to Protocol No. 232.

HPTLC : High Performance Thin Layer Chromatography
HPTLC Densitogram

No. 207

Cl OH • 2HCl N O O

Levocetirizine dihydrochlolride

O O S HN CH_3 O NO_2

Nimesulide

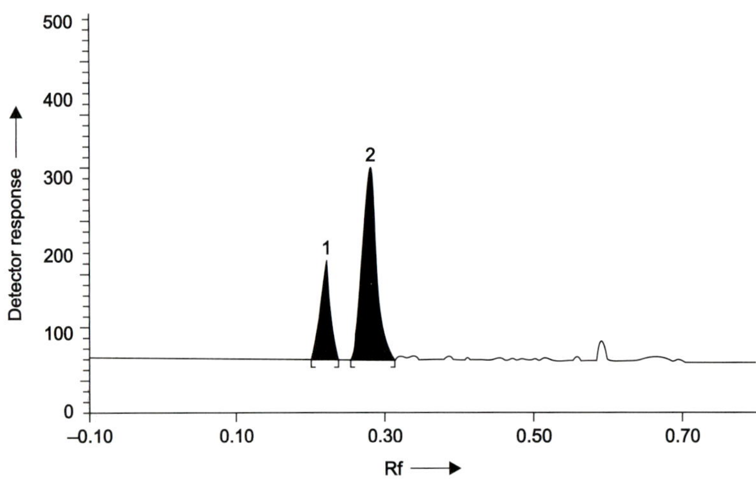

Typical densitogram of the standard containing nimesulide and levocetirizine HCl. For detailed experimental and chromatographic conditions, refer to Protocol No. 207. Peaks identification: 1. Levocetirizine HCl; 2. Nimesulide.

PROTOCOL FOR HPTLC ANALYSIS OF PHARMACEUTICAL FORMULATION

Protocol No. 207

Formulation: Nimesulide, Levocetirizine hydrochloride

Classification: Musculoskeletal Disorders **Dosage form:** Tablets

Standard preparation: Prepare 1 mg/ml solution of nimesulide and 50 μg/ml solution of levocetirizine hydrochloride, both in methanol. Carry out further dilutions to get 100 μg/ml of nimesulide and 5 μg/ml of levocetirizine. Apply 2–7 μl of each solution for linearity profile.

Sample preparation: Powdered sample equivalent to 5 mg of levocetirizine suspended in 30–35 ml of methanol, sonicated for 30 min, diluted to 50 ml, centrifuged (3000 rpm) for 5 min, dilute 5 ml of supernatant to get 50 and 1000 μg/ml of levocetirizine and nimesulide respectively and apply suitable volumes for assay.

Chromatographic equipments:

Sample applicator: Camag Linomat–V

Development chamber: Camag twin–trough glass chamber, 20 × 10 cm

Densitometric scanner: Camag TLC Scanner–III

Chromatographic conditions:

1. Stationary phase: Silica gel $60F_{254}$ pre-coated TLC plates, 20 × 10 cm (250 μm) – Merck, pre-washed with methanol, activated at 110°C for 5 min prior to use
2. Mobile phase (MP): Toluene–ethyl acetate–methanol–25% ammonia (9 : 1 : 1 : 0.5 v/v)
3. Standard/Sample application:
   Band length: 6 mm Volume applied: 2–7 μl Spacing: 6 mm
4. Chamber saturation: 30 min (MP)
5. RH (%): 60 ± 5
6. Temperature °C: 25 ± 2
7. Separation technique: Ascending
8. Quantity of mobile phase: 23 ml
9. Migration distance: 80 mm
10. Migration time: —

Densitometric evaluation:

Wavelength: UV–238 nm Scanning mode: Reflectance/Absorbance

HRF: Levocetirizine HCl—21; Nimesulide—26

Linearity (ng/band): Nimesulide—400–1400; Levocetirizine HCl—100–350

Recovery (%): 99.48–100.06 for both the compounds

References: Sunil R. Dhaneshwar, K.S. Rasal, Vidya K. Bhusari, Janaki V. Salunkhe and Amruta L. Suryan, *Der Pharmacia Sinica* (*Pelagia Research Library*), **2(4)**, 117–124, 2011.

Comments: The method validated for accuracy, precision, linearity, LOD, LOQ, specificity and robustness as per ICH guidelines.

HPTLC : High Performance Thin Layer Chromatography
HPTLC Densitogram

No. 208

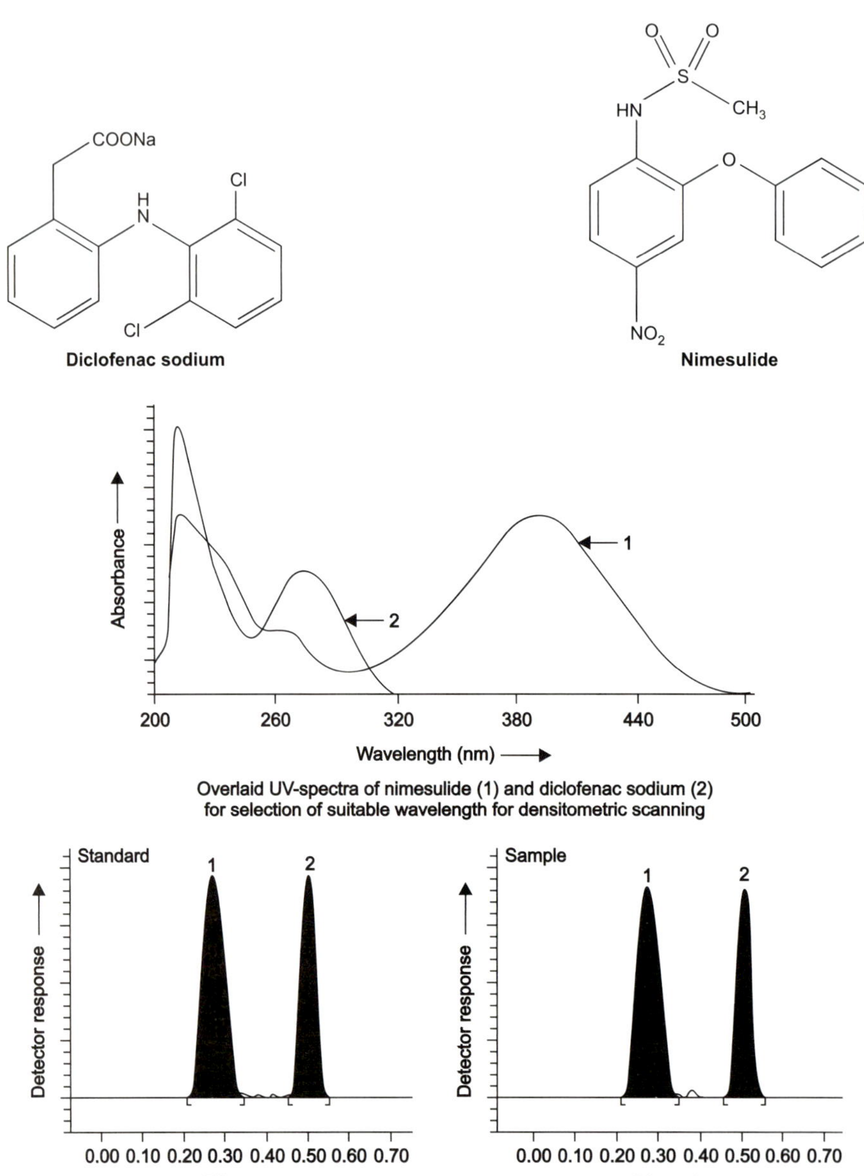

Overlaid UV-spectra of nimesulide (1) and diclofenac sodium (2) for selection of suitable wavelength for densitometric scanning

Typical densitogram of the sample and standard containing diclofenac sodium and nimesulide. For detailed experimental and chromatographic conditions, refer to Protocol No. 208. Peaks identification: 1. Nimesulide; 2. Diclofenac sodium.

PROTOCOL FOR HPTLC ANALYSIS OF PHARMACEUTICAL FORMULATION

Protocol No. 208

Formulation: Diclofenac sodium, Nimesulide

Classification: Musculoskeletal Disorders **Dosage form:** Tablets

Standard preparation: Prepare solution of each compound in methanol to get 0.5 mg/ml of nimesulide and 0.25 mg/ml of diclofenac sodium. Apply varying volumes of each solution for linearity profile.

Sample preparation: Powdered sample equivalent to 10 mg of nimesulide suspended in methanol, sonicated for 5 min, diluted and filtered. The filtrate suitably diluted for application and chromatographic analysis.

Chromatographic equipments:

Sample applicator: Camag Linomat–IV

Development chamber: Camag twin–trough glass chamber, 10 × 10 cm

Densitometric scanner: Camag TLC Scanner–III

Chromatographic conditions:

1. Stationary phase: Silica gel $60F_{254}$ pre-coated HPTLC plate, 10 × 10 cm (200 μm) – Merck
2. Mobile phase (MP): n-hexane–ethyl acetate–chloroform–glacial acetic acid (8 : 1 : 1.5 : 0.5 v/v)
3. Standard/Sample application:
   Band length: 6 mm Volume applied: 1–6 μl Spacing: 5 mm
4. Chamber saturation: 10 min (MP)
5. RH (%): 55 ± 5
6. Temperature °C: 22 ± 2
7. Separation technique: Ascending
8. Quantity of mobile phase: 11 ml
9. Migration distance: 70 mm
10. Migration time: 15 min

Densitometric evaluation:

Wavelength: UV–256 nm Scanning mode: Reflectance/Absorbance

HRF: Nimesulide—28; Diclofenac sodium—50

Linearity (ng/band): Diclofenac sodium—500–1600; Nimesulide—200–500

Recovery (%): 99.14–100.99 for both the compounds

References: Sanjay G. Walode et al., *Asian J. Chem.*, **18(2)**, 1078–1084, 2006.

Comments:

- The method validated for accuracy, precision, linearity, LOD, LOQ, specificity, robustness and ruggedness.
- The method is stability indicating (acid, base, oxidative, thermal, photolytic). The degradation products were separated from the main compounds.

HPTLC : High Performance Thin Layer Chromatography
HPTLC Densitogram

No. 209

Drotaverine

Nimesulide

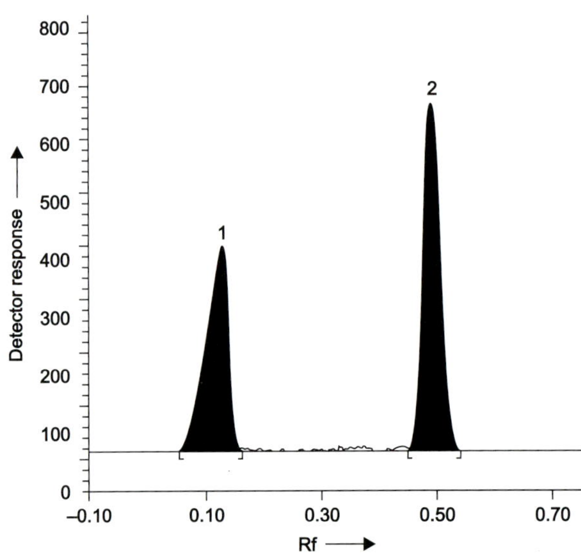

Typical densitogram of the sample containing drotaverine HCl and nimesulide. For detailed experimental and chromatographic conditions, refer to Protocol No. 209. Peaks identification: 1. Drotaverine HCl; 2. Nimesulide.

PROTOCOL FOR HPTLC ANALYSIS OF PHARMACEUTICAL FORMULATION

Protocol No. 209

Formulation: **Drotaverine hydrochloride, Nimesulide**

Classification: Musculoskeletal Disorders **Dosage form:** Tablets

Standard preparation: Dissolve separately 40 mg of drotaverine and 100 mg of nimesulide in methanol. Further dilutions made to get 10 μg/ml of each. Apply varying volumes of each for linearity profile.

Sample preparation: Weigh appropriate quantity of the powdered sample, suspend in methanol, sonicate, dilute, filter and apply sufficient quantity to get 400–600 ng/band and carry out the chromatographic analysis.

Chromatographic equipments:

Sample applicator: Camag Linomat–V

Development chamber: Camag twin–trough glass chamber, 10 × 10 cm

Densitometric scanner: Camag TLC Scanner–III

Chromatographic conditions:

1. Stationary phase: Silica gel 60F_{254} pre-coated TLC plates, 10 × 10 cm (250 μm) – Merck
2. Mobile phase (MP): Cyclohexane–methanol–ethyl acetate (6 : 2 : 2 v/v)
3. Standard/Sample application:
   Band length: 5 mm Volume applied: 5 μl Spacing: 5 mm
4. Chamber saturation: 30 min (MP)
5. RH (%): 55 ± 5
6. Temperature °C: 25 ± 2
7. Separation technique: Ascending
8. Quantity of mobile phase: 10 ml
9. Migration distance: 70 mm
10. Migration time: 20 min

Densitometric evaluation:

Wavelength: UV–295 nm Scanning mode: Reflectance/Absorbance

HRF: Drotaverine HCl—12; Nimesulide—49

Linearity (ng/band): Drotaverine HCl—100–600; Nimesulide—200–700

Recovery (%): Drotaverine HCl—99.53–99.83; Nimesulide—99.83–99.90

References: Sohan Chitlange, Nitin Kumar, Parag Kulkarni and Sagar Wankhede, *Der Pharma Chemica*, **1(2)**, 50–58, 2009.

Comments:

- The method validated for accuracy, precision, linearity, LOD, LOQ, specificity, robustness and ruggedness.
- The method is stability indicating (acid, base, oxidative, thermal, photolytic). The degradation products were separated from the main compounds.

HPTLC : High Performance Thin Layer Chromatography
HPTLC Densitogram

No. 211

Aceclofenac **Drotaverine**

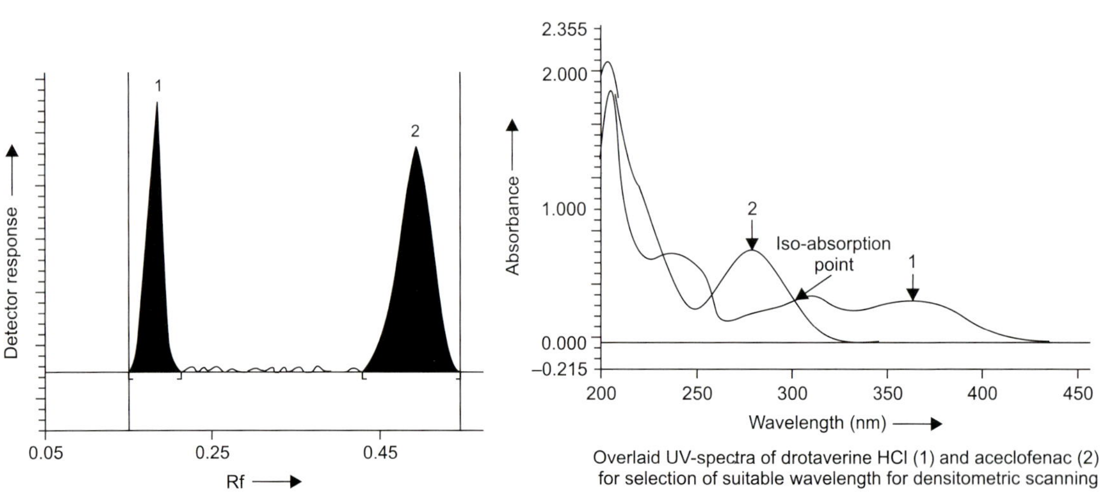

Overlaid UV-spectra of drotaverine HCl (1) and aceclofenac (2) for selection of suitable wavelength for densitometric scanning

Typical densitogram of the sample containing aceclofenac and drotaverine HCl. For detailed experimental and chromatographic conditions, refer to Protocol No. 211. Peaks identification: 1. Drotaverine HCl; 2. Aceclofenac.

PROTOCOL FOR HPTLC ANALYSIS OF PHARMACEUTICAL FORMULATION

Protocol No. 211

Formulation: **Drotaverine hydrochloride, Aceclofenac sodium**

Classification: Musculoskeletal Disorders **Dosage form:** Tablets

Standard preparation: Prepare standard solution of both the compounds separately in methanol to get 80 μg/ml drotaverine hydrochloride and 100 μg/ml aceclofenac. Apply 1–7 μl of each solution for linearity profile.

Sample preparation: Powdered sample equivalent to 80 mg of drotaverine hydrochloride suspended in methanol, sonicated for 5 min, diluted, filtered and the filtrate suitably diluted with methanol. Apply 5 μl for assay.

Chromatographic equipments:

Sample applicator: Camag Linomat–IV

Development chamber: Camag twin–trough glass chamber, 10 × 10 cm

Densitometric scanner: Camag TLC Scanner–III

Chromatographic conditions:

1. Stationary phase: Silica gel 60F_{254} pre-coated HPTLC plates, 10 × 10 cm (200 μm) – Merck, pre-washed with methanol, dried at 105°C for 5 min prior to use
2. Mobile phase (MP): Ethyl acetate–methanol–glacial acetic acid (9 : 1 : 0.01 v/v)
3. Standard/Sample application:
   Band length: 10 mm Volume applied: 1–7 μl Spacing: 10 mm
4. Chamber saturation: 10 min (MP)
5. RH (%): 55 ± 5
6. Temperature °C: 25 ± 2
7. Separation technique: Ascending
8. Quantity of mobile phase: 10 ml
9. Migration distance: 85 mm
10. Migration time: 25 min

Densitometric evaluation:

Wavelength: UV–300 nm (iso-absorption point)

Scanning mode: Reflectance/Absorbance

HRF: Drotaverine HCl—18; Aceclofenac—51

Linearity (ng/band): Aceclofenac—100–700; Drotaverine hydrochloride—80–560

Recovery (%): 99.65–99.8 for both the compounds

References: Suganthi Azhlwar and T.K. Ravi, *Der Pharmacia Lettre*, **2(2)**, 328–332, 2010.

Comments: The method validated for accuracy, precision, linearity, LOD, LOQ, specificity, robustness and ruggedness.

HPTLC : High Performance Thin Layer Chromatography
HPTLC Densitogram

No. 212

Drotaverine

Aceclofenac

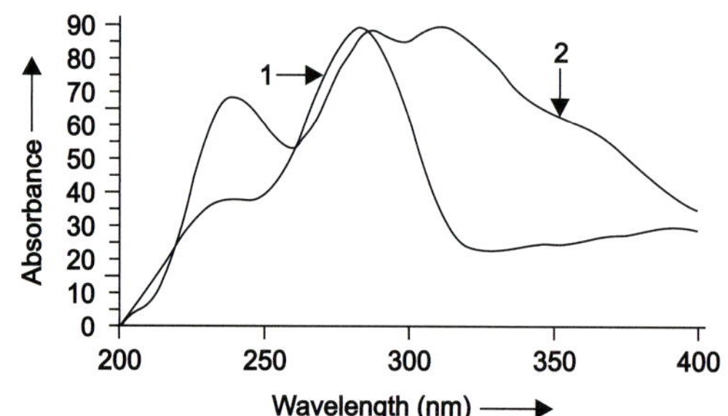

Overlaid UV-spectra of aceclofenac (1) and drotaverine HCl (2) for selection of suitable wavelength for densitometric scanning

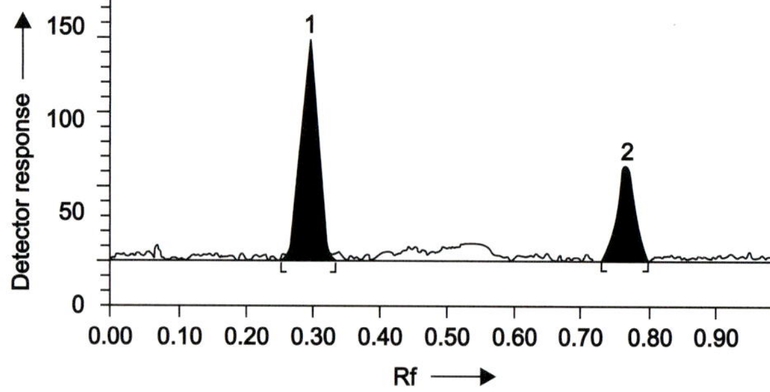

Typical densitogram of the standard containing drotaverine hydrochloride and aceclofenac. For detailed experimental and chromatographic conditions, refer to Protocol No. 212. Peaks identification: 1. Aceclofenac; 2. Drotaverine HCl.

PROTOCOL FOR HPTLC ANALYSIS OF PHARMACEUTICAL FORMULATION

Protocol No. 212

Formulation: Drotaverine hydrochloride, Aceclofenac

Classification: Musculoskeletal Disorders **Dosage form:** Tablets

Standard preparation: Prepare 50 μg/ml solution of each compound in methanol. Apply varying volumes of each solution (2–10 μl) for linearity profile.

Sample preparation: Powdered sample equivalent to 10 mg of aceclofenac suspended in 7 ml of methanol, sonicated for 5 min, diluted to 10 ml with methanol, filter and apply 4 μl for chromatographic analysis.

Chromatographic equipments:

Sample applicator: Camag Linomat–V

Development chamber: Camag twin–trough glass chamber, 20 × 10 cm

Densitometric scanner: Camag TLC Scanner–III

Chromatographic conditions:

1. Stationary phase: Silica gel $60F_{254}$ pre-coated HPTLC plates, 20 × 10 cm (200 μm) – Merck
2. Mobile phase (MP): Ethyl acetate–methanol–triethylamine (7.5 : 2 : 0.5 v/v)
3. Standard/Sample application:
   Band length: 6 mm Volume applied: 4 μl Spacing: 5 mm
4. Chamber saturation: 25 min (MP)
5. RH (%): 55 ± 5
6. Temperature °C: 22 ± 2
7. Separation technique: Ascending
8. Quantity of mobile phase: 20 ml
9. Migration distance: 90 mm
10. Migration time: 20 min

Densitometric evaluation:

Wavelength: UV–284 nm Scanning mode: Reflectance/Absorbance

HRF: Aceclofenac—29; Drotaverine HCl—76

Linearity: 100–500 ng/band for both the drugs

Recovery (%): Drotaverine HCl—98.99–100.50; Aceclofenac—99.30–100.85

References: Santosh V. Gandhi, Padmanabh Deshpande, Rajmane Vivek and Sagar Chaudhari, *Int. Res. J. Pharma* (IRJP), **1(1)**, 189–193, 2010.

Comments: The method validated for accuracy, precision, linearity, LOD, LOQ, specificity, robustness and ruggedness.

HPTLC : High Performance Thin Layer Chromatography
HPTLC Densitogram

No. 213

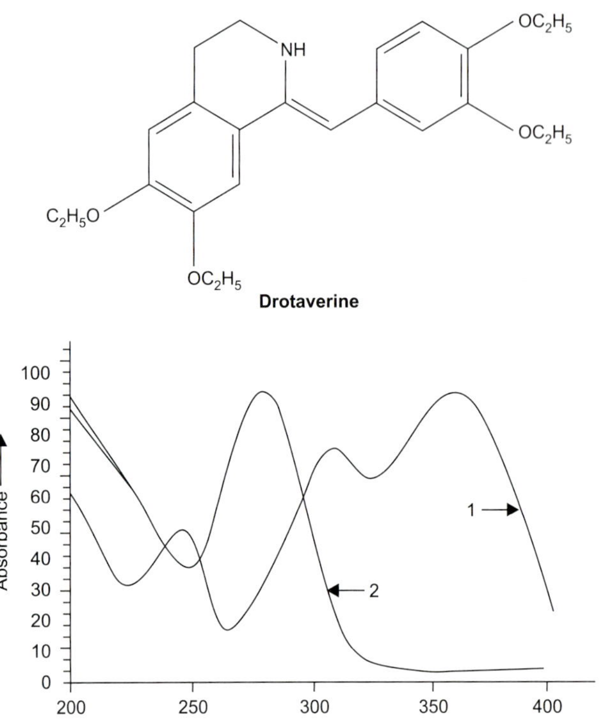

Overlaid UV-spectra of drotaverine hydrochloride (1) and diclofenac potassium (2) for selection of suitable wavelength for densitometric scanning

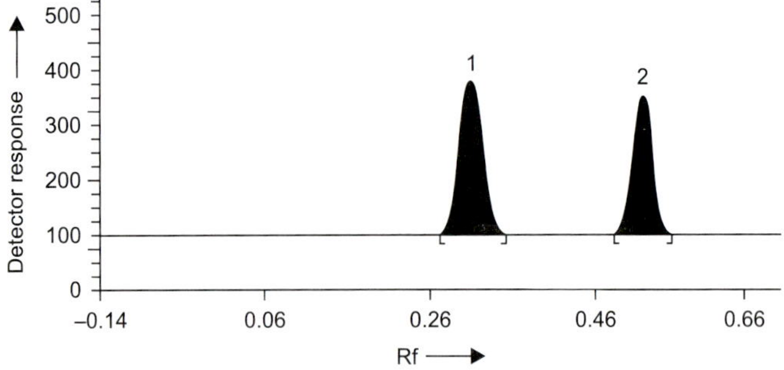

Typical densitogram of the standard containing drotaverine hydrochloride and diclofenac potassium. For detailed experimental and chromatographic conditions, refer to Protocol No. 213. Peaks identification: 1. Drotaverine HCl; 2. Diclofenac K^+.

PROTOCOL FOR HPTLC ANALYSIS OF PHARMACEUTICAL FORMULATION

Protocol No. 213

Formulation: **Drotaverine hydrochloride, Diclofenac potassium**

Classification: Musculoskeletal Disorders **Dosage form:** Tablets

Standard preparation: Prepare solution of both the drugs in methanol to get 80 μg/ml of drotaverine hydrochloride and 50 μg/ml of diclofenac potassium. Apply varying volumes of each solution for linearity studies.

Sample preparation: Powdered sample equivalent to 50 mg of diclofenac potassium suspended in 40 ml of methanol, sonicated for 10 min, diluted to 50 ml with methanol. Filter and dilute suitably to get 50 μg/ml. Apply adequate volume to get 600 ng of drotaverine and 400 ng of diclofenac and carry out the chromatographic analysis.

Chromatographic equipments:

Sample applicator: Camag Linomat–V

Development chamber: Camag twin–trough glass chamber, 20 × 10 cm

Densitometric scanner: Camag TLC Scanner–III

Chromatographic conditions:

1. Stationary phase: Silica gel $60F_{254}$ pre-coated TLC plates, 20 × 10 cm (250 μm) – Merck, pre-washed with methanol, activated at 110°C for 5 min prior to use
2. Mobile phase (MP): Toluene–ethyl acetate–methanol (2 : 8 : 2 v/v)
3. Standard/Sample application:
   Band length: 6 mm Volume applied: 1–10 μl Spacing: 11.2 mm
4. Chamber saturation: 30 min (MP)
5. RH (%): 60 ± 5
6. Temperature °C: 25 ± 2
7. Separation technique: Ascending
8. Quantity of mobile phase: 24 ml
9. Migration distance: 85 mm
10. Migration time: 18 min

Densitometric evaluation:

Wavelength: UV–298 nm Scanning mode: Reflectance/Absorbance

HRF: Drotaverine HCl—28; Diclofenac K^+—51

Linearity (ng/band): Drotaverine hydrochloride—160–1280; Diclofenac K^+—100–800

Recovery (%): 99.39–101.42 for both the drugs

References: Snehl S Ingale, Dipali D. Tajane, Vikram G. Modak, Sacchidanand R Gile, Vishnu P. Choudhari and Bhanudas S. Kuchekar, *Der Pharma Chemica*, **2(5)**, 126–132, 2010.

Comments: The method validated for accuracy, precision, linearity, LOD, LOQ, specificity, robustness and ruggedness.

HPTLC : High Performance Thin Layer Chromatography
HPTLC Densitogram

No. 214

Drotaverine

Etoricoxib

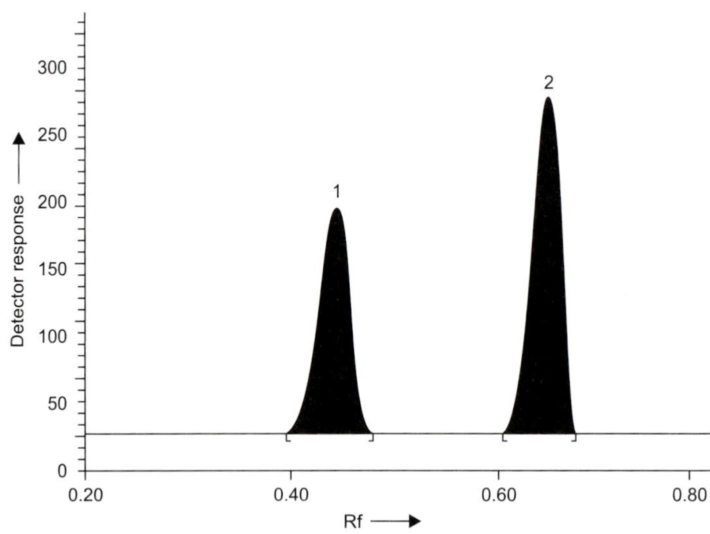

Typical densitogram of the standard containing drotaverine hydrochloride and etoricoxib. For detailed experimental and chromatographic conditions, refer to Protocol No. 214. Peaks identification: 1. Drotaverine HCl; 2. Etoricoxib.

PROTOCOL FOR HPTLC ANALYSIS OF PHARMACEUTICAL FORMULATION

Protocol No. 214

Formulation: Drotaverine hydrochloride, Etoricoxib

Classification: Musculoskeletal Disorders **Dosage form:** Tablets

Standard preparation: Prepare 1 mg/ml solution of each compound in methanol. Further dilutions made with methanol to get 100 μg/ml. Apply varying volumes to establish linearity range.

Sample preparation: Powdered sample equivalent to 80 mg of drotaverine hydrochloride suspended in 40 ml of methanol, sonicated for 10 min, diluted to 50 ml with methanol. Filtered and diluted suitably for chromatographic analysis.

Chromatographic equipments:

Sample applicator: Camag Linomat–V

Development chamber: Camag twin–trough glass chamber, 20 × 10 cm

Densitometric scanner: Camag TLC Scanner–III

Chromatographic conditions:

1. Stationary phase: Silica gel $60F_{254}$ pre-coated TLC plates, 20 × 10 cm (250 μm) – Merck, pre-washed with methanol, activated at 110°C for 5 min prior to use
2. Mobile phase (MP): Toluene–ethyl acetate–methanol (2 : 8 : 2 v/v)
3. Standard/Sample application:
   Band length: 6 mm Volume applied: 1–10 μl Spacing: 4.5 mm
4. Chamber saturation: 20 min (MP)
5. RH (%): 55 ± 5
6. Temperature °C: 22 ± 2
7. Separation technique: Ascending
8. Quantity of mobile phase: 24 ml
9. Migration distance: 85 mm
10. Migration time: 18 min

Densitometric evaluation:

Wavelength: UV–304 nm Scanning mode: Reflectance/Absorbance

HRF: Drotaverine HCl—45; Etoricoxib—66

Linearity (ng/band): Drotaverine HCl—200–700; Etoricoxib—225–787

Recovery (%): Drotaverine HCl—99.87–101.20; Etoricoxib—99.39–100.92

References: Abstract No F-339, 62nd IPC-2010 and Personal communication, Prof. B.S. Kuchekar, Maharashtra Institute of Pharmacy, Pune, India.

Comments: The method validated for accuracy, precision, linearity, LOD, LOQ, specificity, robustness and ruggedness.

HPTLC : High Performance Thin Layer Chromatography
HPTLC Densitogram

No. 215

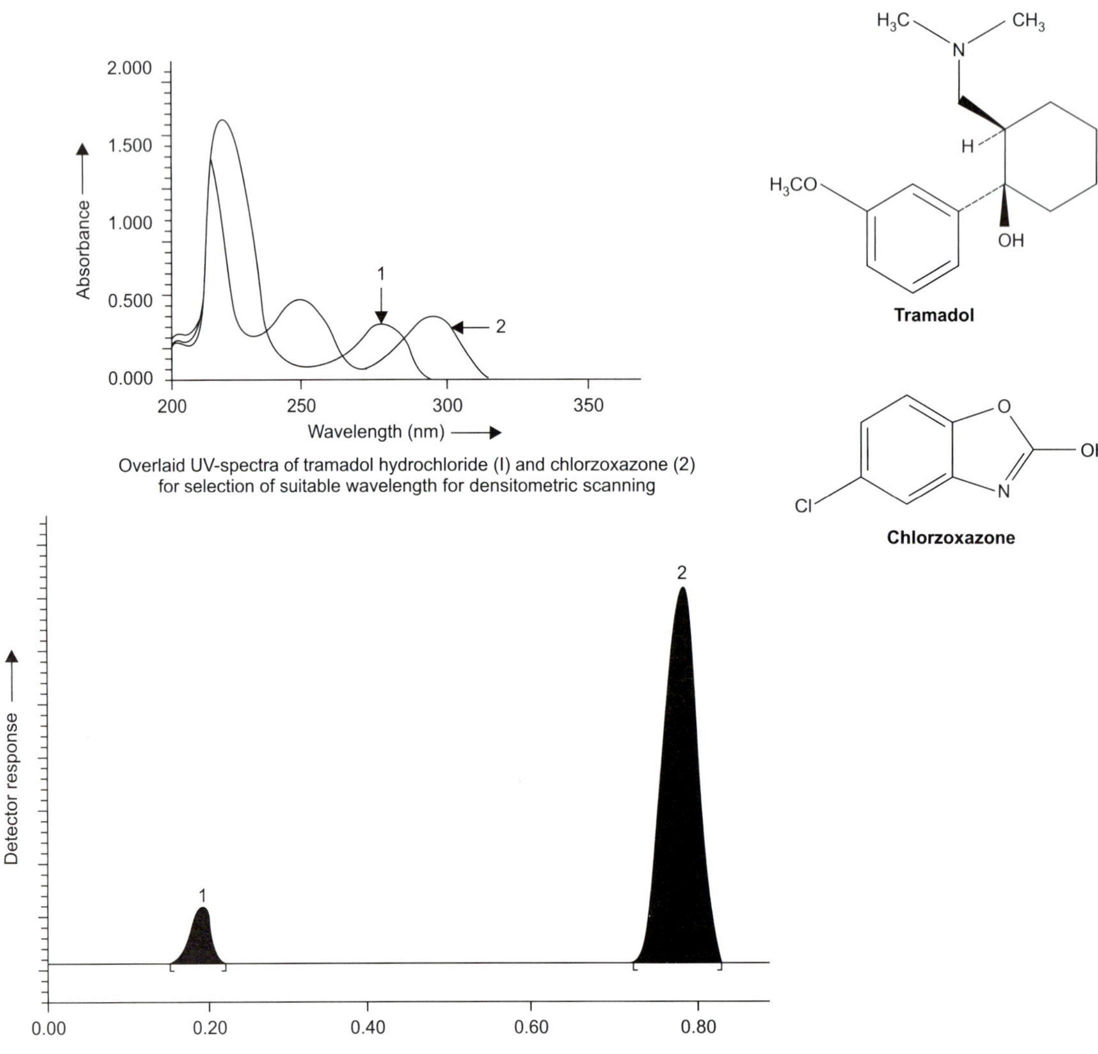

Typical densitogram of the sample containing tramadol HCl and chlorzoxazone. For detailed experimental and chromatographic conditions, refer to Protocol No. 215. Peaks identification: 1. Tramadol HCl; 2. Chlorzoxazone.

PROTOCOL FOR HPTLC ANALYSIS OF PHARMACEUTICAL FORMULATION

Protocol No. 215

Formulation: Tramadol hydrochloride, Chlorzoxazone

Classification: Musculoskeletal Disorders **Dosage form:** Tablets

Standard preparation: Prepare solution of each compound separately in methanol to get 1 mg/ml of tramadol and 5 mg/ml of chlorzoxazone. Further dilutions made with methanol. Apply varying volumes for linearity profile.

Sample preparation: Powdered sample equivalent to 10 mg of tramadol HCl suspended in methanol, sonicated for 10 min, diluted to 10 ml, filtered. The filtrate suitably diluted to get 0.3 mg/ml of tramadol and 1.5 mg/ml of chlorzoxazone and used for analysis.

Chromatographic equipments:

Sample applicator: Camag Linomat–IV

Development chamber: Camag twin–trough glass chamber, 10 × 10 cm

Densitometric scanner: Camag TLC Scanner–III

Chromatographic conditions:

1. Stationary phase: Silica gel $60F_{254}$ pre-coated HPTLC plates, 10 × 10 cm (200 μm) – Merck, pre-washed with methanol, dried at 105°C for 5 min prior to use
2. Mobile phase (MP): Ethyl acetate–toluene–25% ammonia (7 : 3 : 0.2 v/v)
3. Standard/Sample application:
   Band length: 5 mm Volume applied: 0.5–2.5 μl Spacing: 10 mm
4. Chamber saturation: 10 min (MP)
5. RH (%): 55 ± 5
6. Temperature °C: 25 ± 1
7. Separation technique: Ascending
8. Quantity of mobile phase: 10 ml
9. Migration distance: 85 mm
10. Migration time: 20 min

Densitometric evaluation:

Wavelength: UV–273 nm Scanning mode: Reflectance/Absorbance

HRF: Tramadol hydrochloride—19; Chlorzoxazone—78

Linearity (ng/band): Tramadol HCl—150–750; Chlorzoxazone—750–3750

Recovery (%): 98.72–102.46 for both the compounds

References: M. Gandhimathi and T.K. Ravi, *J. Planar Chromatogr.*, **21(4)**, 305–307, 2008.

Comments: The method validated for accuracy, precision, linearity, LOD, LOQ, specificity, robustness and ruggedness.

HPTLC : High Performance Thin Layer Chromatography
HPTLC Densitogram

No. 216

Pentazocine hydrochloride

Tramadol

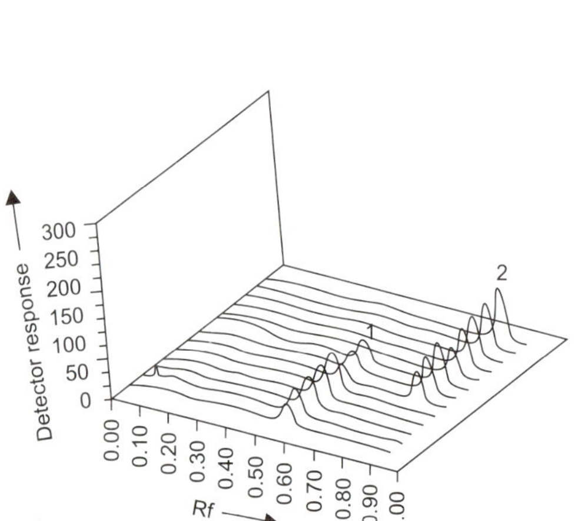

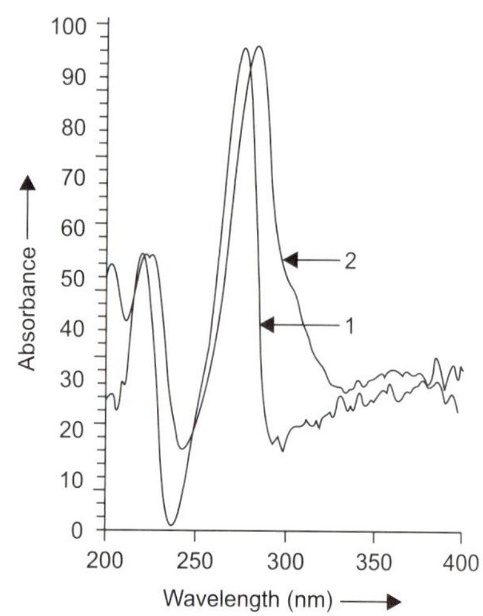

Overlaid UV-spectra of tramadol HCl (1) and pentazocine HCl (2) for selection of suitable wavelength for densitometric scanning

Typical densitogram of the standard containing tramadol HCl and pentazocine HCl. For detailed experimental and chromatographic conditions, refer to Protocol No. 216. Peaks identification: 1. Tramadol HCl; 2. Pentazocine HCl.

PROTOCOL FOR HPTLC ANALYSIS OF PHARMACEUTICAL FORMULATION

Protocol No. 216

Formulation: Tramadol hydrochloride, Pentazocine hydrochloride

Classification: Musculoskeletal Disorders **Dosage form:** Analyte mixture

Standard preparation: Prepare 1 mg/ml solution of each compound in ethanol. Apply varying volumes of each solution for linearity profile.

Sample preparation: Powdered sample equivalent to 50 mg of pentazocine suspended in ethanol, sonicated, diluted to 50 ml, filtered and the filtrate used for chromatographic evaluation.

Chromatographic equipments:

Sample applicator: Camag Linomat–V

Development chamber: Camag twin–trough glass chamber, 10 × 10 cm

Densitometric scanner: Camag TLC Scanner–III

Chromatographic conditions:

1. Stationary phase: Silica gel $60F_{254}$ pre-coated TLC plates, 10 × 10 cm (250 μm) – Merck
2. Mobile phase (MP): Acetic acid–n-butanol–water (1 : 4 : 1 v/v)
3. Standard/Sample application:
   Band length: 10 mm Volume applied: 4–12 μl Spacing: 10 mm
4. Chamber saturation: —
5. RH (%): 55 ± 5
6. Temperature °C: 22 ± 2
7. Separation technique: Ascending
8. Quantity of mobile phase: 12 ml
9. Migration distance: —
10. Migration time: —

Densitometric evaluation:

Wavelength: UV–254 nm Scanning mode: Reflectance/Absorbance

HRF: Tramadol HCl—54; Pentazocine HCl—82

Linearity (ng/band): —

Recovery (%): —

References: Zainab Abdul Jalil Ebrahim et al., *Farmacia*, **59(3)**, 381–387, 2011.

Comments: —

HPTLC : High Performance Thin Layer Chromatography
HPTLC Densitogram

No. 218

Ketoprofen

Propyphenazone

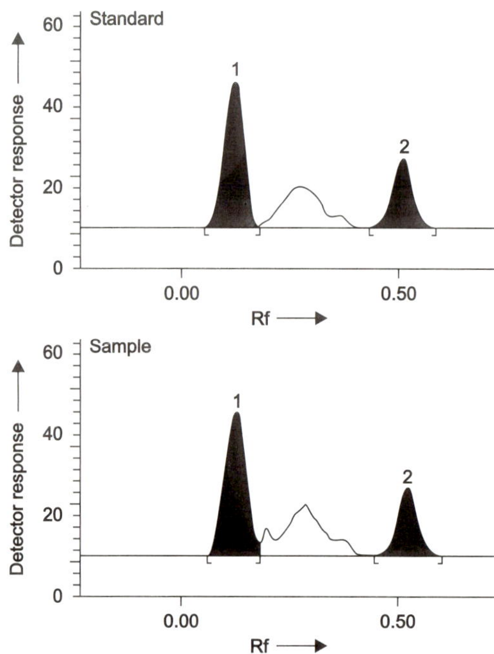

Typical densitogram of the sample and standard containing ketoprofen and propyphenazone. For detailed experimental and chromatographic conditions, refer to Protocol No. 218. Peaks identification: 1. Propyphenazone; 2. Ketoprofen.

PROTOCOL FOR HPTLC ANALYSIS OF PHARMACEUTICAL FORMULATION

Protocol No. 218

Formulation: Ketoprofen, Propyphenazone

Classification: Musculoskeletal Disorders **Dosage form:** Tablets

Standard preparation: Prepare 1 mg/ml solution in methanol each of ketoprofen (K) and propyphenazone (P). Mix 0.2 ml of solution (K) and 0.6 ml of solution (P) and dilute to 10 ml with methanol and use for analysis.

Sample preparation: Weigh accurately sample equivalent to 20 mg of ketoprofen, add 70–80 ml of methanol, sonicate for 5 min, make up to 100 ml, filter and dilute 1 ml to 10 ml for chromatographic analysis.

Chromatographic equipments:

Sample applicator: Camag Linomat–IV

Development chamber: Camag twin–trough glass chamber, 10 × 10 cm

Densitometric scanner: Camag TLC Scanner–II

Chromatographic conditions:

1. Stationary phase: Silica gel 60 RP-18F_{254s} pre-coated HPTLC plates, 10 × 10 cm (200 μm) – Merck
2. Mobile phase (MP): 0.5 M sodium chloride–methanol–glacial acetic acid (12 : 8 : 0.01 v/v)
3. Standard/Sample application:
   Band length: 5 mm Volume applied: 5 μl Spacing: 5 mm
4. Chamber saturation: 30 min (MP)
5. RH (%): 55 ± 5
6. Temperature °C: 22 ± 2
7. Separation technique: Ascending
8. Quantity of mobile phase: 20 ml
9. Migration distance: 50 mm
10. Migration time: 40 min

Densitometric evaluation:

Wavelength: UV–265 nm Scanning mode: Reflectance/Absorbance

HRF: Propyphenazone—12; Ketoprofen—51

Linearity: —

Recovery (%): 96.95–97.80 for both the compounds

References: —

Comments:

- The method was optimized and analytical work carried out at **Anchrom's HPTLC Application Laboratory**, Mumbai, India.
- Several market samples of similar composition were analysed by the proposed method with reproducible results.
- Reversed-phase chromatography resulted in reversal of retention order as compared to normal-phase chromatography.

HPTLC : High Performance Thin Layer Chromatography
HPTLC Densitogram

No. 219

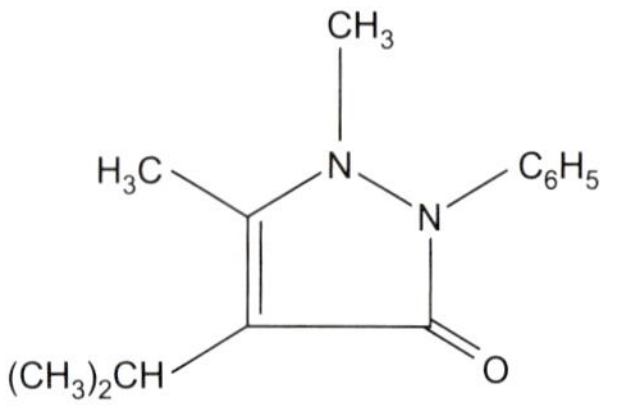

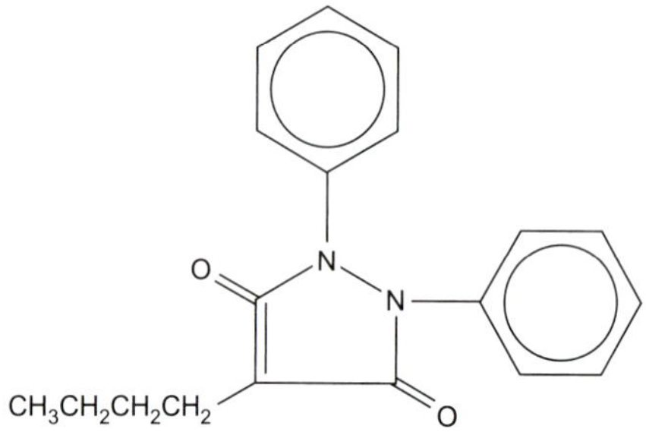

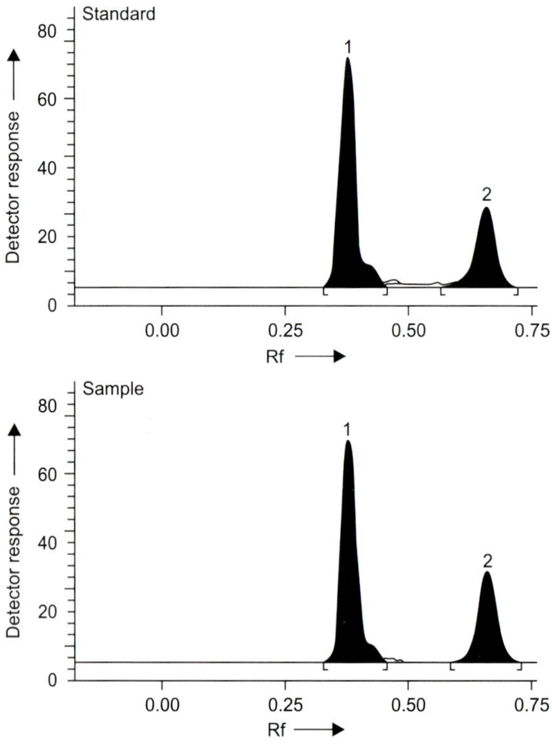

Propyphenazone

Phenylbutazone

Typical densitogram of the sample and standard containing phenylbutazone and propyphenazone. For detailed experimental and chromatographic conditions, refer to Protocol No. 219. Peaks identification: 1. Propyphenazone; 2. Phenylbutazone

PROTOCOL FOR HPTLC ANALYSIS OF PHARMACEUTICAL FORMULATION

Protocol No. 219

Formulation: **Phenylbutazone, Propyphenazone**

Classification: Musculoskeletal Disorders **Dosage form:** Tablets

Standard preparation: Weigh accurately about 25 mg each of phenylbutazone and propyphenazone. Dissolve in methanol to make 10 ml. Dilute 0.5 ml to 10 ml with methanol and use for application.

Sample preparation: Weigh accurately powdered tablets equivalent to 125 mg of phenylbutazone, suspend in 70–80 methanol, sonicate for 5 min, and dilute to 100 ml, filter and dilute 1 ml to 10 ml for chromatographic application.

Chromatographic equipments:

Sample applicator: Camag Linomat–IV

Development chamber: Camag twin–trough glass chamber, 10 × 10 cm

Densitometric scanner: Camag TLC Scanner–II

Chromatographic conditions:

1. Stationary phase: Silica gel 60F_{254} pre-coated HPTLC plates, 7 × 10 cm (200 μm) – Merck
2. Mobile phase (MP): Toluene–acetone–glacial acetic acid (8 : 2 : 0.1 v/v)
3. Standard/Sample application:
   Band length: 5 mm Volume applied: 5 μl Spacing: 5 mm
4. Chamber saturation: 10 min (MP)
5. RH (%): 55 ± 5
6. Temperature °C: 22 ± 2
7. Separation technique: Ascending
8. Quantity of mobile phase: 10 ml
9. Migration distance: 50 mm
10. Migration time: 16 min

Densitometric evaluation:

Wavelength: UV–245 nm or 272 nm Scanning mode: Reflectance/Absorbance

HRF: Propyphenazone—40; Phenylbutazone—70

Linearity: 200–1000 ng/band for both the compounds

Recovery (%): 99.60–101.90 for both the compounds

References: —

Comments:

- The method was optimized and analytical work carried out at **Anchrom's HPTLC Application Laboratory**, Mumbai, India.
- Several market samples of similar composition were analysed by the proposed method with reproducible results.

HPTLC : High Performance Thin Layer Chromatography
HPTLC Densitogram

No. 220

CH3
H3C
N
N
C6H5
(CH3)2CH
O

Propyphenazone

O
N
N
CH3CH2CH2CH2
O

Phenylbutazone

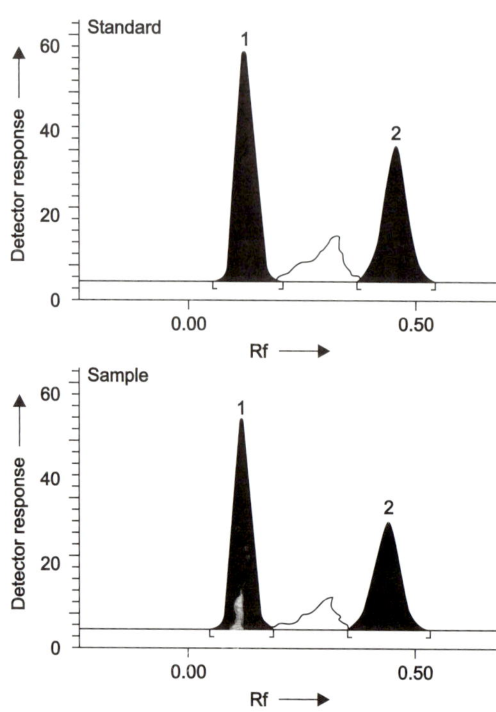

Typical densitogram of the sample and standard containing phenylbutazone and propyphenazone. For detailed experimental and chromatographic conditions, refer to Protocol No. 220. Peaks identification: 1. Propyphenazone; 2. Phenylbutazone.

PROTOCOL FOR HPTLC ANALYSIS OF PHARMACEUTICAL FORMULATION

Protocol No. 220

Formulation: Phenylbutazone, Propyphenazone

Classification: Musculoskeletal Disorders **Dosage form:** Tablets

Standard preparation: Weigh accurately about 25 mg each of phenylbutazone and propyphenazone. Dissolve in methanol to make 10 ml. Dilute 0.5 ml to 10 ml with methanol and use for application.

Sample preparation: Weigh accurately powdered tablets equivalent to 125 mg of phenylbutazone, suspend in 70–80 methanol, sonicate for 5 min, and dilute to 100 ml, filter and dilute 1 ml to 10 ml for chromatographic application.

Chromatographic equipments:

Sample applicator: Camag Linomat–IV

Development chamber: Camag twin–trough glass chamber, 10 × 10 cm

Densitometric scanner: Camag TLC Scanner–II

Chromatographic conditions:

1. Stationary phase: Silica gel 60 RP-18F_{254s} pre-coated HPTLC plates, 10 × 10 cm (200 μm) – Merck
2. Mobile phase (MP): 0.5 M sodium chloride–methanol–glacial acetic acid (12 : 8 : 0.01 v/v)
3. Standard/Sample application:
   Band length: 5 mm Volume applied: 5 μl Spacing: 5 mm
4. Chamber saturation: —
5. RH (%): 55 ± 5
6. Temperature °C: 22 ± 2
7. Separation technique: Ascending
8. Quantity of mobile phase: 20 ml
9. Migration distance: 50 mm
10. Migration time: 40 min

Densitometric evaluation:

Wavelength: UV–245 nm or 272 nm Scanning mode: Reflectance/Absorbance

HRF: Propyphenazone—12; Phenylbutazone—46

Linearity: 200–1000 ng/band for both the compounds

Recovery (%): 97.50–99.25 for both the compounds

References: —

Comments:

- The method was optimized and analytical work carried out at **Anchrom's HPTLC Application Laboratory**, Mumbai, India.
- Several market samples of similar composition were analysed by the proposed method with reproducible results.
- No reversal of retention order was observed in RP-chromatography.

HPTLC : High Performance Thin Layer Chromatography
HPTLC Densitogram

No. 221

OH | O — CH_2 — CH — CH_2 — O · CO · NH_2, OCH_3

Methocarbamol

CH_3, CH_3, COOH, H_3C

Ibuprofen

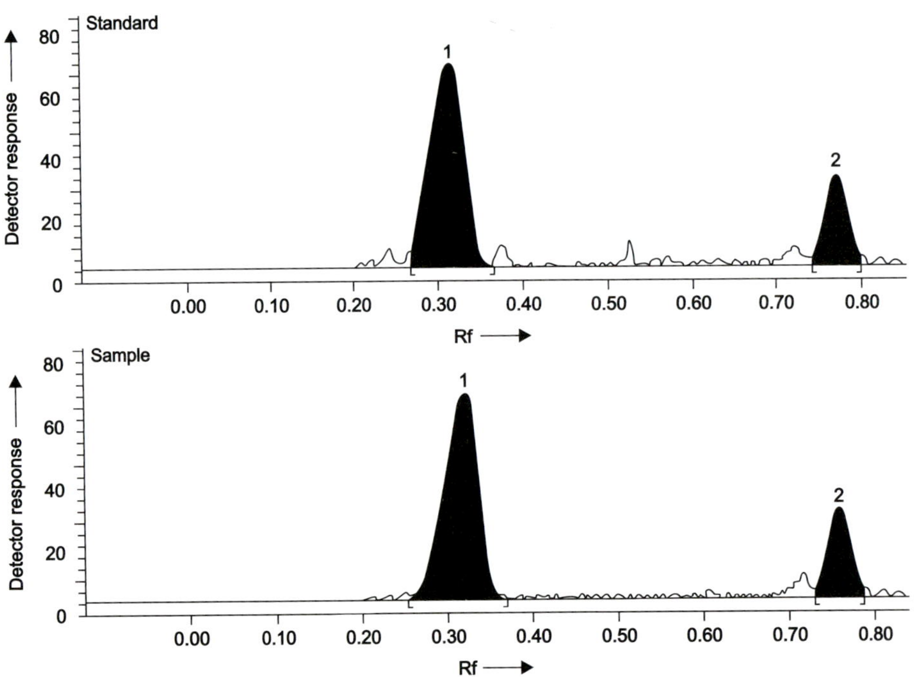

Typical densitogram of the sample and standard containing methocarbamol and ibuprofen. For detailed experimental and chromatographic conditions, refer to Protocol No. 221. Peaks identification: 1. Methocarbamol; 2. Ibuprofen.

PROTOCOL FOR HPTLC ANALYSIS OF PHARMACEUTICAL FORMULATION

Protocol No. 221

Formulation: **Methocarbamol, Ibuprofen**

Classification: Musculoskeletal Disorders **Dosage form:** Tablets

Standard preparation: Weigh accurately 20 mg of ibuprofen and 75 mg of methocarbamol, dissolve in methanol to make 25 ml. Dilute 1 ml to 10 ml with methanol for analysis.

Sample preparation: Weigh accurately powdered sample equivalent to 40 mg of ibuprofen, suspend in 30–40 methanol, sonicate for 5 min, make up to 50 ml, filter and dilute 1 ml to 10 ml with methanol for chromatographic analysis.

Chromatographic equipments:

Sample applicator: Camag Linomat–IV

Development chamber: Camag twin–trough glass chamber, 10 × 10 cm

Densitometric scanner: Camag TLC Scanner

Chromatographic conditions:

1. Stationary phase: Silica gel 60F_{254} pre-coated HPTLC plates, 10 × 10 cm (200 μm) – Merck
2. Mobile phase (MP): Toluene–ethyl acetate–glacial acetic acid (6 : 3 : 1 v/v)
3. Standard/Sample application:
   Band length: 10 mm Volume applied: 5 μl Spacing: 10 mm
4. Chamber saturation: 10 min (MP)
5. RH (%): 55 ± 5
6. Temperature °C: 22 ± 2
7. Separation technique: Ascending
8. Quantity of mobile phase: 10 ml
9. Migration distance: 50 mm
10. Migration time: 14 min

Densitometric evaluation:

Wavelength: UV–254 nm Scanning mode: Reflectance/Absorbance

HRF: Methocarbamol—31; Ibuprofen—77

Linearity (ng/band): Ibuprofen—100–1000; Methocarbamol—500–2000

Recovery (%): 97.40–101.10 for both the compounds

References: —

Comments:

- The method was optimized and analytical work carried out at **Anchrom's HPTLC Application Laboratory**, Mumbai, India.
- Several market samples of similar composition were analysed by the proposed method with reproducible results.

HPTLC : High Performance Thin Layer Chromatography
HPTLC Densitogram

No. 222

Methocarbamol

Nimesulide

Overlaid UV-spectra of methocarbamol (1) and nimesulide (2) for selection of suitable wavelength for densitometric scanning

Typical densitogram of the sample and standard containing methocarbamol and nimesulide. For detailed experimental and chromatographic conditions, refer to Protocol No. 222. Peaks identification: 1. Methocarbamol; 2. Nimesulide.

PROTOCOL FOR HPTLC ANALYSIS OF PHARMACEUTICAL FORMULATION

Protocol No. 222

Formulation: Methocarbamol, Nimesulide

Classification: Musculoskeletal Disorders **Dosage form:** Tablets

Standard preparation: Prepare 100 μg/ml solution of methocarbamol and 10 μg/ml of nimesulide. Further suitable dilutions made with methanol for linearity profile.

Sample preparation: Powdered sample equivalent to 50 mg of methocarbamol suspended in methanol, sonicated, diluted to 50 ml, filtered and filtrate suitably diluted for assay. Apply 5 μl.

Chromatographic equipments:

Sample applicator: Camag Linomat–IV

Development chamber: Camag twin–trough glass chamber, 10 × 10 cm

Densitometric scanner: Camag TLC Scanner–III

Chromatographic conditions:

1. Stationary phase: Silica gel $60F_{254}$ pre-coated HPTLC plates, 10 × 10 cm (200 μm) – Merck
2. Mobile phase (MP): Toluene–0.05 M methanolic ammonia (8 : 2 v/v)
3. Standard/Sample application:
   Band length: 4 mm Volume applied: 5 μl Spacing: 10 mm
4. Chamber saturation: 10 min (MP)
5. RH (%): 55 ± 5
6. Temperature °C: 22 ± 2
7. Separation technique: Ascending
8. Quantity of mobile phase: 10 ml
9. Migration distance: 70 mm
10. Migration time: 15 min

Densitometric evaluation:

Wavelength: UV–276 nm Scanning mode: Reflectance/Absorbance

HRF: Methocarbamol—38; Nimesulide—60

Linearity (ng/band): Methocarbamol—900–9500; Nimesulide—200–1000

Recovery (%): 99.66–99.93 for both the compounds

References: S.B. Bagade, D.B. Meshram, J.V. Manwar and M.R. Tajne, *J. Pharm. Research*, **5(4)**, 137–140, 2006.

Comments: The method validated for accuracy, precision, linearity, LOD, LOQ, specificity, robustness and ruggedness.

HPTLC : High Performance Thin Layer Chromatography
HPTLC Densitogram

No. 223

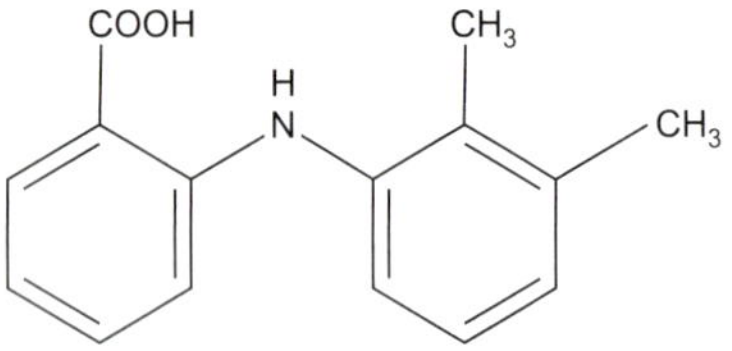

COOH H N CH3 CH3

Mefenamic acid

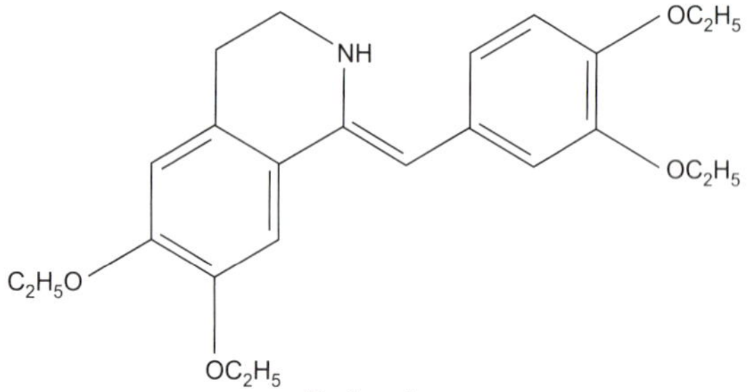

NH OC2H5 OC2H5 C2H5O OC2H5

Drotaverine

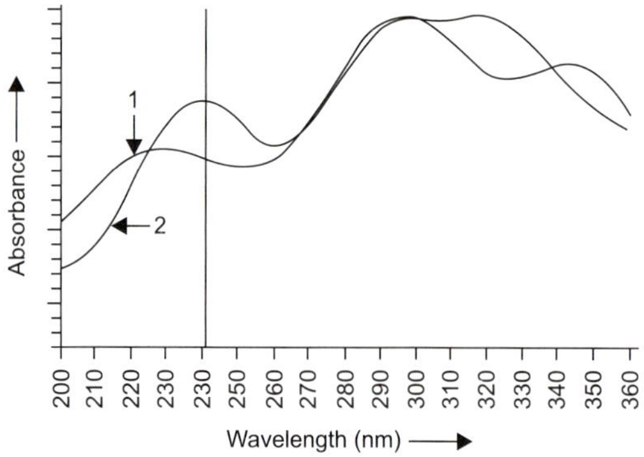

Absorbance
1
2
200 210 220 230 230 250 260 270 280 290 300 310 320 330 340 350 360
Wavelength (nm)

Overlaid UV-spectra of mefenamic acid (1) and drotaverine HCl (2) for selection of suitable wavelength for densitometric scanning

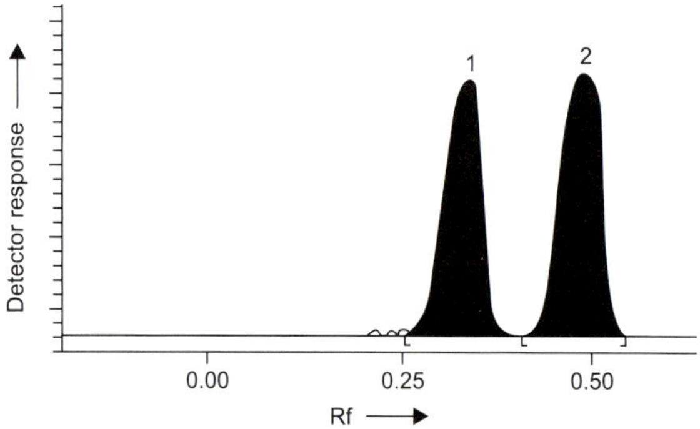

Detector response
1
2
0.00 0.25 0.50
Rf

Typical densitogram of the sample containing mefenamic acid and drotaverine HCl. For detailed experimental and chromatographic conditions, refer to Protocol No. 223. Peaks identification: 1. Mefenamic acid: 2. Drotaverine HCl.

PROTOCOL FOR HPTLC ANALYSIS OF PHARMACEUTICAL FORMULATION

Protocol No. 223

Formulation: Mefenamic acid, Drotaverine hydrochloride

Classification: Musculoskeletal Disorders **Dosage form:** Tablets

Standard preparation: Prepare solution of each compound separately in methanol to get 1 mg/ml of mefenamic acid and 0.32 mg/ml of drotaverine hydrochloride. Further serial dilutions made for linearity studies.

Sample preparation: Powdered sample equivalent to 25 mg of mefenamic acid suspended in methanol, sonicated for 15 min, diluted to 25 ml. Filtered and used the filtrate for chromatographic separation after suitable dilution.

Chromatographic equipments:

Sample applicator: Camag Linomat–IV

Development chamber: Camag twin–trough glass chamber, 10 × 10 cm

Densitometric scanner: Camag TLC Scanner–III

Chromatographic conditions:

1. Stationary phase: Silica gel $60F_{254}$ pre-coated HPTLC plates, 10 × 10 cm (200 μm) – Merck
2. Mobile phase (MP): Methanol–toluene–triethylamine (1 : 7.5 : 0.2 v/v)
3. Standard/Sample application:
   Band length: 6 mm Volume applied: 6 μl Spacing: 10 mm
4. Chamber saturation: 10 min (MP)
5. RH (%): 55 ± 5
6. Temperature °C: 25 ± 2
7. Separation technique: Ascending
8. Quantity of mobile phase: 17 ml
9. Migration distance: 70 mm
10. Migration time: 15 min

Densitometric evaluation:

Wavelength: UV–231 nm Scanning mode: Reflectance/Absorbance

HRF: Mefenamic acid—30; Drotaverine HCl—47

Linearity (ng/band): Mefenamic acid—3800–5400; Drotaverine HCl—1300–2600

Recovery (%): 99.08–100.86 for both the compounds

References: Amit N. Maliye, Sanjay G. Walode, A.V. Kasture and S.G. Wadodkar, *Asian J. Chem.*, **18(1)**, 667–672, 2006.

Comments: The method validated for accuracy, precision, linearity, LOD, LOQ, specificity, robustness and ruggedness.

HPTLC : High Performance Thin Layer Chromatography
HPTLC Densitogram

No. 224

Mefenamic acid

Ethamsylate

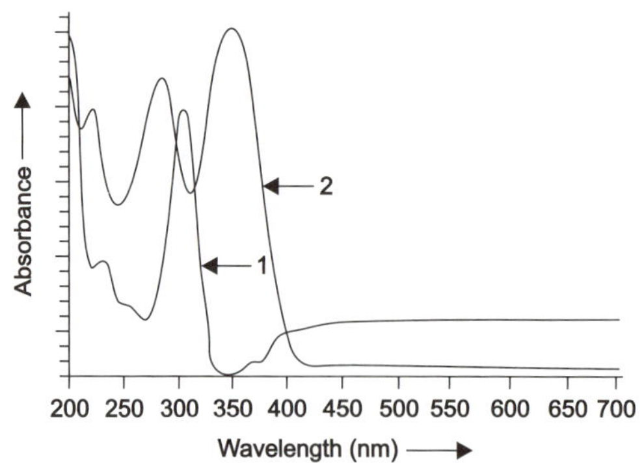

Overlaid UV-spectra of ethamsylate (1) and mefenamic acid (2) for selection of suitable wavelength for densitometric scanning

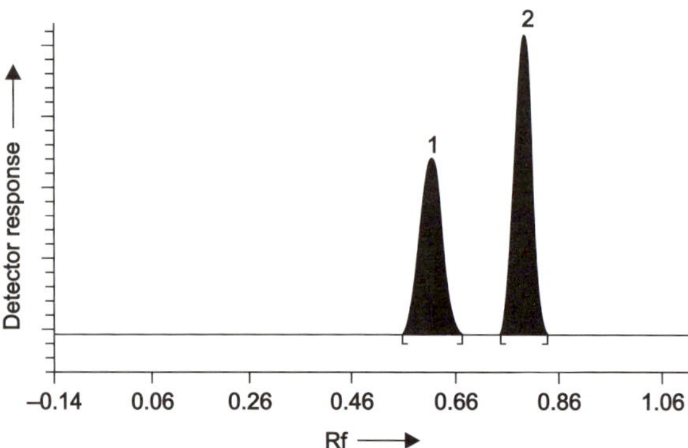

Typical densitogram of the standard containing ethamsylate and mefenamic acid. For detailed experimental and chromatographic conditions, refer to Protocol No. 224. Peaks identification: 1. Ethamsylate; 2. Mefenamic acid.

PROTOCOL FOR HPTLC ANALYSIS OF PHARMACEUTICAL FORMULATION

Protocol No. 224

Formulation: Mefenamic acid, Ethamsylate

Classification: Musculoskeletal Disorders **Dosage form:** Tablets

Standard preparation: Prepare 1 mg/ml solution of each compound in methanol. Further serial dilutions made to cover the range of linearity. Apply 2–10 µl for analysis.

Sample preparation: Powdered sample equivalent to 10 mg of either drug suspended in methanol, sonicated for 10 min, diluted and filtered, the filtrate suitably diluted to get 100 ng/µl. Apply 10 µl for chromatographic separation and analysis.

Chromatographic equipments:

Sample applicator: Camag Linomat–IV

Development chamber: Camag twin–trough glass chamber, 20 × 10 cm

Densitometric scanner: Camag TLC Scanner–III

Chromatographic conditions:

1. Stationary phase: Silica gel $60F_{254}$ pre-coated HPTLC plates, 20 × 10 cm (200 µm) – Merck, pre-washed with methanol and dried prior to use
2. Mobile phase (MP): Chloroform–methanol–acetic acid (10 : 8 : 0.2 v/v)
3. Standard/Sample application:
   Band length: 6 mm Volume applied: 10 µl Spacing: 15 mm
4. Chamber saturation: 10 min (MP)
5. RH (%): 55 ± 5
6. Temperature °C: 25 ± 2
7. Separation technique: Ascending
8. Quantity of mobile phase: 18 ml
9. Migration distance: 70 mm
10. Migration time: 15 min

Densitometric evaluation:

Wavelength: UV–300 nm Scanning mode: Reflectance/Absorbance

HRF: Ethamsylate—56; Mefenamic acid—75

Linearity: 500–2500 ng/band for both the drugs

Recovery (%): Ethamsylate—98.99–99.83; Mefenamic acid—99.36–99.80

References: Yogini S. Jaiswal, Gokul S. Talete and Sanjay J. Surane, *J. Planar Chromatogr.*, **18(6)**, 460–464, 2005.

Comments: The method validated for accuracy, precision, linearity, LOD, LOQ, specificity, robustness and ruggedness.

HPTLC : High Performance Thin Layer Chromatography
HPTLC Densitogram

No. 225

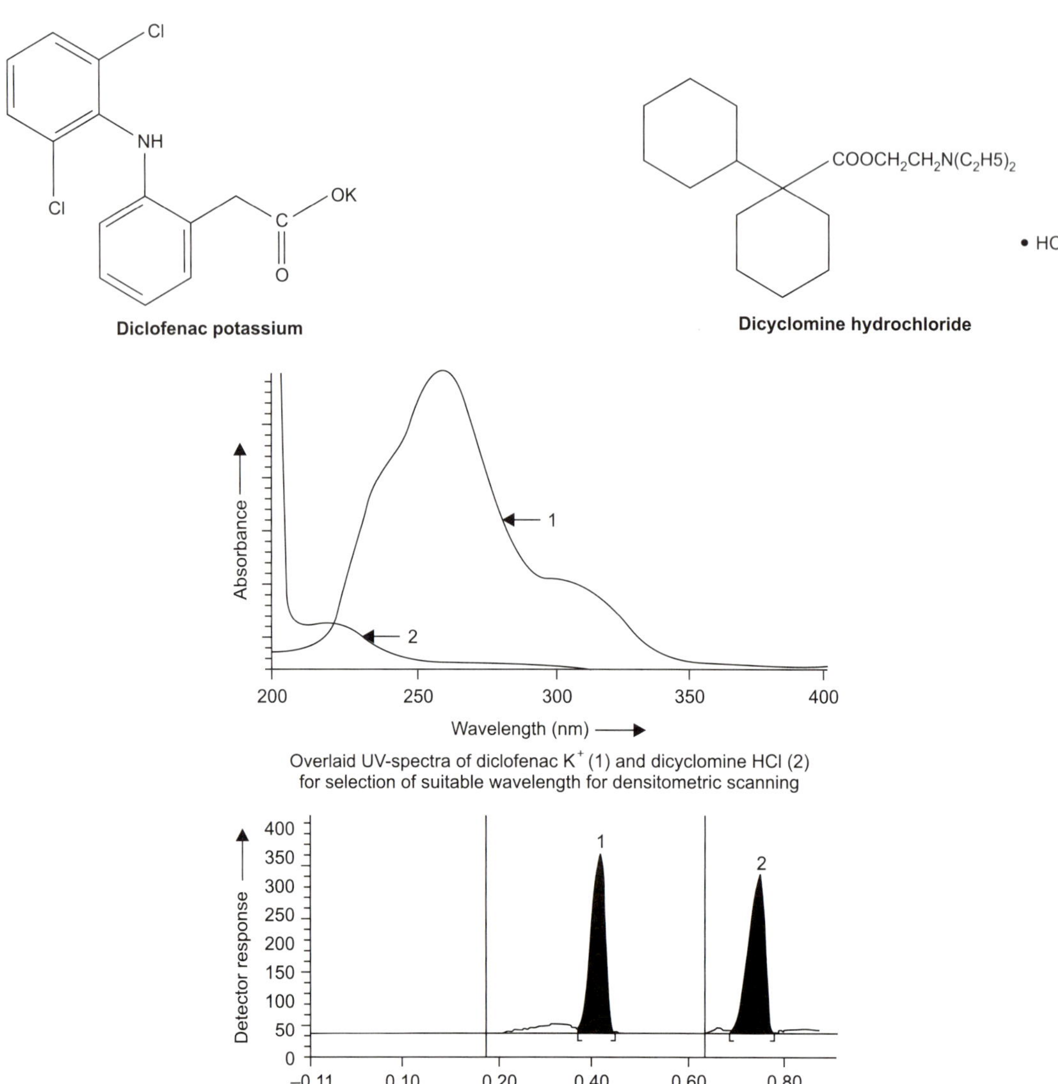

Typical densitogram of the standard containing diclofenac potassium and dicyclomine HCl. For detailed experimental and chromatographic conditions, refer to Protocol No. 225. Peaks identification: 1. Diclofenac potassium; 2. Dicyclomine HCl.

PROTOCOL FOR HPTLC ANALYSIS OF PHARMACEUTICAL FORMULATION

Protocol No. 225

Formulation: Diclofenac potassium, Dicyclomine hydrochloride

Classification: Musculoskeletal Disorders **Dosage form:** Tablets

Standard preparation: Prepare solution of both the compounds in methanol to get 2 mg/ml of dicyclomine HCl and 5 mg/ml of diclofenac potassium. Carry out further dilutions and apply varying volumes of each solution for linearity profile.

Sample preparation: Powdered sample equivalent to 20 mg of dicyclomine HCl suspended in 20 ml of methanol, sonicated for 45 min, diluted to 25 ml, centrifuged (3000 rpm) for 5 min. Further dilute suitably and apply 5 μl of the resulting solution for assay of both the compounds.

Chromatographic equipments:

Sample applicator: Camag Linomat–V

Development chamber: Camag twin–trough glass chamber, 10 × 10 cm

Densitometric scanner: Camag TLC Scanner–II

Chromatographic conditions:

1. Stationary phase: Silica gel $60F_{254}$ pre-coated TLC plates, 10 × 10 cm (250 μm) – Merck, pre-washed with methanol and activated at 80°C for 5 min prior to use
2. Mobile phase (MP): Toluene–acetone–methanol–25% ammonia (5 : 2 : 1 : 0.02 v/v)
3. Standard/Sample application:
   Band length: — Volume applied: 5 μl Spacing: —
4. Chamber saturation: 30 min (MP)
5. RH (%): 60 ± 5
6. Temperature °C: Ambient
7. Separation technique: Ascending
8. Quantity of mobile phase: 16 ml
9. Migration distance: 80 mm
10. Migration time: 18 min

Densitometric evaluation:

Wavelength: UV–260 nm (Diclofenac potassium) and 523 nm (Dicyclomine HCl)

Scanning mode: Reflectance/Absorbance

HRF: Diclofenac potassium—41; Dicyclomine hydrochloride—72

Linearity (ng/band): Diclofenac potassium—1800–9000; Dicyclomine HCl—1300–6500

Recovery (%): 99.10–99.92 for both the compounds

References: Sunil R. Dhaneshwar, Amey R. Keer, Shweta S. Havele and Kiran H. Gopani, *Res. J. Pharm. Biol. Chemical Sciences*, **2(4)**, 314–324, 2011.

Comments:

- The method validated for accuracy, precision, linearity, LOD, LOQ, specificity and robustness.
- For detection of dicyclomine HCl, see Protocol No. 232.

HPTLC : High Performance Thin Layer Chromatography
HPTLC Densitogram

No. 230

OH

O — CH_2 — CH — CH_2 — O · CO · NH_2

OCH_3

Methocarbamol

CH_3

CH_3

COOH

H_3C

Ibuprofen

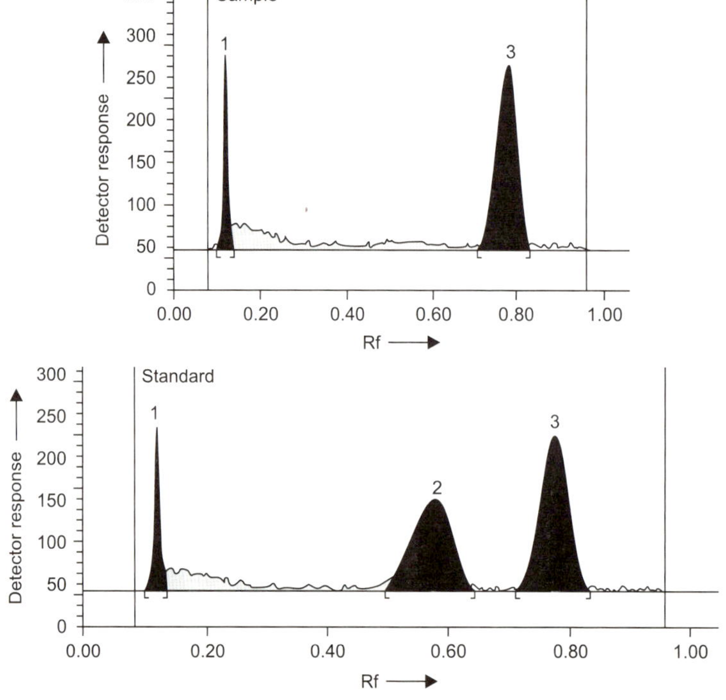

Typical densitogram of the standard and the sample containing methocarbamol and ibuprofen. For detailed experimental and chromatographic conditions, refer to Protocol No. 230. Peaks identification: 1. Ibuprofen; 2. Guaiphenesin (degradation product of methocarbamol); 3. Methocarbamol.

PROTOCOL FOR HPTLC ANALYSIS OF PHARMACEUTICAL FORMULATION

Protocol No. 230

Formulation: Methocarbamol, Ibuprofen

Classification: Musculoskeletal Disorders **Dosage form:** Tablets

Standard preparation: Prepare 1 mg/ml solution of each compound in methanol, carryout further dilution with methanol to get 100 μg/ml. Apply varying volumes for linearity profile.

Sample preparation: Powdered sample equivalent to 750 mg of methocarbamol and 40 mg of ibuprofen suspended in 50 ml of methanol, stirred for 10 min, dilute to 100 ml with methanol and filtered. The filtrate-suitably diluted with methanol and used for chromatographic evaluation.

Chromatographic equipments:

Sample applicator: Camag Linomat–V

Development chamber: Camag twin–trough glass chamber, 20 × 20 cm

Densitometric scanner: Camag TLC Scanner–III

Chromatographic conditions:

1. Stationary phase: Silica gel $60F_{254}$ pre-coated plates, 20 × 20 cm (200 μm) – M&N
2. Mobile phase (MP): Ethyl acetate–acetone–triethylamine–formic acid (12.4 : 7 : 1.2 : 0.06 v/v), pre-washed with methanol, dried at 60°C for 5 min prior to sample application
3. Standard/Sample application:
   Band length: 4 mm Volume applied: 10 μl Spacing: 20 mm
4. Chamber saturation: 60 min (MP)
5. RH (%): —
6. Temperature °C: Ambient
7. Separation technique: Ascending
8. Quantity of mobile phase: 20 ml
9. Migration distance: 90 mm
10. Migration time: —

Densitometric evaluation:

Wavelength: UV–222 nm Scanning mode: Reflectance/Absorbance

HRF: Ibuprofen—14; Guaiphenesin—54; Methocarbamol—78

Linearity (μg/band): Methocarbamol—2–12; Ibuprofen—4–20

Recovery (%): Ibuprofen—99.50–100.90; Methocarbamol—98.50–101.60

References: Nouruddin W. Ali, Maha A. Hagazy, Mohammed Abdelkawy and Eglal A. Abdelaleem. *J. Planar Chromatogr.*, **25(2)**, 150–155, 2012.

Comments: The method validated as per ICH guidelines.

HPTLC : High Performance Thin Layer Chromatography
HPTLC Densitogram

No. 231

COONa, H N, Cl, Cl

Diclofenac sodium

O, COOCH$_3$, H_3C, OH, HO

MIsoprostol

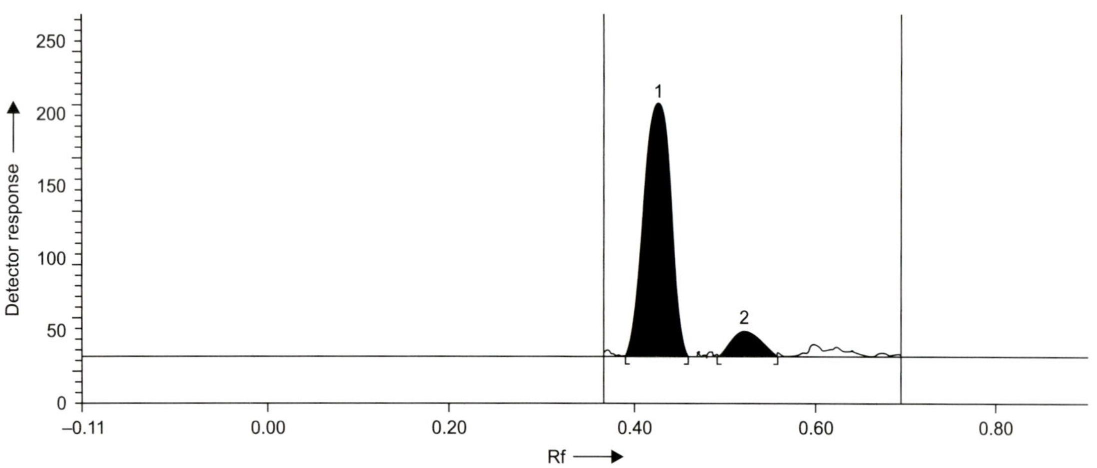

Typical densitogram of the sample containing diclofenac sodium and misoprostol. For detailed experimental and chromatographic conditions, refer to Protocol No. 231. Peaks identification: 1. Diclofenac Na^+; 2. Misoprostol.

PROTOCOL FOR HPTLC ANALYSIS OF PHARMACEUTICAL FORMULATION

Protocol No. 231

Formulation: Diclofenac sodium, Misoprostol

Classification: Musculoskeletal Disorders **Dosage form:** Tablets

Standard preparation: Prepare solution of both the compounds separately in methanol to get 5000 μg/ml of diclofenac sodium and 20 μg/ml of misoprostol. Further diluted to get 200 μg/ml of diclofenac sodium and 0.8 μg/ml of misoprostol. Apply varying volumes for linearity profile.

Sample preparation: Powdered sample equivalent to 50 mg of diclofenac suspended in 40 ml of water, sonicated for 30 min, diluted to 50 ml with water and centrifuged (3000 rpm) for 5 min. Apply 2 μl of the supernatant for analysis.

Chromatographic equipments:

Sample applicator: Camag Linomat–V

Development chamber: Camag twin–trough glass chamber, 20 × 10 cm

Densitometric scanner: Camag TLC Scanner–III

Chromatographic conditions:

1. Stationary phase: Silicagel $60F_{254}$ pre-coated TLC plate 20 × 10 cm (250 μm) – Merck, pre-washed with methanol, activated at 110°C for 5 min prior to chromatography
2. Mobile phase (MP): Toluene–ethylacetate–ethanol–glacial acetic acid (8 : 2 : 1 : 0.1 v/v)
3. Standard/Sample application:
   Band length: 6 mm Volume applied: 10 μl Spacing: 10 mm
4. Chamber saturation: 30 min (MP)
5. RH (%): 60 ± 5
6. Temperature °C: 25 ± 2
7. Separation technique: Ascending
8. Quantity of mobile phase: 22 ml
9. Migration distance: 80 mm
10. Migration time: 25 min

Densitometric evaluation:

Wavelength: UV–220 nm Scanning mode: Reflectance/Absorbance

HRF: Diclofenac sodium—43; Misoprostol—52

Linearity (ng/band): Diclofenac sodium—40–240; Misoprostol—8–48

Recovery (%): Diclofenac sodium—99.87–100.52; Misoprostol—100.25–101.13

References: Sunil R. Dhaneshwar and Vidya K. Bhusari, *Asian J. Pharm. Biol. Res.*, **1(1)**, 15–21, 2011.

Comments: The method validated for accuracy, precision, linearity, LOD, LOQ, specificity, robustness and ruggedness.

HPTLC : High Performance Thin Layer Chromatography
HPTLC Densitogram

No. 232

COOH H N CH_3 CH_3

Mefenamic acid

$COOCH_2CH_2N(C_2H5)_2$ • HCl

Dicyclomine hydrochloride

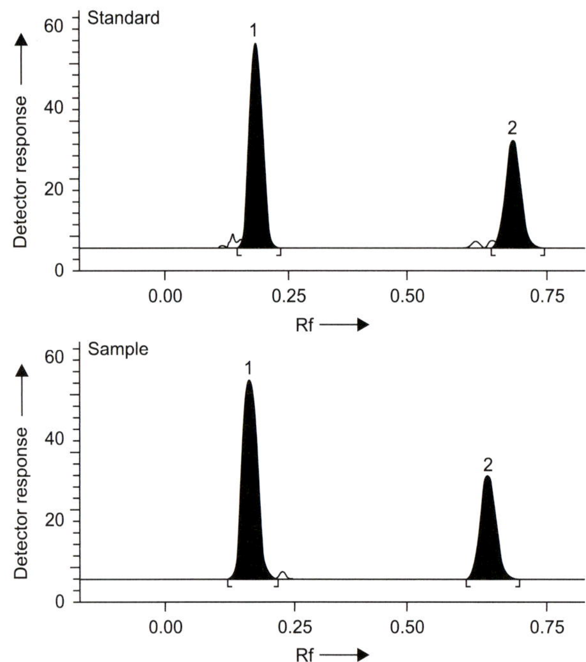

Typical densitogram of the sample and standard containing mefenamic acid and dicyclomine HCl. For detailed experimental and chromatographic conditions, refer to Protocol No. 232. Peaks identification: 1. Mefenamic acid; 2. Dicyclomine HCl.

PROTOCOL FOR HPTLC ANALYSIS OF PHARMACEUTICAL FORMULATION

Protocol No. 232

Formulation: Mefenamic acid, Dicyclomine hydrochloride

Classification: Musculoskeletal Disorders **Dosage form:** Tablets

Standard preparation: (a) Prepare 400 μg/ml solution of dicyclomine HCl in methanol; (b) Prepare 50 μg/ml solution of mefenamic acid in methanol. Carry out the chromatographic separation and analysis.

Sample preparation: Weigh accurately powdered sample equivalent to 10 mg of dicyclomine HCl, suspend in 20 ml methanol, sonicate for 5 min, make up to 25 ml. Dilute 0.25 ml of solution to 100 ml with methanol and use for analysis.

Chromatographic equipments:

Sample applicator: Camag Linomat–IV

Development chamber: Camag twin–trough glass chamber, 10 × 10 cm

Densitometric scanner: Camag TLC Scanner–II

Chromatographic conditions:

1. Stationary phase: Silica gel $60F_{254}$ pre-coated HPTLC plates, 10 × 10 cm (200 μm) – Merck
2. Mobile phase (MP): Toluene–acetone–methanol–25% ammonia (7 : 2 : 1 : 0.05 v/v)
3. Standard/Sample application:
   Band length: 10 mm Volume applied: 5 and 10 μl
   Spacing: 10 mm
4. Chamber saturation: 10 min (MP)
5. RH (%): 55 ± 5
6. Temperature °C: 25 ± 2
7. Separation technique: Ascending
8. Quantity of mobile phase: 10 ml
9. Migration distance: 50 mm
10. Migration time: 15 min

Densitometric evaluation:

Wavelength: UV–287 nm and 623 nm Scanning mode: Reflectance/Absorbance

HRF: Mefenamic acid—19; Dicyclomine HCl—72

Linearity (ng/band): Mefenamic acid—100–500; Dicyclomine HCl—500–500

Recovery (%): 98.60–101.54 for both the compounds

References: —

HPTLC : High Performance Thin Layer Chromatography
HPTLC Densitogram

No. 233

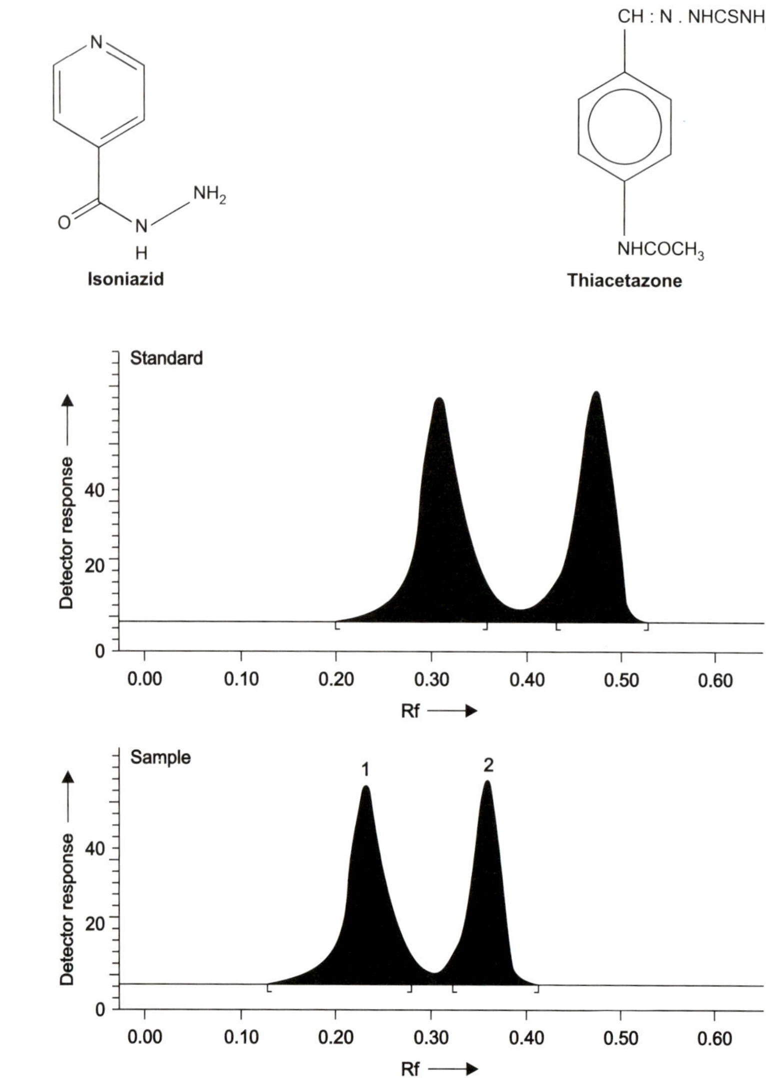

Typical densitogram of the standard and the sample containing isoniazid and thiacetazone. For detailed experimental and chromatographic conditions, refer to Protocol No. 233. Peaks identification: 1. Isoniazid; 2. Thiacetazone.

PROTOCOL FOR HPTLC ANALYSIS OF PHARMACEUTICAL FORMULATION

Protocol No. 233

Formulation: Isoniazid, Thiacetazone

Classification: Antibiotics **Dosage form:** Tablets

Standard preparation: Prepare 1 mg/ml solution of each compound in methanol. Mix 1.2 ml of isoniazide solution and 0.6 ml of thiacetazone solution and dilute to 10 ml with methanol. Apply varying volumes for linearity profile.

Sample preparation: Powdered sample equivalent to 300 mg of isoniazide is suspended in 50–60 ml of methanol, sonicated for 10 min, dilute to 100 ml, filter and dilute 0.4 ml of filtrate to 10 ml with methanol and use for chromatographic application.

Chromatographic equipments:

Sample applicator: Camag Linomat–IV

Development chamber: Camag twin-trough glass chamber, 10 × 10 cm

Denistometric scanner: Camag TLC Scanner–II

Chromatographic conditions:

1. Stationary phase: Silica gel $60F_{254}$ pre-coated HPTLC plates, 10 × 10 cm (200 μm) – Merck
2. Mobile phase (MP): Chloroform–methanol–glacial acetic acid (9 : 1 : 0.1 v/v)
3. Standard/Sample application:
   Band length: 5 mm Volume applied: 4 μl Spacing: 5 mm
4. Chamber saturation: 20 min (MP)
5. RH (%): 55 ± 5
6. Temperature °C: 22 ± 2
7. Separation technique: Ascending
8. Quantity of mobile phase: 10 ml
9. Migration distance: 50 mm
10. Migration time: 10 min

Densitometric evaluation:

Wavelength: UV–272 nm Scanning mode: Reflectance/Absorbance

HRF: Isoniazid—32; Thiacetazone—48

Linearity: 100–1000 ng/band for both the compounds

Recovery (%): 100.90–101.10 for both the compounds

References: —

Comments:

- The method was optimized and analytical work carried out at **Anchrom's HPTLC Application Laboratory**, Mumbai, India.
- Several market samples of similar composition were analysed by the proposed method and found to give reproducible results.

HPTLC : High Performance Thin Layer Chromatography
HPTLC Densitogram

No. 237

Isoniazid

$C_2H_5—C(H)(CH_2OH)—NH—CH_2CH_2—NH—C(CH_2OH)(H)—C_2H_5 \cdot HCl$

Ethambutol hydrochloride

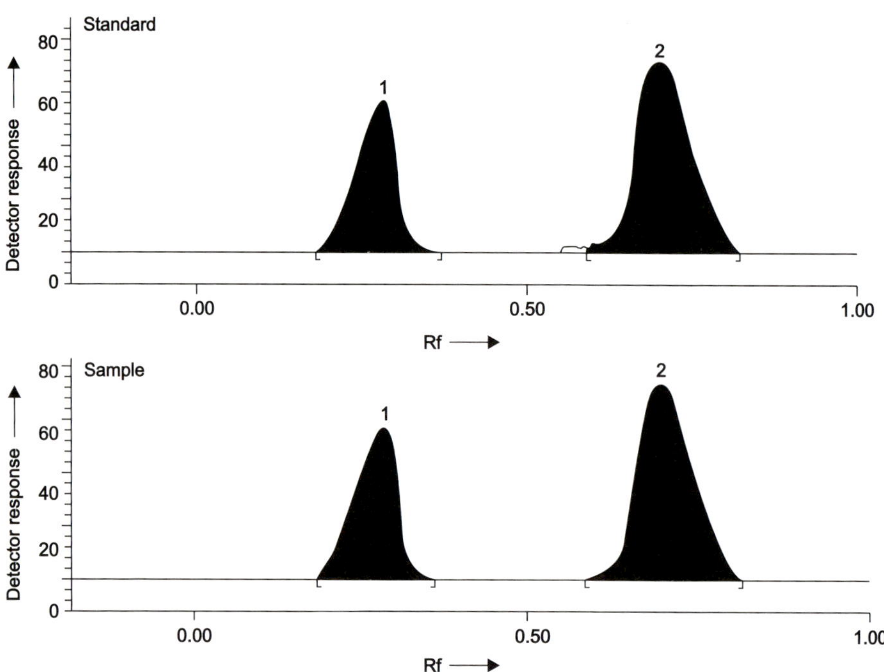

Typical densitogram of the standard and the sample containing isoniazid and ethambutol. For detailed experimental and chromatographic conditions, refer to Protocol No. 237. Peaks identification: 1. Ethambutol hydrochloride; 2. Isoniazid.

PROTOCOL FOR HPTLC ANALYSIS OF PHARMACEUTICAL FORMULATION

Protocol No. 237

Formulation: Isoniazid, Ethambutol hydrochloride

Classification: Antibiotics **Dosage form:** Tablets

Standard preparation: Prepare 1 mg/ml solution of both the compounds in methanol. Mix 4 ml of ethambutol and 1 ml of isoniazid solution and dilute to 10 ml with methanol and use for chromatographic application.

Sample preparation: Weigh accurately powdered sample equivalent to 30 mg of isoniazid, suspend in 50–60 ml of methanol, sonicate for 10 min, dilute to 100 ml, filter and dilute 0.5 ml of filtrate to 10 ml and use for application.

Chromatographic equipments:

Sample applicator: Camag Linomat–IV

Development chamber: Camag twin-trough glass chamber, 10 × 10 cm

Densitometric scanner: Camag TLC Scanner–II

Chromatographic conditions:

1. Stationary phase: Silica gel 60F_{254} pre-coated HPTLC plates, 10 × 10 cm (200 μm) – Merck
2. Mobile phase (MP): Methanol–25% ammonia (10 : 0.15 v/v)
3. Standard/Sample application:
   Band length: 10 mm Volume applied: 10 μl Spacing: 10 mm
4. Chamber saturation: 20 min (MP)
5. RH (%): 55 ± 5
6. Temperature °C: 22 ± 2
7. Separation technique: Ascending
8. Quantity of mobile phase: 10 ml
9. Migration distance: 50 mm
10. Migration time: 11 min

Densitometric evaluation:

Wavelength: UV–282 nm Scanning mode: Reflectance/Absorbance

HRF: Ethambutol—28; Isoniazid—70

Linearity: Isoniazid—100–2000 ng/band; Ethambutol—1–20 μg/band

Recovery (%): 99.40–100.33 for both the compound

References: —

Comments:

- The method was optimized and analytical work carried out at **Anchrom's HPTLC Application Laboratory**, Mumbai, India.
- Although ethambutol is a non-UV-absorbing compound, but on exposure to iodine (vapours), it forms an ion-pair complex exhibiting absorption maxima at 282 nm. Isoniazid also showed significant absorpotion at 282 nm, hence both compounds were scanned at 282 nm.

HPTLC : High Performance Thin Layer Chromatography
HPTLC Densitogram

No. 238

Pyrazinamide

Ethambutol hydrochloride

Isoniazid

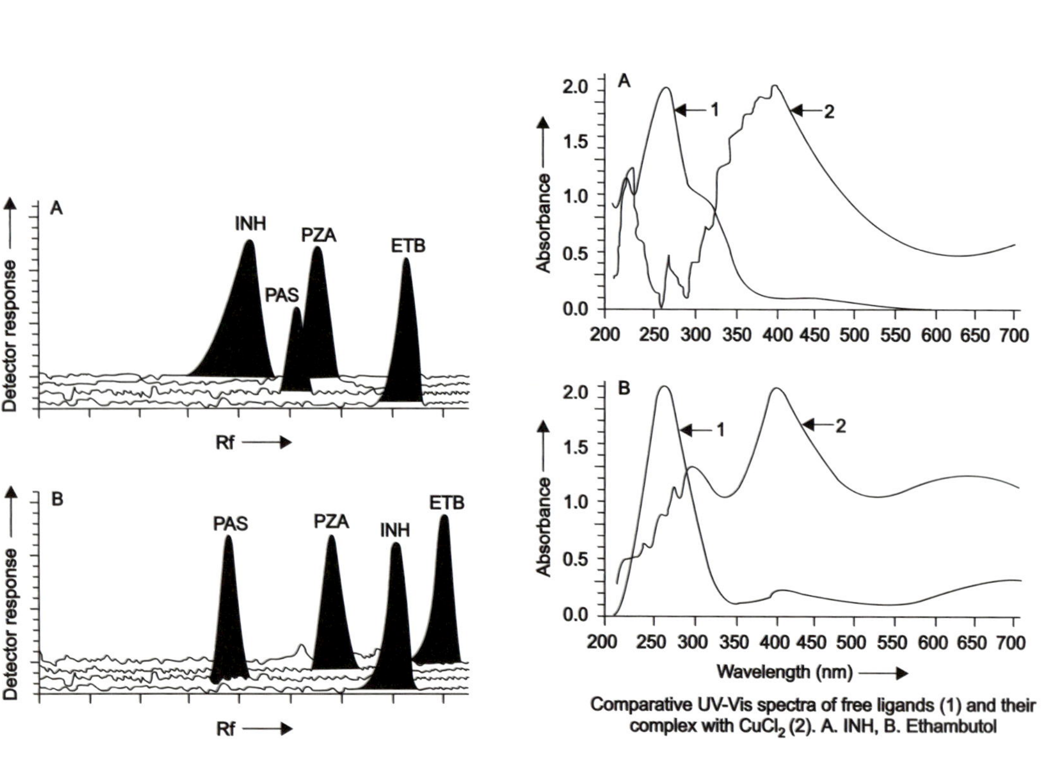

Comparative UV-Vis spectra of free ligands (1) and their complex with $CuCl_2$ (2). A. INH, B. Ethambutol

Typical densitograms (A and B) of the standard solutions of isoniazid (INH), aminosalicylate (PAS), ethambutol (ETB) and pyrazinamide (PZA).(A) Without $CuCl_2$; (B) with 0.05 M $CuCl_2$ in mobile phase (acetonitrile–water – 3 : 7). For detailed experimental and chromatographic conditions, refer to Protocol No.238. Peaks identification: See densitograms.

PROTOCOL FOR HPTLC ANALYSIS OF PHARMACEUTICAL FORMULATION

Protocol No. 238

Formulation: Isoniazid, Ethambutol

Classification: Antibiotics **Dosage form:** Tablets

Standard preparation: Standard solution of both the compounds prepared in methanol (3 mg/ml). Further suitable dilutions made with methanol for chromatographic analysis.

Sample preparation: The sample was prepared in methanol, filtered and used for analysis. Apply 10 μl on the plate for chromatographic separation and evaluation.

Chromatographic equipments:

Sample applicator: —

Development chamber: Horizontal Teflon DS Chamber (Chromdes-Poland)

Densitometric scanner: J and M TLC–HPTLC Scanner (Germany)

Chromatographic conditions:

1. Stationary phase: Silica gel RP–18F_{254} pre-coated HPTLC plates, 10 × 10 cm (200 μm) – Merck
2. Mobile phase (MP): Acetonitrile–water (3 : 7 v/v) containing 0.05 M Copper (II) chloride
3. Standard/Sample application:
   Band length: 10 mm Volume applied: 10 μl Spacing: 15 mm
4. Chamber saturation: —
5. RH (%): 55 ± 5
6. Temperature °C: 20 ± 2
7. Separation technique: Ascending
8. Quantity of mobile phase: 10 ml
9. Migration distance: 90 mm
10. Migration time: 40 min

Densitometric evaluation:

Wavelength: UV–254 nm Scanning mode: Reflectance/Absorbance

HRF: See densitograms

Linearity: —

Recovery (%): —

References: Jolanta Flieger, Piotr Paneth, Krystyna Gietzak-Kotwin and Maigorrata Tatarizak, *J. Planar Chromatogr.*, **22(2)**, 83-88, 2009.

Comments: Copper ligand of both the compounds were isolated by micro-preparative TLC and estimated by electron paramagnetic resonance (EPR).

HPTLC : High Performance Thin Layer Chromatography
HPTLC Densitogram

No. 239

Isoniazid

Pyrazinamide

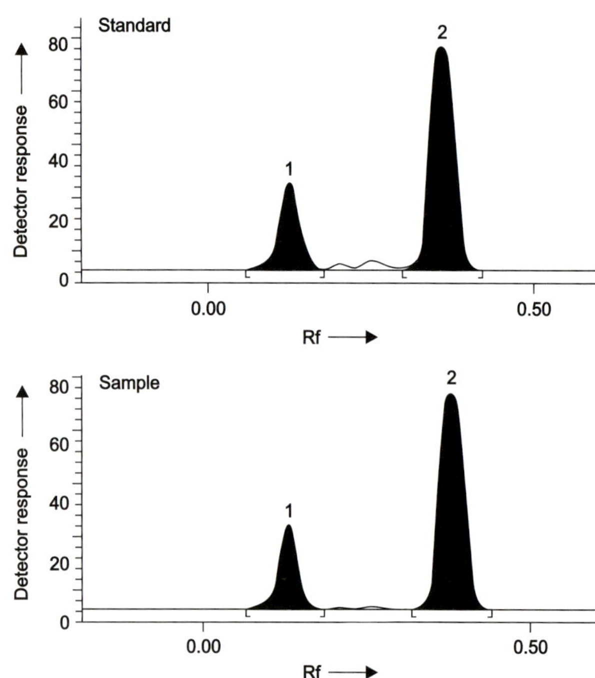

Typical densitogram of the standard and the sample containing isoniazid and pyrazinamide. For detailed experimental and chromatographic conditions, refer to Protocol No. 239. Peaks identification: 1. Isoniazid; 2. Pyrazinamide.

PROTOCOL FOR HPTLC ANALYSIS OF PHARMACEUTICAL FORMULATION

Protocol No. 239

Formulation: **Isoniazid, Pyrazinamide**

Classification: Antibiotics **Dosage form:** Tablets

Standard preparation: Prepare 1 mg/ml solution of isoniazid and 5 mg/ml solution of pyrazinamide, both in methanol. Dilute 0.5 ml of each solution to 10 ml with methanol. Apply varying volumes of each solution for linearity.

Sample preparation: Powdered sample equivalent to 500 mg of pyrazinamide suspended in 50 ml of methanol, sonicated for 5 min, diluted to 100 ml, filtered and 0.5 ml of the filtrate diluted to 10 ml with methanol and used for chromatographic application.

Chromatographic equipments:

Sample applicator: Camag Linomat–IV

Development chamber: Camag twin-trough glass chamber, 10 × 10 cm

Denistometric scanner: Camag TLC Scanner–II

Chromatographic conditions:

1. Stationary phase: Silica gel 60F$_{254}$ pre-coated HPTLC plates, 10 × 10 cm (200 μm) – Merck
2. Mobile phase (MP): Chloroform-methanol (9.5 : 0.5 v/v)
3. Standard/Sample application:
   Band length: 5 mm Volume applied: 5 μml Spacing: 5 mm
4. Chamber saturation: 20 min (MP)
5. RH (%): 55 ± 5
6. Temperature °C: 22 ± 2
7. Separation technique: Ascending
8. Quantity of mobile phase: 10 ml
9. Migration distance: 50 mm
10. Migration time: 20 min

Densitometric evaluation:

Wavelength: UV–266 nm Scanning mode: Reflectance/Absorbance

HRF: Isoniazid—12; Pyrazinamide—37

Linearity (ng/band): Isoniazid—100–1000; Pyrazinamide—100–1500

Recovery (%): 99.30–99.31 for both the compound

References: —

Comments:

- The method was optimized and analytical work carried out at **Anchrom's HPTLC Application Laboratory**, Mumbai, India.
- Several market samples of similar composition were analysed by the proposed method and found to give reproducable results.

HPTLC : High Performance Thin Layer Chromatography
HPTLC Densitogram

No. 240

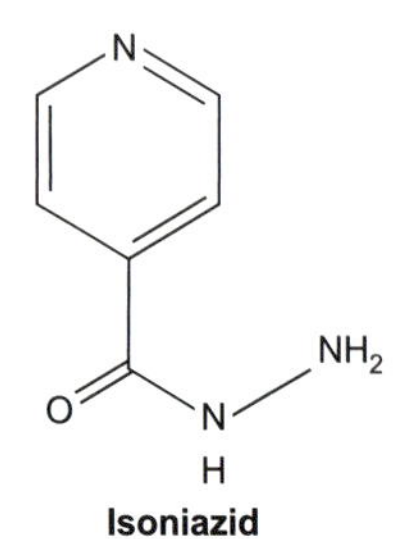

Isoniazid

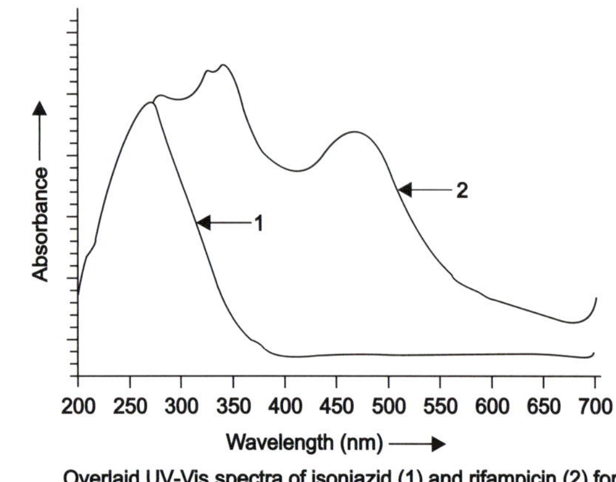

Overlaid UV-Vis spectra of isoniazid (1) and rifampicin (2) for selection of suitable wavelength for densitometric scanning

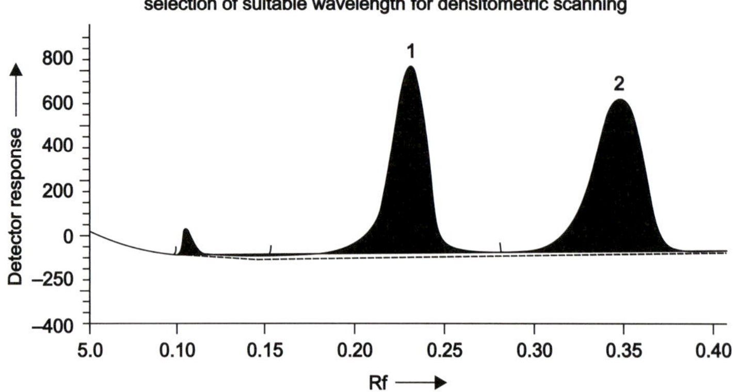

Typical densitogram of the standard containing isoniazid and rifampicin. For detailed experimental and chromatographic conditions, refer to Protocol No. 240. Peaks identification: 1. Rifampicin; 2. Isoniazid.

PROTOCOL FOR HPTLC ANALYSIS OF PHARMACEUTICAL FORMULATION

Protocol No. 240

Formulation: Isoniazid, Rifampicin

Classification: Antibiotics **Dosage form:** Capsule

Standard preparation: Prepare stock solution of both the compounds in methanol to get different concentrations i.e isoniazid—2.7–7.5 mg/ml; rifampicin—5–15 mg/ml. Further dilutions suitably made for application to study linearity profile. Apply 1 μl of each solution.

Sample preparation: Suspend the contents of one capsule containing 150 mg of isoniazid and 300 mg of rifampicin in 20 ml of methanol, sonicate, dilute and filter. Dilute 1.5 ml of the filtrate to 10 ml with methanol and use for chromatographic evaluation.

Chromatographic equipments:

Sample applicator: Desaga AS30

Development chamber: Horizontal Teflon DS chamber

Denistometric scanner: Desaga CD 60 densitometer

Chromatographic conditions:

1. Stationary phase: Silica gel $60F_{254}$ pre-coated HPTLC plates, 10 × 10 cm (200 μm) – Merck, pre-washed with methanol, dried prior to use
2. Mobile phase (MP): Ethyl acetate–methanol–acetone–glacial acetic acid (5 : 2 : 2 : 1 v/v)
3. Standard/Sample application:
   Band length: 5 mm Volume applied: 1 μl Spacing: 5 mm
4. Chamber saturation: 30 min (MP)
5. RH (%): 55 ± 5
6. Temperature °C: 22 ± 2
7. Separation technique: Ascending
8. Quantity of mobile phase: 10 ml
9. Migration distance: 70 mm
10. Migration time: 15 min

Densitometric evaluation:

Wavelength: UV–270 nm (isoniazid), 345 nm (rifampicin)

Scanning mode: Reflectance/Absorbance

HRF: Rifampicin—23; Isoniazid—35

Linearity (μg/band): Isoniazid—0.5–1.0; Rifampicin—1–2.5

Recovery (%): 98.94–102.48 for both the compound

References: Malgorzata Tatarczak, Jolanta Flieger and Halina Szumilo, *J. Planar Chromatogr.*, **18**, 207–211, 2005.

Comments: Chromatographic conditions were suitable for separation of other antitubercular drugs i.e. Pyrazinamide (Rf – 0.48), Ethambutol (Rf – 0.17), and PAS (Rf – 0.46).

HPTLC : High Performance Thin Layer Chromatography
HPTLC Densitogram

No. 241

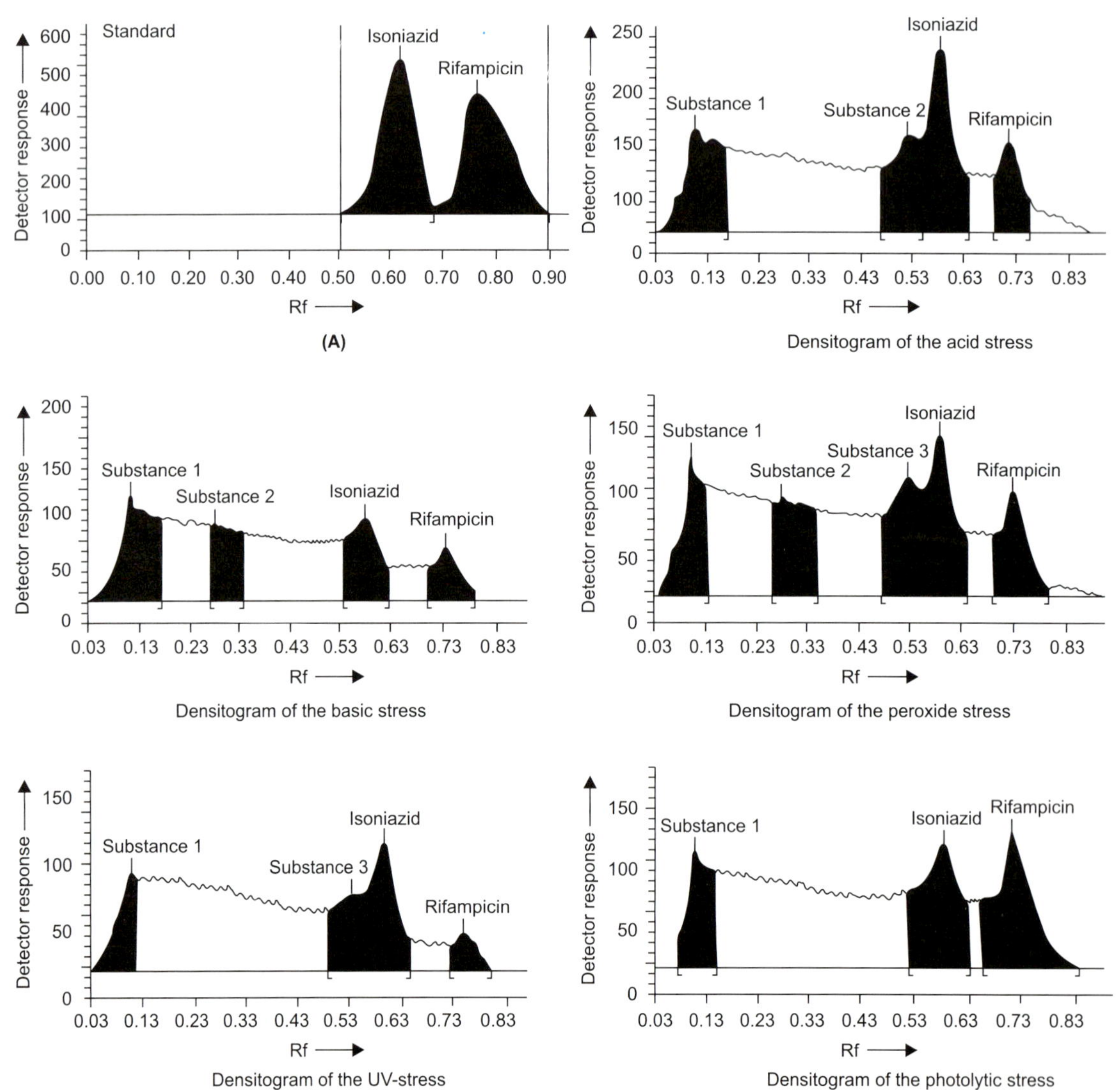

Typical densitogram of the standard (A) containing isoniazid and rifampicin. For detailed experimental and chromatographic conditions, refer to Protocol No. 241. Peaks identification: 1. Isoniazid; 2. Rifampicin. Other densitograms are related to stability studies.

PROTOCOL FOR HPTLC ANALYSIS OF PHARMACEUTICAL FORMULATION

Protocol No. 241

Formulation: Isoniazid, Rifampicin

Classification: Antibiotics **Dosage form:** Tablets

Standard preparation: Prepare 100 μg/ml solution of each compound in methanol–chloroform (1 : 1 v/v). Apply varying volumes of each solution for linearity profile.

Sample preparation: Powdered sample equivalent to 10 mg of INH was extracted with methanol–chloroform (1 : 1 v/v) with sonication, diluted to 100 ml. Apply 5 μl of the final solution for assay.

Chromatographic equipments:

Sample applicator: Camag Linomat–V

Development chamber: Camag twin-trough glass chamber, 10 × 10 cm

Denistometric scanner: Camag TLC Scanner–III

Chromatographic conditions:

1. Stationary phase: Silica gel $60F_{254}$ pre-coated HPTLC plates, 10 × 10 cm (200 μm) – Merck
2. Mobile phase (MP): n-hexane-2–prepanol–acetone-25% ammonia-formic acid (3 : 3.8 : 2.8 : 0.3 : 0.1 v/v)
3. Standard/Sample application:
   Band length: 4 mm Volume applied: 5 μl Spacing: 5 mm
4. Chamber saturation: 10 min (MP)
5. RH (%): 55 ± 5
6. Temperature °C: 22 ± 2
7. Separation technique: Ascending
8. Quantity of mobile phase: 10 ml
9. Migration distance: 80 mm
10. Migration time: 30 min

Densitometric evaluation:

Wavelength: UV–254 nm Scanning mode: Reflectance/Absorbance

HRF: Isoniazid—59; Rifampicin—73

Linearity: 100–700 ng/band for both the compounds

Recovery (%): 100.68–100.48 for both the compounds

References: J. Ali, N. Ali, Y. Sultana and S. Faiyaz, *Acta Chromatographia*, **18**, 168–179, 2007.

Comments:

- The method validated for accuracy, precision, linearity, LOD, LOQ and robustness.
- The method is stability indicating (acid, base, oxidative, UV, photolytic).

HPTLC : High Performance Thin Layer Chromatography
HPTLC Densitogram

No. 242

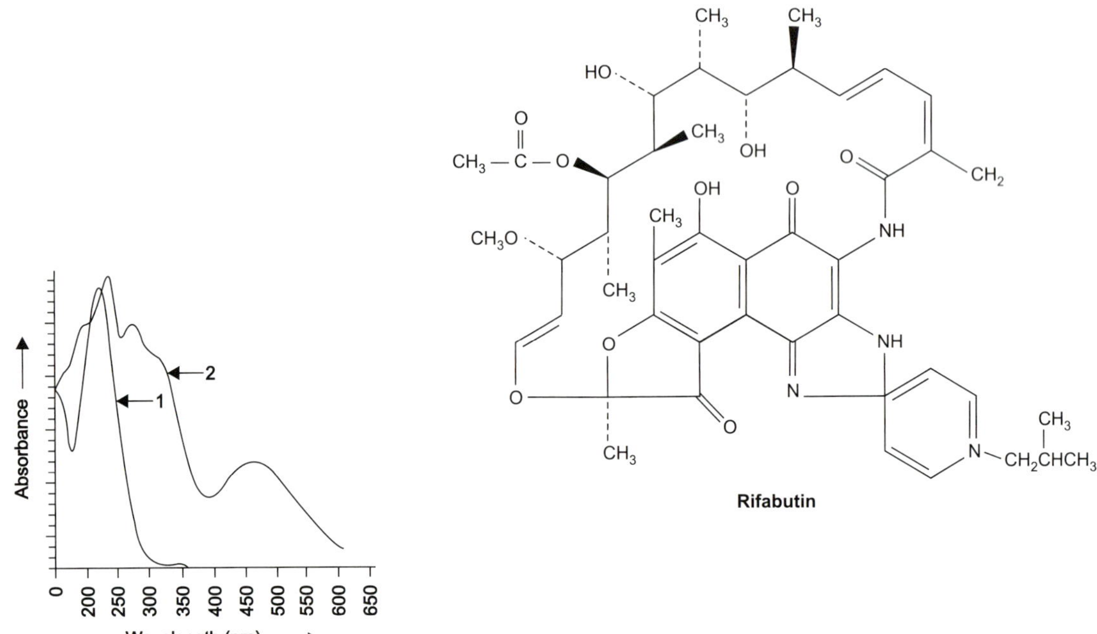

Overlaid UV spectra of isoniazid (1) and rifabutin (2) for selection of suitable wavelength for densitometric scanning

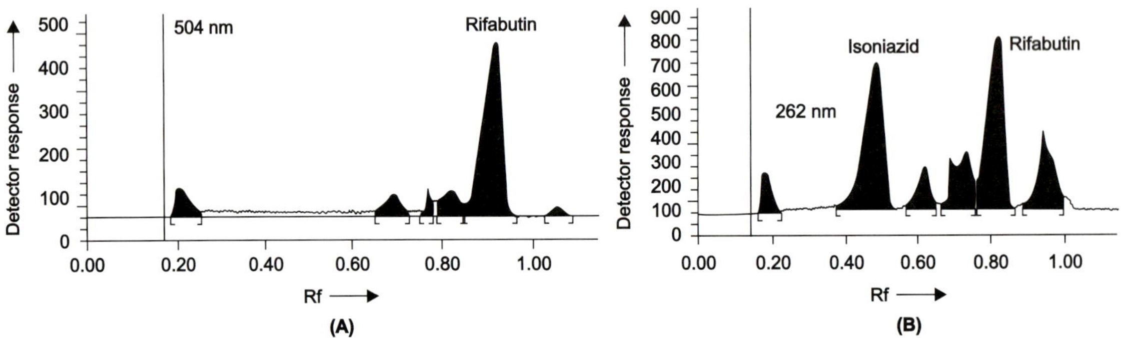

Typical densitogram obtained with isoniazid and rifabutin and their impurities and degradation products (A) at 504 nm and (B) at 262 nm scanned. For detailed experimental and chromographic conditions, refer to Protocol No. 242. Peaks identification see densitogram.

PROTOCOL FOR HPTLC ANALYSIS OF PHARMACEUTICAL FORMULATION

Protocol No. 242

Formulation: Isoniazid, Rifabutin

Classification: Antibiotics **Dosage form:** Suspension

Standard preparation: Prepare stock solution of both the compounds in solvent to get 100 μg/ml (rifabutin) and 50 μg/ml (isoniazid). Further serial dilutions made with solvent for linearity profile by applying varying volumes of each solution.

Sample preparation: Sample equivalent to 75 mg of isoniazid extracted with solvent, suitably diluted, filtered after sonication (20 min). The filtrate suitably diluted for analysis.

Solvent: Methanol–acetone (1 : 1 v/v).

Chromatographic equipments:

Sample applicator: Camag Linomat–IV sample application

Development chamber: Camag twin-trough glass chamber, 10 × 20 cm

Densitometric scanner: Camag TLC Scanner–IV

Chromatographic conditions:

1. Stationary phase: Silica gel $60F_{254}$ pre-coated HPTLC plates, 10 × 20 cm (200 μm) – Merck
2. Mobile phase (MP): Dichloromethane–acetone–methanol (20 : 7 : 2 v/v)
3. Standard/Sample application:
   Band length: 5 mm Volume applied: 10 μl Spacing: 15 mm
4. Chamber saturation: 25 min (MP)
5. RH (%): 55 ± 5
6. Temperature °C: 22 ± 2
7. Separation technique: Ascending
8. Quantity of mobile phase: 29 ml
9. Migration distance: 80 mm
10. Migration time: 35 min

Densitometric evaluation:

Wavelength: UV–262 nm (INH); 504 nm (rifabutin)

Scanning mode: Reflectance/Absorbance

HRF: Isoniazid—48; Rifabutin–84

Linearity (ng/band): Isoniazid—50–350; Rifabutin—100–700

Recovery (%): 99.96–99.78 for both the compound

References: Amalia M. Avachar and Satish B. Bhise, *J. Planar Chromatogr.*, **23(2)**, 123–128, 2010.

Comments:

- The method validated for accuracy, precision, linearity, LOD, LOQ and robustness.
- The method is stability indicating (acid, base, oxidative, thermal, photolytic). The degradation products are well separated from main compounds.

HPTLC : High Performance Thin Layer Chromatography
HPTLC Densitogram

No. 243

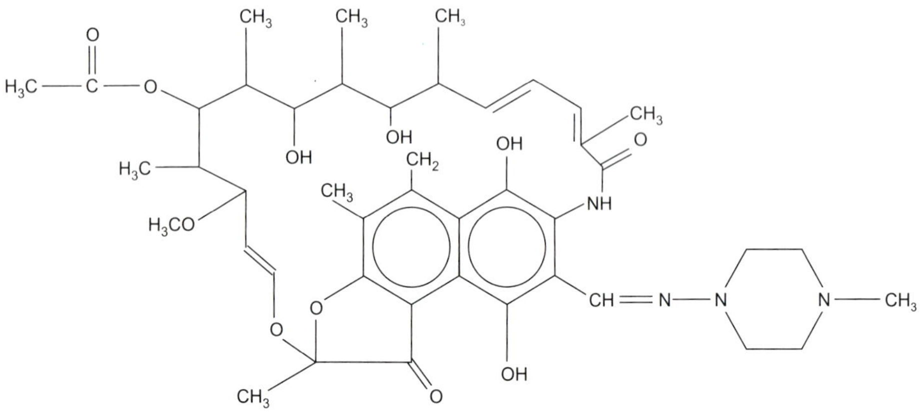

Rifampicin

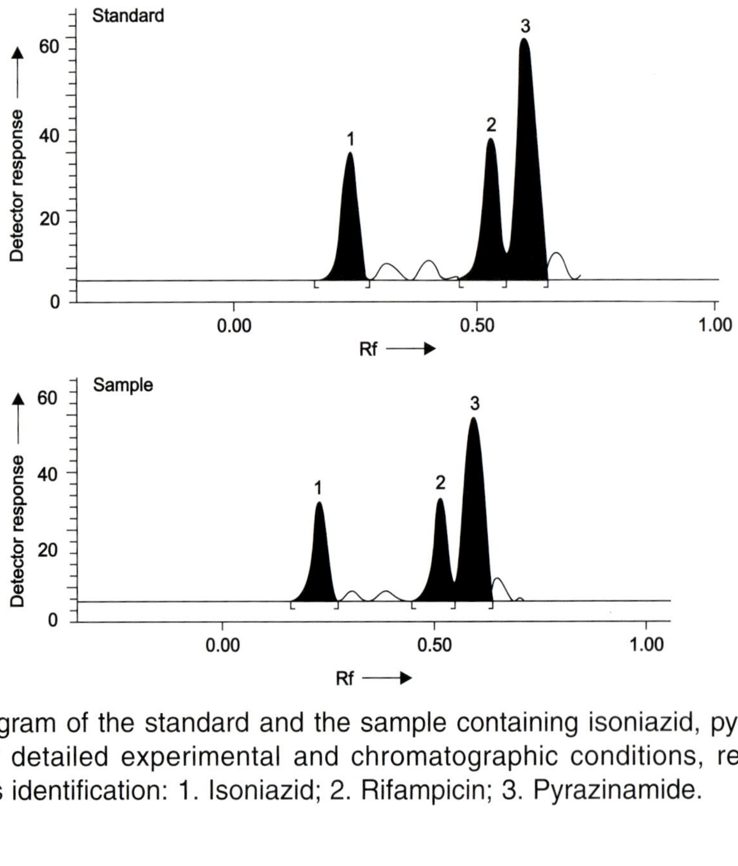

Standard

Sample

Typical densitogram of the standard and the sample containing isoniazid, pyrazinamide and rifampicin. For detailed experimental and chromatographic conditions, refer to Protocol No. 243. Peaks identification: 1. Isoniazid; 2. Rifampicin; 3. Pyrazinamide.

PROTOCOL FOR HPTLC ANALYSIS OF PHARMACEUTICAL FORMULATION

Protocol No. 243

Formulation: **Isoniazid, Pyrazinamide, Rifampicin**

Classification: Antibiotics **Dosage form:** Tablets, Capsules

Standard preparation: Weigh accurately 12 mg of rifampicin (R), 8 mg of isoniazid (I) and 30 mg of pyrazinamide (P) and dissolve in methanol to produce 10 ml. Further dilute 1 ml to 10 ml for chromatographic application.

Sample preparation: Powdered sample equivalent to 10 mg of pyrazinamide suspended in 30–40 ml methanol, sonicated for 5 min, diluted to 50 ml, filtered and 1 ml of the filtrate diluted to 10 ml with methanol and used for chromatographic evolution.

Chromatographic equipments:

Sample applicator: Camag Linomat–IV

Development chamber: Camag twin-trough glass chamber, 10 × 10 cm

Densitometric scanner: Camag TLC Scanner–II

Chromatographic conditions:

1. Stationary phase: Silica gel $60F_{254}$ pre-coated HPTLC plates, 10 × 10 cm (200 μm) – Merck
2. Mobile phase (MP): Chloroform–methanol (9 : 1 v/v)
3. Standard/Sample application:
   Band length: 5 mm Volume applied: 5 μl Spacing: 5 mm
4. Chamber saturation: 20 min (MP)
5. RH (%): 55 ± 5
6. Temperature °C: 22 ± 2
7. Separation technique: Ascending
8. Quantity of mobile phase: 10 ml
9. Migration distance: 50 mm
10. Migration time: 15 min

Densitometric evaluation:

Wavelength: UV-254 nm Scanning mode: Reflectance/Absorbance

HRF: Isoniazid—19; Rifampicin—52; Pyrazinamide—60

Linearity (ng/band): Isoniazid—100–200; Pyrazinamide—300–3000; Rifampicin—100–1000

Recovery (%): 97.90–99.30 for all the three compounds

References: —

Comments:

- The method was optimized and analytical work carried out at **Anchrom's HPTLC Application Laboratory**, Mumbai, India.
- Several market samples of similar composition were analysed by the proposed method with reproducible results.

HPTLC : High Performance Thin Layer Chromatography
HPTLC Densitogram

No. 244

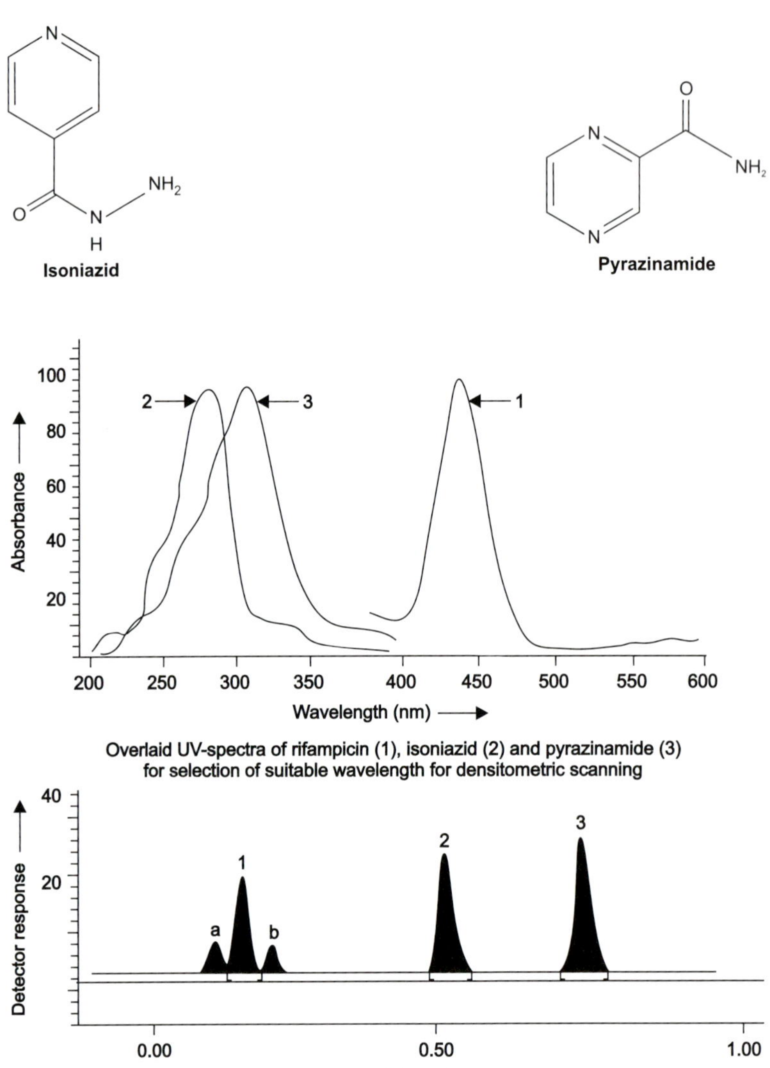

Typical densitogram of the sample containing rifampicin, isoniazid and pyrazinamide. For detailed experimental and chromatographic conditions, refer to Protocol No. 244. Peaks identification: 1. Rifampicin; 2. Isoniazid; 3. Pyrazinamide; (a) 25-Desacetyl rifampicin; (b) Rifampicin quinone.

PROTOCOL FOR HPTLC ANALYSIS OF PHARMACEUTICAL FORMULATION

Protocol No. 244

Formulation: Isoniazid, Pyrazinamide, Rifampicin

Classification: Antibiotics **Dosage form:** Tablets

Standard preparation: Accurately weighed quantity of each substance separately dissolved in mixture of chloroform–methanol (60 : 40) to get stock solution. Further serial dilutions made with solvent. Apply varying volumes of each solution for linearity profile.

Sample preparation: Powdered sample equivalent to average weight of one tablet suspended in solvent, sonicated for 20 min, diluted, filtered and filtrate suitably diluted with solvent and used for chromatographic analysis.

Solvent: Mixture of chloroform–methanol (60 : 40 v/v).

Chromatographic equipments:

Sample applicator: Camag Linomat–IV sample applicator

Development chamber: Camag twin-trough glass chamber, 10 × 20 cm

Densitometric scanner: Camag TLC Scanner–II

Chromatographic conditions:

1. Stationary phase: Silica gel $60F_{254}$ pre-coated TLC plate, 10 × 20 cm (250 μm) – Merck
2. Mobile phase (MP): Ethyl acetate–6.75 M ammonia–ethyl alcohol–cyclohexane (20 : 9 : 4.5 : 5 v/v)
3. Standard/Sample application:
   Band length: 8 mm Volume applied: 1–10 μl Spacing: 10 mm
4. Chamber saturation: 20 min (MP)
5. RH (%): 55 ± 5
6. Temperature °C: 22 ± 2
7. Separation technique: Ascending
8. Quantity of mobile phase: 17 ml
9. Migration distance: 90 mm
10. Migration time: 40 min

Densitometric evaluation:

Wavelength: Rifampicin—440 nm; Isoniazid and Pyrazinamide—275 nm

Scanning mode: Reflectance/Absorbance

HRF: 25-Desacetyl rifampicin—07; Rifampicin—12; Rifampicin quinone—25; Isoniazid—52; Pyrazinamide—75

Linearity (ng/band): Rifampicin—120–400; Isoniazid—40–200; Pyrazinamide—40–200

Recovery (%): Rifampicin—99.98; Isoniazid—101.74; Pyrazinamide—100.01

References: A.P. Argekar, S.S. Kunjir and K.S. Purandare, *J. Pharm. and Biomed. Analysis*, **14**, 1645–1650, 1996. MP consisting of toluene-methanol–25% ammonia (5 : 6 : 0.25 v/v) gave excellant separation all the three compounds with HRF values of Isoniazid—45; Pyrazinamide–56; Rifampicin—71; (GPHF-minilab manual-2nd supplement to Vol. II of TLC, p-34-37).

Comments:

- The method validated for accuracy, precision, linearity, LOD and LOQ.
- The method is comparble with HPLC method.

HPTLC : High Performance Thin Layer Chromatography
HPTLC Densitogram

No. 245

CH3
N
• HCl
HO
OH
OH
Pyridoxine hydrochloride

N
NH2
O
N
H
Isoniazid

Standard
Detector response
40
20
0
1
2
0.00 0.10 0.20 0.30 0.40 0.50 0.60 0.70 0.80
Rf

Sample
Detector response
40
20
0
1
2
0.00 0.10 0.20 0.30 0.40 0.50 0.60 0.70 0.80
Rf

Typical densitogram of the standard and the sample containing isoniazid and pyridoxine HCl. For detailed experimental and chromatographic conditions, refer to Protocol No. 245. Peaks identification: 1. Pyridoxine HCl; 2. Isoniazid.

PROTOCOL FOR HPTLC ANALYSIS OF PHARMACEUTICAL FORMULATION

Protocol No. 245

Formulation: **Isoniazid, Pyridoxine hydrochloride**

Classification: Antibiotics **Dosage form:** Tablets

Standard preparation: (a) Prepare 1 mg/ml solution of pyridoxine hydrochloride in methanol. Weigh 30 mg of isoniazid, add 5–6 ml of methanol and 1 ml of solution (a) and dilute to 10 ml with methanol. Dilute 1 ml of the resulting solution to 10 ml and use for chromatographic application.

Sample preparation: Powdered sample equivalent to 10 mg of pyridoxine HCl is suspended in 50–60 ml of methanol, sonicated for 5 min, diluted to 100 ml and filtered. Dilute 0.4 ml of the filtrate to 10 ml with methanol and use for chromatographic evolution.

Chromatographic equipments:

Sample applicator: Camag Linomat–IV

Development chamber: Camag twin-trough glass chamber, 10 × 10 cm

Densitometric scanner: Camag TLC Scanner–II

Chromatographic conditions:

1. Stationary phase: Silica gel $60F_{254}$ pre-coated HPTLC plates, 7 × 10 cm (200 μm) – Merck
2. Mobile phase (MP): Toluene–acetone–methanol–25% ammonia (2.5 : 7.0 : 0.5 : 0.1 v/v)
3. Standard/Sample application:
   Band length: 10 mm Volume applied: 10 μl Spacing: 10 mm
4. Chamber saturation: 20 min (MP)
5. RH (%): 55 ± 5
6. Temperature °C: 22 ± 2
7. Separation technique: Ascending
8. Quantity of mobile phase: 10 ml
9. Migration distance: 50 mm
10. Migration time: 10 min

Densitometric evaluation:

Wavelength: UV–271 nm (isoniazid); 306 nm (vit. B_6)

Scanning mode: Reflectance/Absorbance

HRF: Pyridoxine HCl—32; Isoniazid—54

Linearity: 100–200 ng/band for both the compounds

Recovery (%): 98.75–99.60 for both the compounds

References: —

Comments:

- The method was optimized and analytical work carried out at **Anchrom's HPTLC Application Laboratory**, Mumbai, India.
- Several market sample of similar composition were analysed by the proposed method and found to give reproducable results.

HPTLC : High Performance Thin Layer Chromatography
HPTLC Densitogram

No. 246

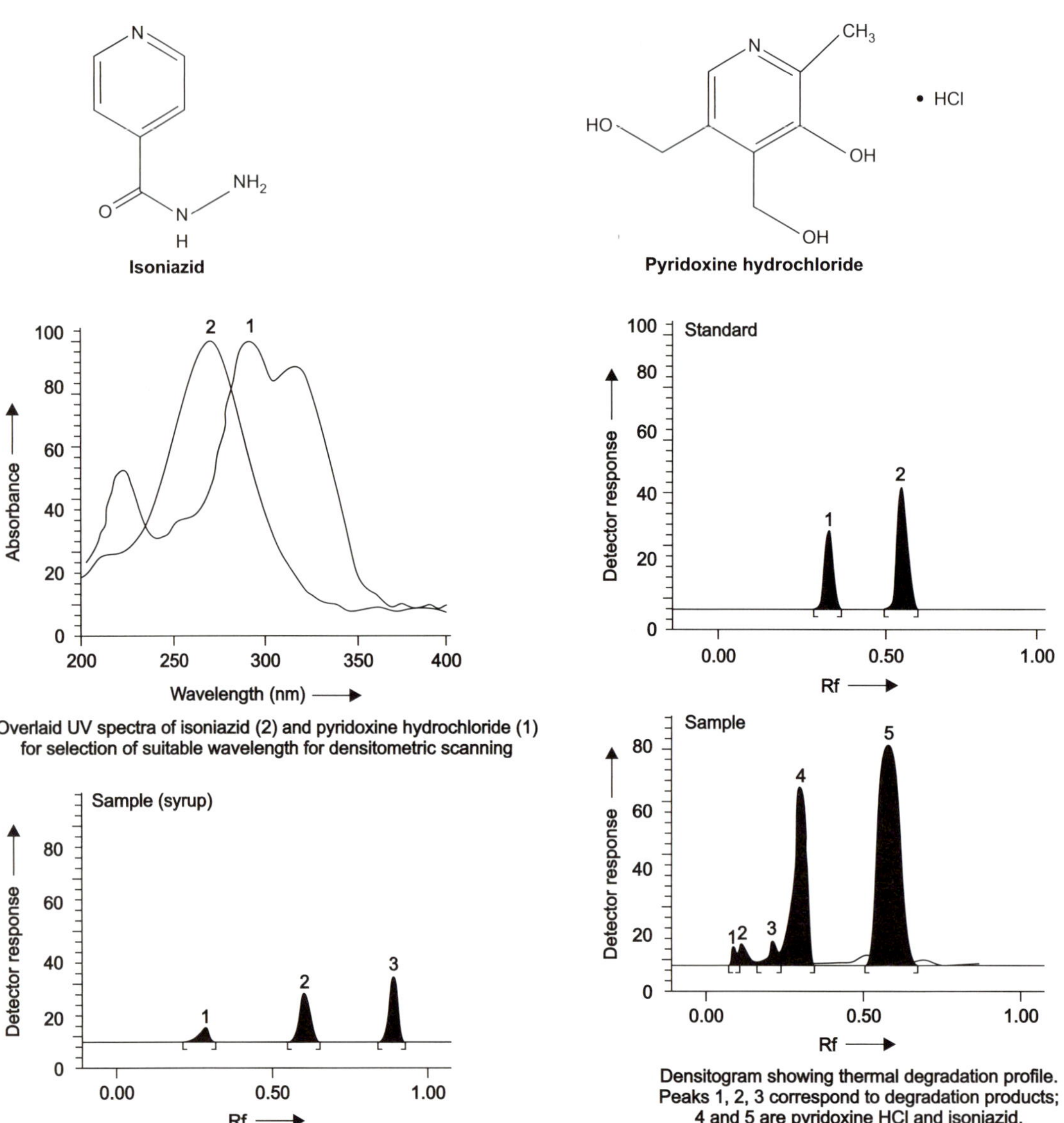

Typical densitogram of the standard and the sample containing isoniazid and pyridoxine HCl. For detailed experimental and chromatographic conditions, refer to Protocol No. 246. Peaks identification: 1. Pyridoxine HCl; 2. Isoniazid; 3. Methyl paraben.

PROTOCOL FOR HPTLC ANALYSIS OF PHARMACEUTICAL FORMULATION

Protocol No. 246

Formulation: Isoniazid, Pyridoxine hydrochloride
Classification: Antibiotics **Dosage form:** Tablets, Syrup
Standard preparation: Prepare 1 mg/ml solution of each compound in methanol. Further dilutions made to get 20 μg/ml solution and used for chromatographic application.
Sample preparation: Powdered sample equivalent to 100 mg of isoniazid suspended in methanol, sonicated for 20 min, diluted to 100 ml, filtered through 0.45 μm membrane filter and filtrate suitably diluted for chromatographic analysis. For syrups, dilute 5 ml to 100 ml with methanol, further dilutions made as for tablets sample preparation.
Chromatographic equipments:
Sample applicator: Camag Linomat–IV
Development chamber: Camag twin-trough glass chamber, 10 × 10 cm
Densitometric scanner: Camag TLC Scanner–II
Chromatographic conditions:
1. Stationary phase: Silica gel $60F_{254}$ pre-coated HPTLC plates, 10 × 10 cm (200 μm) – Merck, pre-washed with ammonical methanol and dried prior to use
2. Mobile phase (MP): Acetone–carbon tetrachloride–6.5 M ammonia (10.5 : 3.5 : 1 v/v)
3. Standard/Sample application:
   Band length: 10 mm Volume applied: 5 and 20 μl Spacing: 10 mm
4. Chamber saturation: 20 min (MP)
5. RH (%): 55 ± 5
6. Temperature °C: 22 ± 2
7. Separation technique: Ascending
8. Quantity of mobile phase: 15 ml
9. Migration distance: 90 mm
10. Migration time: 30 min

Densitometric evaluation:
Wavelength: UV–275 nm Scanning mode: Reflectance/Absorbance
HRF: Pyridoxine HCl—34; Isoniazid—56; Methyl paraben—80
Linearity (ng/band): Isoniazid—100–600; Pyridoxine hydrochloride—250–750
Recovery (%): 99.05–101.55 for both the compounds
References: A.R. Argekar and S.S. Kunjir, *J. Planar Chromatogr.*, **9**, 390–94, 1996.
Comments:
- The method validated for accuracy precision, linearity, LOD and LOQ.
- The method is stability indicating (acid, base, oxidative, thermal, photolytic). The degradation products were separated from main compounds.

HPTLC : High Performance Thin Layer Chromatography
HPTLC Densitogram

No. 247

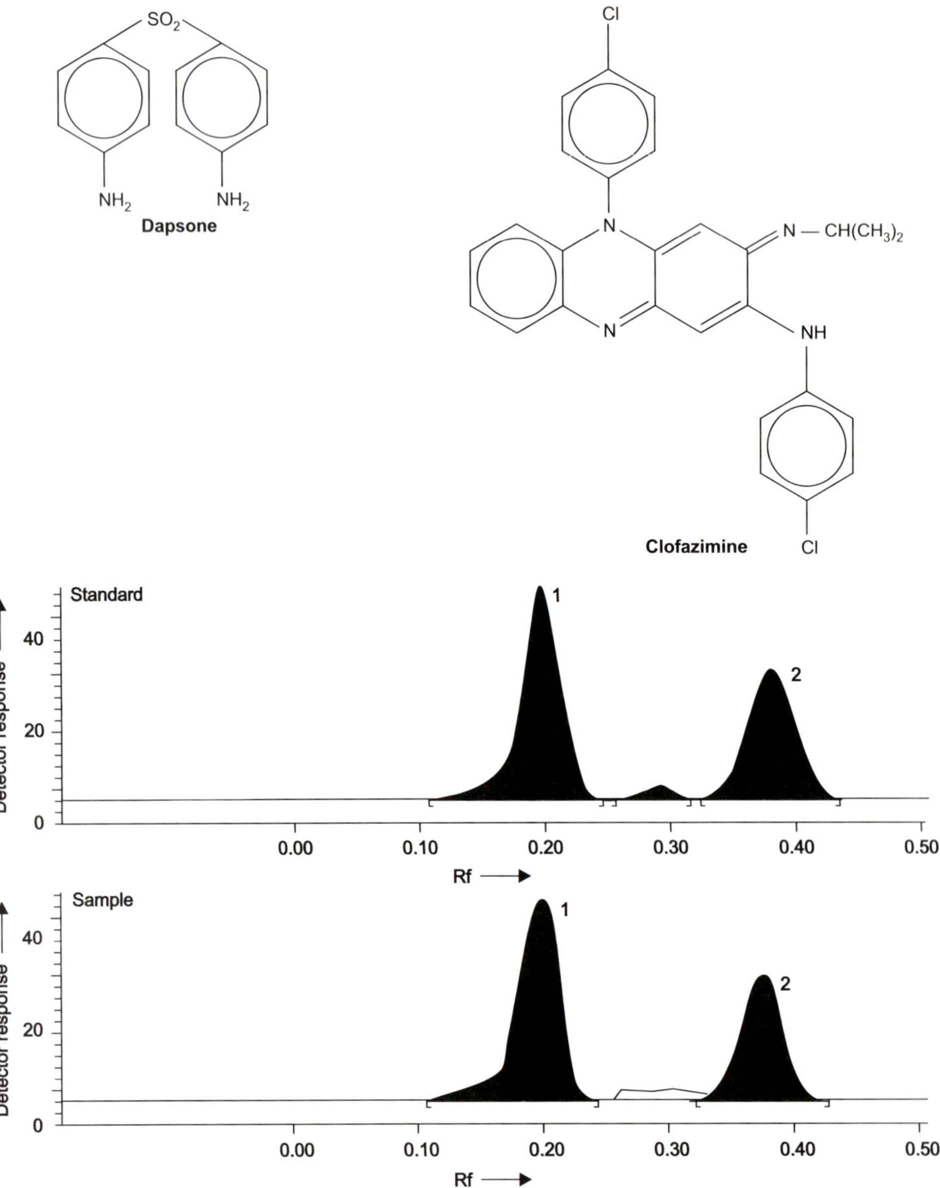

Typical densitogram of the standard and the sample containing dapsone and clofazimine. For detailed experimental and chromatographic conditions, refer to Protocol No. 247. Peaks identification: 1. Dapsone; 2. Clofazimine.

PROTOCOL FOR HPTLC ANALYSIS OF PHARMACEUTICAL FORMULATION

Protocol No. 247

Formulation: Dapsone, Clofazimine

Classification: Antibiotics **Dosage form:** Capsules

Standard preparation: Dissolve 10 mg of clofazimine in 2 ml of DMF, dilute to 10 ml with methanol (a). Prepare 1 mg/ml solution of dapsone in methanol (b). Mix 0.5 ml of (a) and 1 ml of (b), dilute to 10 ml. Further dilute 5 ml to 10 ml with methanol for chromatographic applicaton.

Sample preparation: Powdered sample equivalent to 50 mg of dapsone suspended in 10 ml of DMF, sonicate for 5 min, dilute to 50 ml with methanol. Further dilutions carried out as under standard solution and used for chromatographic analysis.

Chromatographic equipments:

Sample applicator: Camag Linomat–IV

Development chamber: Camag twin-trough glass chamber, 10 × 10 cm

Densitometric scanner: Camag TLC Scanner–II

Chromatographic conditions:

1. Stationary phase: Silica gel $60F_{254}$ pre-coated HPTLC plates, 10 × 10 cm (200 μm) – Merck
2. Mobile phase (MP): Toluene–acetone (8 : 2 v/v)
3. Standard/Sample application:
   Band length: 5 mm Volume applied: 4 μl Spacing: 5 mm
4. Chamber saturation: 20 min (MP)
5. RH (%): 55 ± 5
6. Temperature °C: 22 ± 2
7. Separation technique: Ascending
8. Quantity of mobile phase: 10 ml
9. Migration distance: 50 mm
10. Migration time: 15 min

Densitometric evaluation:

Wavelength: UV–283 nm Scanning mode: Reflectance/Absorbance

HRF: Dapsone—20; Clofazimine—38

Linearity (ng/band): Dapsone—100–600; Clofazimine—50–300

Rccovery (%): 99.65–100.08 for both the compounds

References: —

Comments:

- The method was optimized and analytical work carried out at **Anchrom's HPTLC Application Laboratory**, Mumbai, India.
- Several market samples of similar composition were analysed by the proposed method and found to give reproducible results.

HPTLC : High Performance Thin Layer Chromatography
HPTLC Densitogram

No. 248

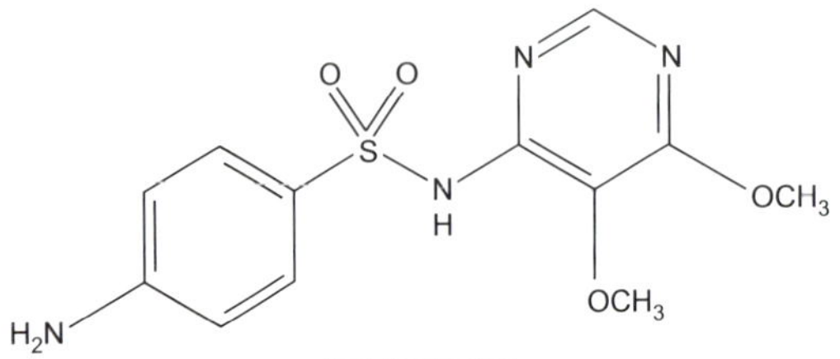

Sulphadoxine

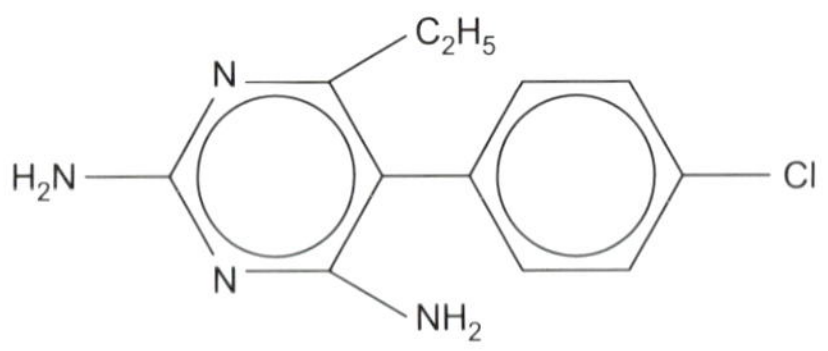

Pyrimethamine

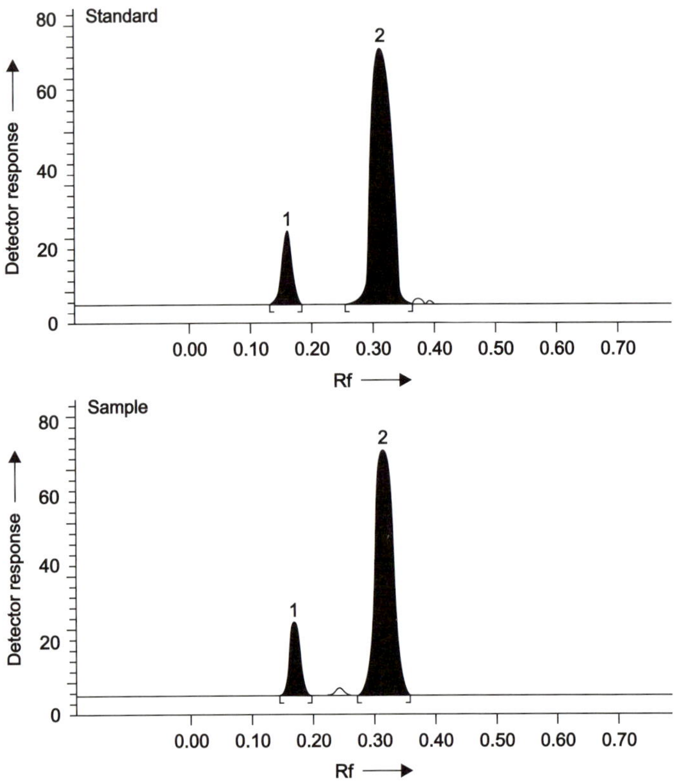

Typical densitogram of the standard and the sample containing sulphadoxine and pyrimethamine. For detailed experimental and chromatographic conditions, refer to Protocol No. 248. Peaks identification: 1. Pyrimethamine; 2. Sulphadoxine

PROTOCOL FOR HPTLC ANALYSIS OF PHARMACEUTICAL FORMULATION

Protocol No. 248

Formulation: Sulphadoxine, Pyrimethamine

Classification: Antibiotics **Dosage form:** Tablets

Standard preparation: Dissolved 25 mg of pyrimethamine in methanol (a). Take 25 mg of sulphadoxine, add 0.5 ml of solution (a) and 0.2 ml of ammonia and dilute to 10 ml with methanol. Further dilute 0.1 ml to 10 ml for chromatographic analysis.

Sample preparation: Powdered sample equivalent to 125 mg of sulphadoxine suspended in 30–35 ml methanol, add 2 ml of 25% ammonia, sonicate for 5 min, dilute to 50 ml with methanol, filter and dilute 0.1 ml of filtrate to 10 ml with methanol for chromatographic application.

Chromatographic equipments:

Sample applicator: Camag Linomat–IV

Development chamber: Camag twin-trough glass chamber, 10 × 10 cm

Densitometric scanner: Camag TLC Scanner–II

Chromatographic conditions:

1. Stationary phase: Silica gel $60F_{254}$ pre-coated HPTLC plates, 10 × 10 cm (200 μm) – Merck
2. Mobile phase (MP): Chlorofom–methanol (12 : 0.5 v/v)
3. Standard/Sample application:
   Band length: 5 mm Volume applied: 6 μl Spacing: 5 mm
4. Chamber saturation: 20 min (MP)
5. RH (%): 55 ± 5
6. Temperature °C: 22 ± 2
7. Separation technique: Ascending
8. Quantity of mobile phase: 12 ml
9. Migration distance: 50 mm
10. Migration time: 22 min

Densitometric evaluation:

Wavelength: UV–235 nm or 260 nm Scanning mode: Reflectance/Absorbance

HRF: Pyrimethamine—17; Sulphadoxine—34

Linearity (ng/band): Sulphadoxine—50–500; Pyrimethamine—10–100

Recovery (%): 99.71–102.76 for both the compounds

References: —

Comments:

- The method was optimized and analytical work carried out at **Anchrom's HPTLC Application Laboratory**, Mumbai, India.
- Several market samples of similar composition were analysed by the proposed method and found to give reproducable results.

HPTLC : High Performance Thin Layer Chromatography
HPTLC Densitogram

No. 249

Sulphadoxine

Pyrimethamine

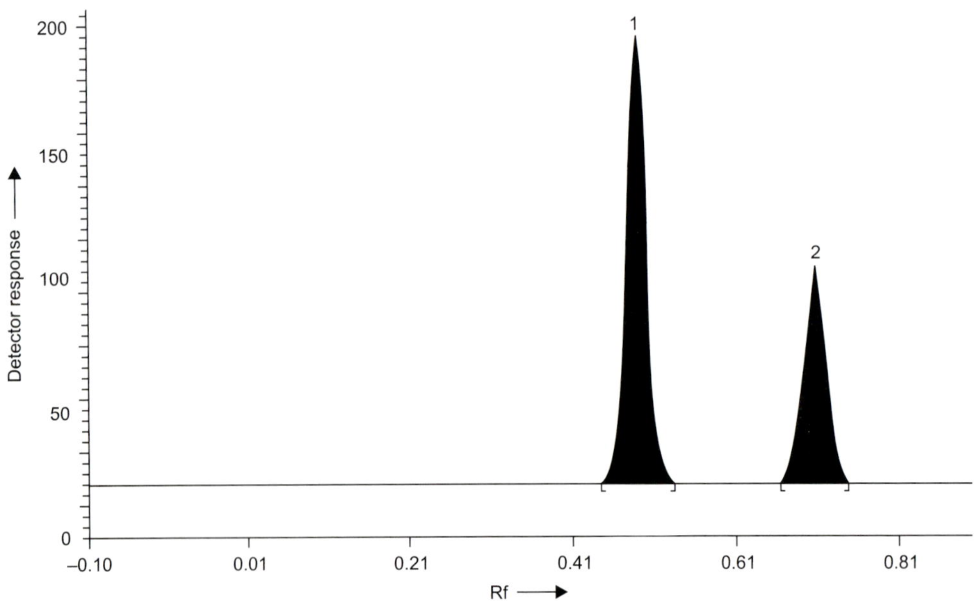

Typical densitogram of the standard containing sulphadoxine and pyrimethamine. For detailed experimental and chromatographic conditions, refer to Protocol No. 249. Peaks identification: 1. Sulphadoxine; 2. Pyrimethamine.

PROTOCOL FOR HPTLC ANALYSIS OF PHARMACEUTICAL FORMULATION

Protocol No. 249

Formulation: Sulphadoxine, Pyrimethamine

Classification: Antibiotics **Dosage form:** Tablets

Standard preparation: Dissolve 25 mg of pyrimethamine (P) in 10 ml of methanol. Take 25 mg of sulphadoxine (S), add 0.5 ml of solution (P) to 0.2 ml of 25% ammonia, dilute to 10 ml with methanol. Further dilute 0.1 ml to 10 ml with methanol for chromatographic evaluation.

Sample preparation: Powdered sample equivalent to 250 mg of sulphadoxine suspended in 70 ml of methanol containing 2 ml of 25% of ammonia, sonicate for 5 min, dilute to 100 ml with methanol, filter and dilute 0.1 ml of filtrate to 10 ml with methanol for analysis.

Chromatographic equipments:

Sample applicator: Camag Linomat–IV

Development chamber: Camag twin-trough glass chamber, 10 × 10 cm

Densitometric scanner: Camag TLC Scanner–II

Chromatographic conditions:

1. Stationary phase: Silica gel 60 RP–18F$_{254s}$ pre-coated HPTLC plates, 10 × 10 cm (200 μm) – Merck
2. Mobile phase (MP): 0.5 M sodium chloride–methanol–acetonitrile–glacial acetic acid (5 : 2 : 3 : 0.1 v/v)
3. Standard/Sample application:
   Band length: 5 mm Volume applied: 6 μl Spacing: 5 mm
4. Chamber saturation: 20 min (MP)
5. RH (%): 55 ± 5
6. Temperature °C: 22 ± 2
7. Separation technique: Ascending
8. Quantity of mobile phase: 10 ml
9. Migration distance: 50 mm
10. Migration time: 25 min

Densitometric evaluation:

Wavelength: UV–235 nm or 260 nm Scanning mode: Reflectance/Absorbance

HRF: Sulphadoxine—48; Pyrimethamine—72

Linearity (ng/band): Sulphadoxine—50–500; Pyrimethamine—10–100

Recovery (%): 101.50–102 for both the compounds

References: —

Comments:

- The method was optimized and analytical work carried out at **Anchrom's HPTLC Application Laboratory**, Mumbai, India.
- RP-chromatography using non-halogenated mobile phase resulted in reversal of retention order as compared to NP-chromatography.
- Several market samples of similar composition were analysed by the proposed method and found to give reproducible results.

HPTLC : High Performance Thin Layer Chromatography
HPTLC Densitogram

No. 250

H_2N—C6H4—SO_2NH—C4H2N2—OCH_3

Sulphamethoxypyrazine

H_2N—pyrimidine(C_2H_5, NH_2)—C6H4—Cl

Pyrimethamine

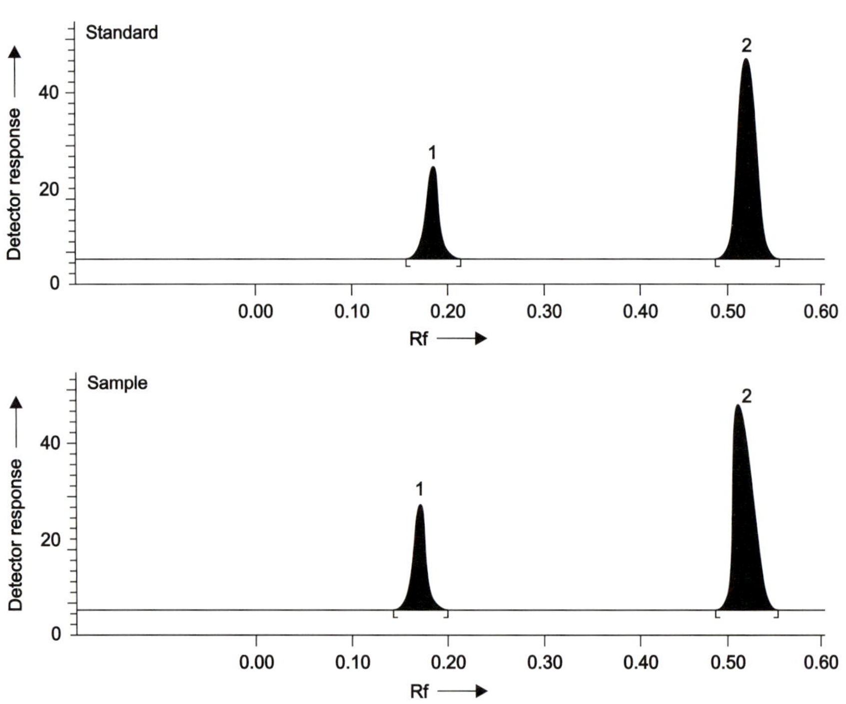

Typical densitogram of the standard and the sample containing sulphamethoxypyrazine and pyrimethamine. For detailed experimental and chromatographic conditions, refer to Protocol No. 250. Peaks identification: 1. Pyrimethamine; 2. Sulphamethoxypyrazine.

PROTOCOL FOR HPTLC ANALYSIS OF PHARMACEUTICAL FORMULATION

Protocol No. 250

Formulation: Sulphamethoxypyrazine, Pyrimethamine

Classification: Antibiotics **Dosage form:** Tablets

Standard preparation: Dissolve 25 mg of pyrimethamine (P) in 10 ml of methanol. Take 25 mg of sulphamethoxypyrazine, add 0.5 ml of solution (P) and 0.2 ml of 25% ammonia, dilute to 10 ml. Further dilute 0.1 ml to 10 ml with methanol for chromatographic application.

Sample preparation: Suspend powdered sample equivalent to 250 mg of sulphamethoxypyrazine in 70 ml of methanol, add 2 ml of 25% ammonia, sonicate for 5 min, dilute to 100 ml, filter and dilute 0.1 ml of filtrate to 10 ml with methanol and use for application.

Chromatographic equipments:

Sample applicator: Camag Linomat–IV
Development chamber: Camag twin-trough glass chamber, 10 × 10 cm
Densitometric scanner: Camag TLC Scanner–II

Chromatographic conditions:

1. Stationary phase: Silica gel $60F_{254}$ pre-coated HPTLC plates, 10 × 10 cm (200 μm) – Merck
2. Mobile phase (MP): Chloroform–methanol (12 : 0.5 v/v)
3. Standard/Sample application:
   Band length: 5 mm Volume applied: 6 μl Spacing: 5 mm
4. Chamber saturation: 20 min (MP)
5. RH (%): 55 ± 5
6. Temperature °C: 22 ± 2
7. Separation technique: Ascending
8. Quantity of mobile phase: 12 ml
9. Migration distance: 50 mm
10. Migration time: 22 min

Densitometric evaluation:

Wavelength: UV–235 nm or 260 nm Scanning mode: Reflectance/Absorbance
HRF: Pyrimethamine—17; Sulphamethoxypyrazine—52
Linearity (ng/band): Pyrimethamine—10–100; Sulphamethoxypyrazine—50–500
Recovery (%): 99.25–100.75 for both the compounds

References: —

Comments:

- The method was optimized and analytical work carried out at **Anchrom's HPTLC Application Laboratory**, Mumbai, India.
- Several market samples of similar composition were analysed by the proposed method and found to give reproducible results.
- The above chromatographic conditions could be used to differentiate different sulphonamides.

HPTLC : High Performance Thin Layer Chromatography
HPTLC Densitogram

No. 251

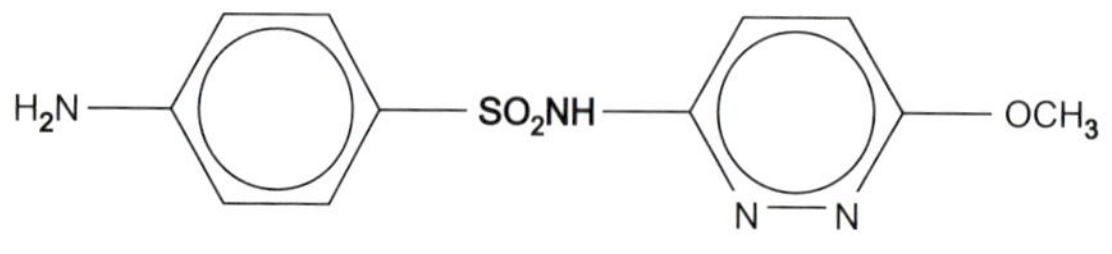

H_2N — SO_2NH — OCH_3 N N

Sulphamethoxypyridazine

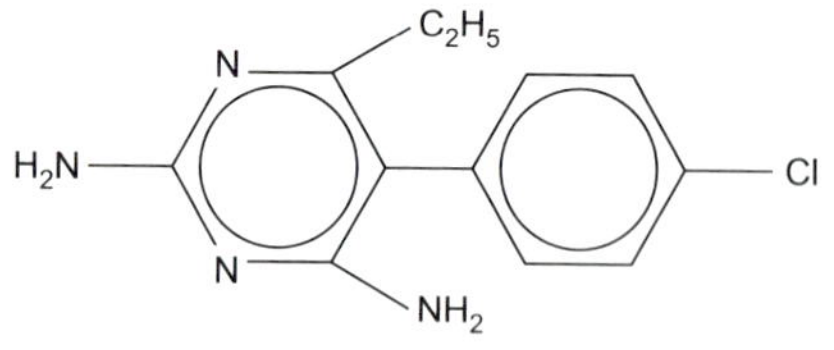

C_2H_5 N H_2N Cl N NH_2

Pyrimethamine

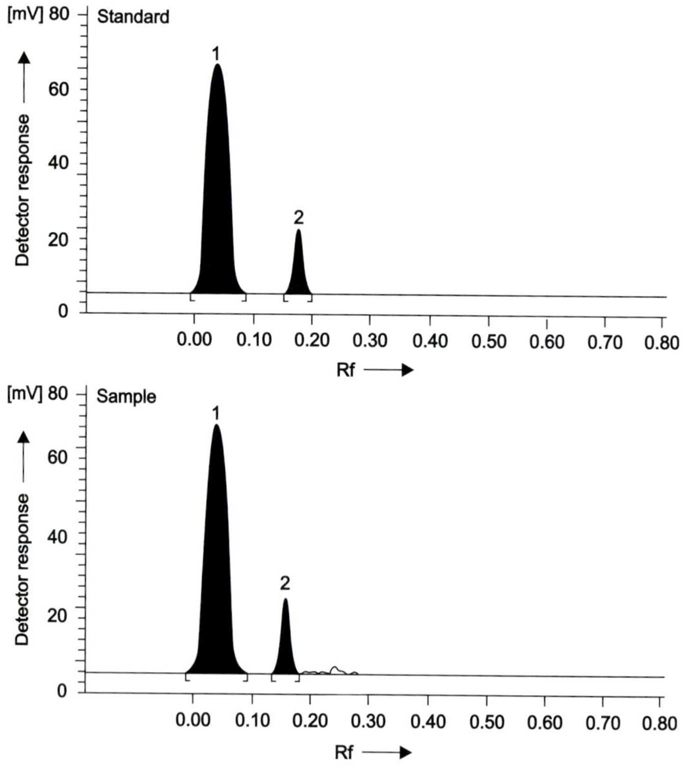

[mV] 80 Standard
Detector response
60 40 20 0
1 2
0.00 0.10 0.20 0.30 0.40 0.50 0.60 0.70 0.80
Rf

[mV] 80 Sample
Detector response
60 40 20 0
1 2
0.00 0.10 0.20 0.30 0.40 0.50 0.60 0.70 0.80
Rf

Typical densitogram of the standard and the sample containing sulphamethoxypyridazine and pyrimethamine. For detailed experimental and chromatographic conditions, refer to Protocol No. 251. Peaks identification: 1. Sulphamethoxypyridazine; 2. Pyrimethamine.

PROTOCOL FOR HPTLC ANALYSIS OF PHARMACEUTICAL FORMULATION

Protocol No. 251

Formulation: Sulphamethoxypyridazine, Pyrimethamine

Classification: Antibiotics **Dosage form:** Tablets

Standard preparation: Dissolve 25 mg of pyrimethamine (P) in 10 ml of methanol. Take 25 mg of sulphamethoxypyridazine, add 0.5 ml of solution P and 0.2 ml of 25% ammonia, dilute to 10 ml. Further dilute 0.1 ml of 10 ml with methanol for chromatographic application.

Sample preparation: Suspend powdered sample equivalent to 250 mg of sulphamethoxypyridazine in 70 ml of methanol, add 2 ml of 25% ammonia, sonicate for 5 min, dilute to 100 ml, filter and dilute 0.1 ml of filtrate to 10 ml with methanol and use for application.

Chromatographic equipments:

Sample applicator: Camag Linomat–IV

Development chamber: Camag twin-trough glass chamber, 10 × 10 cm

Densitometric scanner: Camag TLC Scanner–II

Chromatographic conditions:

1. Stationary phase: Silica gel $60F_{254}$ pre-coated HPTLC plates, 10 × 10 cm (200 μm) – Merck
2. Mobile phase (MP): Chloroform–methanol (12 : 0.5 v/v)
3. Standard/Sample application:
   Band length: 5 mm Volume applied: 6 μl Spacing: 5 mm
4. Chamber saturation: 15 min (MP)
5. RH (%): 55 ± 5
6. Temperature °C: 22 ± 2
7. Separation technique: Ascending
8. Quantity of mobile phase: 12 ml
9. Migration distance: 50 mm
10. Migration time: 22 min

Densitometric evaluation:

Wavelength: UV–235 nm or 260 nm Scanning mode: Reflectance/Absorbance

HRF: Sulphamethoxypyridazine—5; Pyrimethamine—17

Linearity (ng/band): Sulphamethoxypyridazine—50–500; Pyrimethamine—10–100

Recovery (%): 100.50–101.50 for both the compounds

References: —

Comments:

- The method was optimized and analytical work carried out at **Anchrom's HPTLC Application Laboratory**, Mumbai, India.
- Several market samples of similar composition were analysed by the proposed method and found to give reproducible results.

HPTLC : High Performance Thin Layer Chromatography
HPTLC Densitogram

No. 252

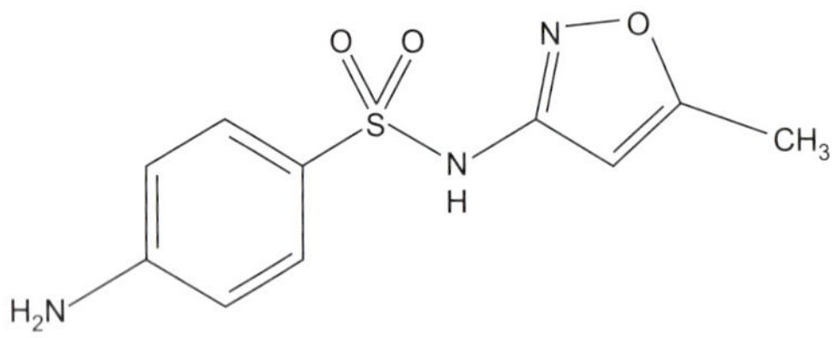

Sulphamethoxazole

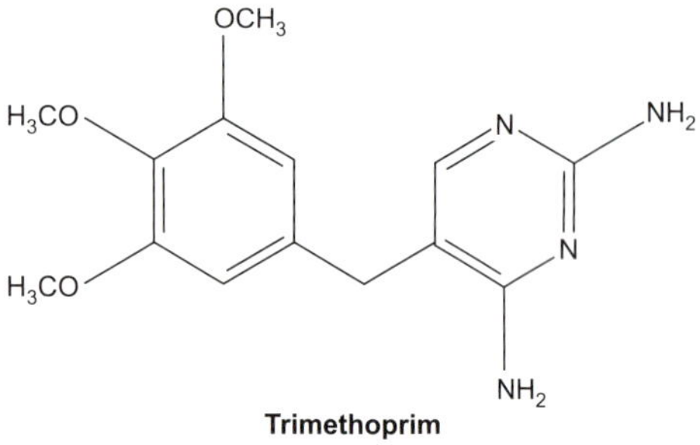

Trimethoprim

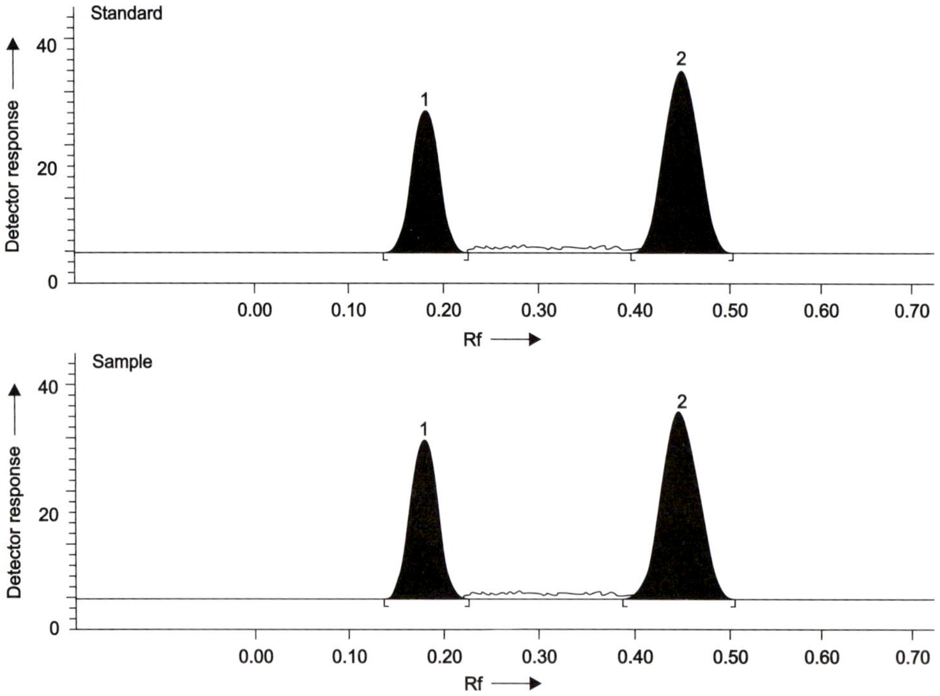

Standard

Sample

Typical densitogram of the standard and the sample containing trimethoprim and sulphamethoxazole. For detailed experimental and chromatographic conditions, refer to Protocol No. 252. Peaks identification: 1. Trimethoprim; 2. Sulphamethoxazole.

PROTOCOL FOR HPTLC ANALYSIS OF PHARMACEUTICAL FORMULATION

Protocol No. 252

Formulation: Sulphamethoxazole, Trimethoprim

Classification: Antibiotics **Dosage form:** Tablets

Standard preparation: (1) 1 mg/ml solution of trimethoprim (TMP) in methanol. (2) 1 mg/ml solution of sulphamethoxazole (SMX) in methanol. Mix 0.2 ml of solution (1) and 1 ml of solution (2) and dilute to 10 ml with methanol. Apply varying volumes for linearity profile.

Sample preparation: Take sample equivalent to 20 mg of TMP, suspend in 50 ml of methanol, sonicate for 10 min, dilute to 100 ml, filter and dilute 1 ml to 10 ml with methanol and use for chromatographic evaluation.

Chromatographic equipments:

Sample applicator: Camag Linomat–IV

Development chamber: Camag twin-trough glass chamber, 10 × 10 cm

Densitometric scanner: Camag TLC Scanner–II

Chromatographic conditions:

1. Stationary phase: Silica gel $60F_{254}$ pre-coated HPTLC plates, 10 × 10 cm (200 μm) – Merck
2. Mobile phase (MP): Chloroform–methanol–DMF (10 : 0.5 : 0.5 v/v)
3. Standard/Sample application:
   Band length: 5 mm Volume applied: 5 μl Spacing: 5 mm
4. Chamber saturation: 15 min (MP)
5. RH (%): 55 ± 5
6. Temperature °C: 22 ± 2
7. Separation technique: Ascending
8. Quantity of mobile phase: 11 ml
9. Migration distance: 50 mm
10. Migration time: 15 min

Densitometric evaluation:

Wavelength: UV–240 nm or 285 nm Scanning mode: Reflectance/Absorbance

HRF: Trimethoprim—18; Sulphamethoxazole—45

Linearity (ng/band): Trimethoprim—50–200; Sulphamethoxazole—250–450

Recovery (%): 98.92–99.74 for both the compounds

References: Camag Application Notes

Comments: Sample could be extracted with chlorofom–methanol mixture (1 : 1 v/v) and chromatographed using methanol–chloroform (1 : 9) as mobile phase in a lined pre-saturated twin-trough chamber (10 × 10 cm), developed for 50 mm (9 min), dried and scanned at 285 mm (HRf: TMP—10, SMX—32).

HPTLC : High Performance Thin Layer Chromatography
HPTLC Densitogram

No. 253

Sulphamethoxazole

Trimethoprim

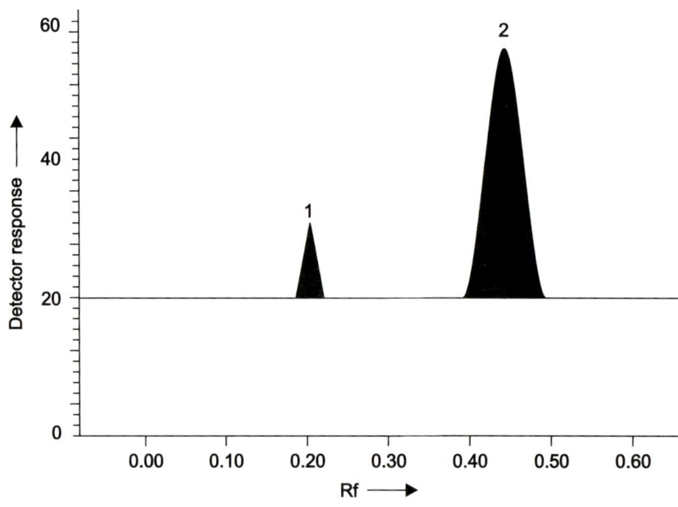

Typical densitogram of the standard containing sulphamethoxazole and trimethoprim. For detailed experimental and chromatographic conditions, refer to Protocol No. 253. Peaks identification: 1. Trimethoprim; 2. Sulphamethoxazole.

PROTOCOL FOR HPTLC ANALYSIS OF PHARMACEUTICAL FORMULATION

Protocol No. 253

Formulation: Sulphamethoxazole, Trimethoprim

Classification: Antibiotics **Dosage form:** Tablets/Suspension

Standard preparation: Prepare 1 mg/ml solution of each drug in methanol. Further serial dilutions made to get range of 10–4000 ng/ml. Apply 10 μl of each solution for analysis.

Sample preparation: An appropriate quantity of the powdered sample suspended in methanol, sonciated for 10 min, filtered and filtrate suitably diluted for chromatographic application and analysis.

Chromatographic equipments:

Sample applicator: Camag Linomat–IV

Development chamber: Camag twin-trough glass chamber, 10 × 10 cm

Densitometric scanner: Camag TLC Scanner–II

Chromatographic conditions:

1. Stationary phase: Silica gel $60F_{254}$ pre-coated HPTLC plates, 10 × 10 cm (200 μm) – Merck
2. Mobile phase (MP): Chloroform–methanol (9 : 1 v/v)
3. Standard/Sample application:
   Band length: 10 mm Volume applied: 10 μl Spacing: 10 mm
4. Chamber saturation: 30 min (MP)
5. RH (%): 55 ± 5
6. Temperature °C: 22 ± 2
7. Separation technique: Ascending
8. Quantity of mobile phase: 10 ml
9. Migration distance: 80 mm
10. Migration time: 40 min

Densitometric evaluation:

Wavelength: UV–254 nm Scanning mode: Reflectance/Absorbance

HRF: Trimethoprim—20; Sulphamethoxazole—45

Linearity (ng/band): Sulphamethoxazole—250–1050; Trimethoprim—50–250

Recovery (%): 98.75–101.25 for both the compounds

References: J.K. Lalla, S.U. Bhat, N.R. Sandhu and M.U. Shah, *Indian Drugs*, **34(5)**, 275–282, 1997.

Comments:

- The method validated for accuracy, precision, linearity, LOD, LOQ, specificity, selectivity and ruggedness.
- The method is suitable for dissolution profile (0.1 N HCl, 37°C, 60 rpm).

HPTLC : High Performance Thin Layer Chromatography
HPTLC Densitogram

No. 254

Sulphamethoxazole

Trimethoprim

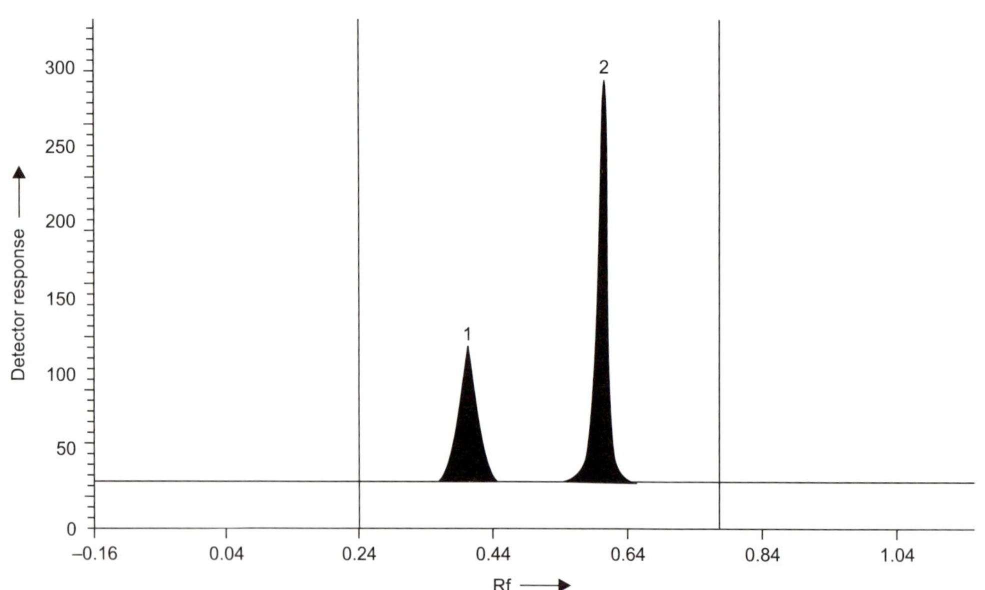

Typical densitogram of the standard containing trimethoprim and sulphamethoxazole. For detailed experimental and chromatographic conditions, refer to Protocol No. 254. Peaks identification: 1. Trimethoprim; 2. Sulphamethoxazole.

PROTOCOL FOR HPTLC ANALYSIS OF PHARMACEUTICAL FORMULATION

Protocol No. 254

Formulation: Sulphamethoxazole, Trimethoprim

Classification: Antibiotics **Dosage form:** Tablets

Standard preparation: Prepare stock solution of each substance in methanol to get 660 μg/ml of sulphamethoxazole and 816 μg/ml of trimethoprim. Further serial dilutions made with methanol for linearity study. Apply 2 μl of each solution for analysis.

Sample preparation: Powdered sample equivalent to 36 mg of trimethoprim suspended in 70 ml of methanol, sonicated for 10 min, diluted to 100 ml with methanol. The resulting solution was filtered and filtrate suitably diluted with methanol and used for assay applying 2 μl of the solution.

Chromatographic equipments:

Sample applicator: Camag Linomat–IV

Development chamber: Camag twin-trough glass chamber, 10 × 20 cm

Densitometric scanner: Camag TLC Scanner–II

Chromatographic conditions:

1. Stationary phase: Silica gel $60F_{254}$ pre-coated HPTLC plates, 10 × 20 cm (200 μm) – Merck
2. Mobile phase (MP): Toluene–ethyl acetate–methanol (50 : 28.5 : 21.5 v/v)
3. Standard/Sample application:
   Band length: 6 mm Volume applied: 2 μl Spacing: 10 mm
4. Chamber saturation: 15 min (MP)
5. RH (%): 55 ± 5
6. Temperature °C: 22 ± 2
7. Separation technique: Ascending
8. Quantity of mobile phase: 20 ml
9. Migration distance: 80 mm
10. Migration time: 25 min

Densitometric evaluation:

Wavelength: UV–254 nm Scanning mode: Reflectance/Absorbance

HRF: Trimethoprim—38; Sulphamethoxazole—61

Linearity (ng/band): Sulphamethoxazole—52.8–264; Trimethoprim—50–400

Recovery (%): 99.0–99.66 for both the compounds

References: D.H. Shewiyo, E-Kaale, P.G. Risha, B. Dejaegher, J. Smeyers-Verbeke, Y. Vander Heyden, *J. Chromatogr. A.*, **1216**, 7102–7107, 2009.

Comments: The method validated for accuracy, precision, linearity, LOD, LOQ, specificity and robustness.

HPTLC : High Performance Thin Layer Chromatography
HPTLC Densitogram

No. 255

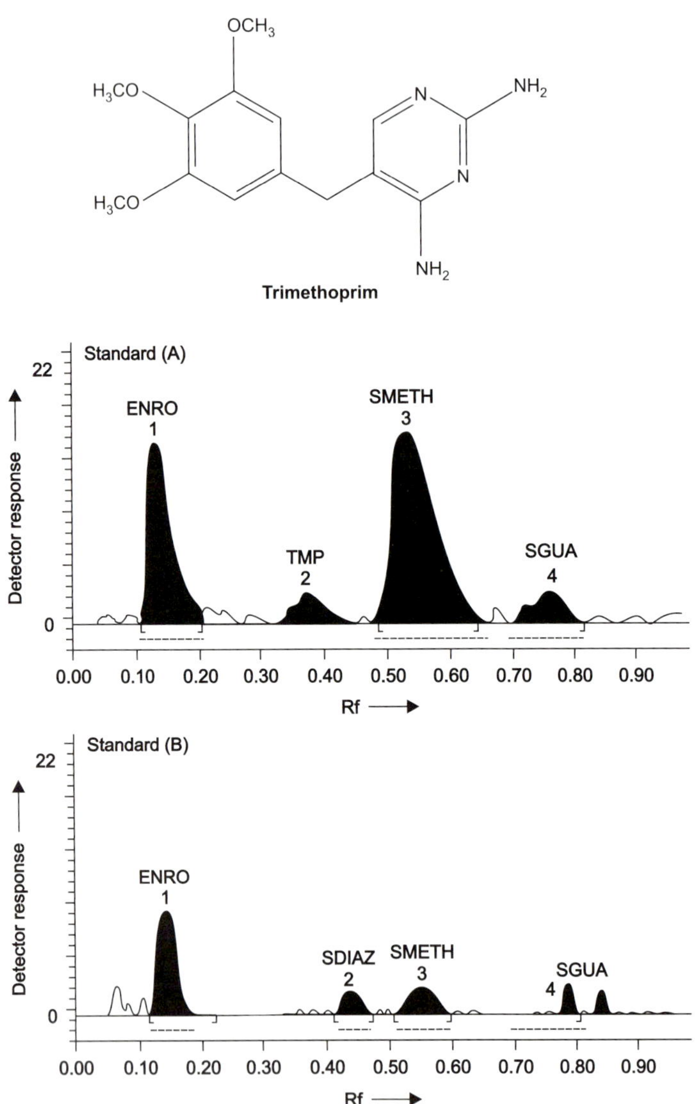

Typical densitogram of the standard (A and B) containing different antibiotics. For detailed experimental and chromatographic conditions, refer to Protocol No. 255. Peaks identification: (A) 1. ENRO; 2. TMP; 3. SMETH; 4. SGUA; (B) 1. ENRO; 2. SDIAZ; 3. SMETH; 4. SGUA.

PROTOCOL FOR HPTLC ANALYSIS OF PHARMACEUTICAL FORMULATION

Protocol No. 255

Formulation: Trimethoprim (TMP), Oxytetracycline (OTC), Enrofloxacin (ENRO), Sulphaguanidine (SGUA), Sulphamethazine (SMETH), Sulphadiazine (SDIAZ), Penicillin G-Procaine (PGP)

Classification: Antibiotics **Dosage form:** Production wash water

Standard preparation: Standard solutions of all the compounds were prepared in methanol to get 0.15–1.5 μg/ml (ENRO); 10–60 μg/ml (OTC, TMP, SDIAZ, SMETH and PGP). Apply 5 μl of each solution for linearity profile.

Sample preparation: The sample was concentrated by passing through 60 mg HLB cartridges (Waters), evaporated and residue taken up in methanol for application.

Chromatographic equipments:

Sample applicator: Camag Linomat–IV

Development chamber: Camag twin-trough glass chamber, 10 × 20 cm

Densitometric scanner: Camag TLC Scanner–III

Chromatographic conditions:

1. Stationary phase: CN modified F_{254} pre-coated HPTLC plates, 10 × 20 cm (200 μm) – Merck
2. Mobile phase (MP): 0.05 M oxalic acid–methanol (16.2 : 3.8 v/v)
3. Standard/Sample application:
   Band length: 7 mm Volume applied: 5 μl Spacing: 15 mm
4. Chamber saturation: 15 min (MP)
5. RH (%): 55 ± 5
6. Temperature °C: 22 ± 2
7. Separation technique: Ascending
8. Quantity of mobile phase: 20 ml
9. Migration distance: 70 mm
10. Migration time: 30 min

Densitometric evaluation:

Wavelength: UV–254 nm (TMP); 366 nm-all other compounds

Scanning mode: Reflectance/Absorbance

HRF: Order of migration distance being ENRO; OTC; TMP; SMETH; SDIM; PGP; SGUA

Linearity (ng/μl): ENRO—1.5–15; OTC—100–500; TMP—150–600; SGUA—300–1100; SDIAZ, PGP, SMETH—100–400 ng

Recovery (%): 91.8–101.2 for all the compounds

References: S. Babic, D. Mutard•ić, D. Ašperger, A.J.M. Harvat and M. Kaštelan, *Chromatographia*, **65(1, 2)**, 105–110, 2007

Comments: —

HPTLC : High Performance Thin Layer Chromatography
HPTLC Densitogram

No. 256

Ampicillin

Cloxacillin sodium

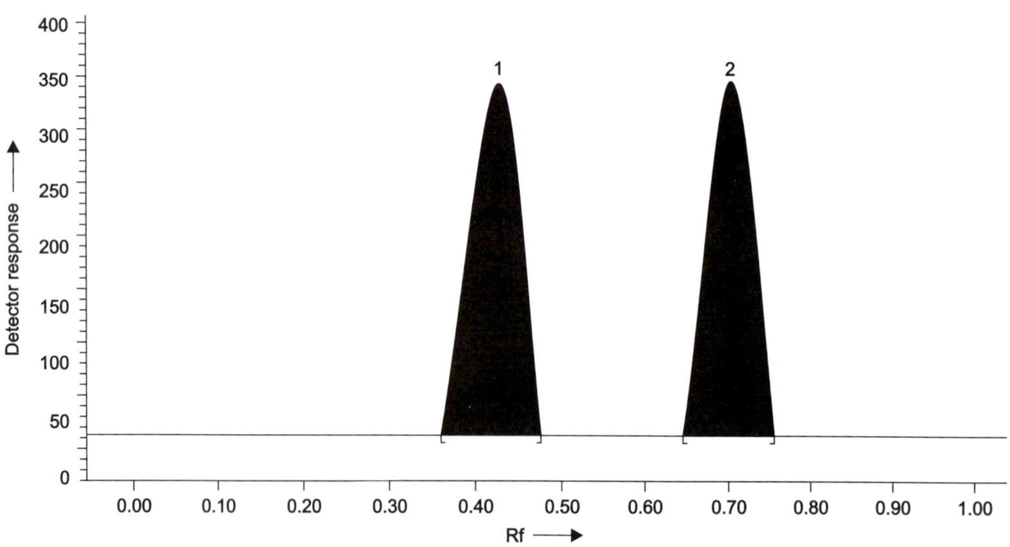

Typical densitogram of the sample containing ampicillin and cloxacillin. For detailed experimental and chromatographic conditions, refer to Protocol No. 256. Peaks identification: 1. Cloxacillin sodium; 2. Ampicillin.

PROTOCOL FOR HPTLC ANALYSIS OF PHARMACEUTICAL FORMULATION

Protocol No. 256

Formulation: **Ampicillin, Cloxacillin sodium**

Classification: Antibiotics

Dosage form: Capsules, Suspension

Standard preparation: Prepare 1 mg/ml solution of each compound in methanol and use for chromatographic application.

Sample preparation: Accurately weighed quantity of the sample equivalent to 100 mg of ampicillin or cloxacillin suspended in methanol, sonicate for 5 min, dilute to 100 ml with methanol. Filter and use for chromatographic analysis.

Chromatographic equipments:

Sample applicator: Camag Linomat–IV

Development chamber: Camag twin-trough glass chamber, 10 × 10 cm

Densitometric scanner: Camag TLC Scanner–III

Chromatographic conditions:

1. Stationary phase: Silica gel RP–$18F_{254s}$ pre-coated HPTLC plates; 10 × 10 cm (250 μm) Whatman
2. Mobile phase (MP): Methanol–0.1 M K_2HPO_4 (5.5 : 4.5 v/v)
3. Standard/Sample application:
   Band length: 5 mm Volume applied: 5 μl Spacing: 5 mm
4. Chamber saturation: —
5. RH (%): 55 ± 5
6. Temperature °C: 22 ± 2
7. Separation technique: Ascending
8. Quantity of mobile phase: 10 ml
9. Migration distance: 100 mm
10. Migration time: 50 min

Densitometric evaluation:

Wavelength: Vis. 490 nm Scanning mode: Reflectance/Absorbance

HRF: Cloxacillin sodium—42; Ampicillin—70

Linearity: 2–10 μg/band both the compounds

Recovery (%): 99.75–101.35 for both the compounds

References: Whatman TLC Technical Series, Application Notes.

Comments:

- Due to possibility of nucelophilic reaction of β-lactam molecule with NP silica gel, it is preferable to analyse the sample on RP-stationary phase.
- After development, the plate air dried and dipped (1 s) in ninhydrin reagent, heated at 105°C and scanned at 490 nm.

HPTLC : High Performance Thin Layer Chromatography
HPTLC Densitogram

No. 257

Cefixime trihydrate

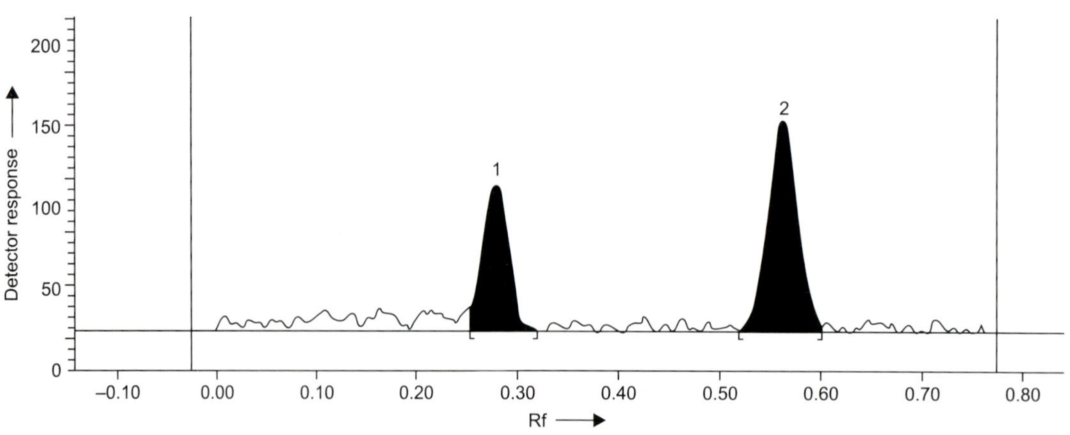

Typical densitogram of the standard containing cefixime trihydrate and dicloxacillin Na^+. For detailed experimental and chromatographic conditions, refer to Protocol No. 257. Peaks identification: 1. Cefixime trihydrate; 2. Dicloxacillin Na^+.

PROTOCOL FOR HPTLC ANALYSIS OF PHARMACEUTICAL FORMULATION

Protocol No. 257

Formulation: Cefixime trihydrate, Dicloxacillin sodium

Classification: Antibiotics **Dosage form:** Tablets

Standard preparation: Prepare solution of both the compounds separately in methanol to get 200 μg/ml of cefixime trihydrate and 500 μg/ml of dicloxacillin sodium. Apply varying volumes of each solution for linearity profile.

Sample preparation: Powdered sample equivalent to 2 mg of cefixime trihydrate and 5 mg of dicloxacillin sodium suspended in 8 ml of methanol, sonicated for 10 min, diluted to 10 ml, filtered and filtrate used for assay of both the ingredients.

Chromatographic equipments:

Sample applicator: Camag Linomat–V

Development chamber: Camag twin-trough glass chamber, 20 × 10 cm

Densitometric scanner: Camag TLC Scanner–III

Chromatographic conditions:

1. Stationary phase: Silica gel $60F_{254}$ pre-coated TLC plates, 10 × 10 cm (250 μm) – Merck, pre-washed with methanol and dried prior to use
2. Mobile phase (MP): Toluene–methanol–triethylamine (5 : 4 : 1 v/v)
3. Standard/Sample application:
   Band length: 5 mm Volume applied: 1–3 μl Spacing: 10 mm
4. Chamber saturation: 15 min (MP)
5. RH (%): 55 ± 5
6. Temperature °C: Ambient
7. Separation technique: Ascending
8. Quantity of mobile phase: 10 ml
9. Migration distance: 80 mm
10. Migration time: 20 min

Densitometric evaluation:

Wavelength: UV–254 nm Scanning mode: Reflectance/Absorbance

HRF: Cefixime trihydrate—26; Cloxacillin Na^+—57

Linearity (ng/band): Cefixime—200–600; Cloxacillin Na^+—500–1500

Recovery (%): 99.40–99.93 for both the compounds

References: Manan B. Tank, Kashyap N. Thumar and Navin R. Sheth, Manuscript submitted for Dr. P.D. Sethi Award, 2011. Data courtesy Prof. Kashyap.

Comments: The method validated for accuracy, precision, linearity, LOD, LOQ, specificity and robustness.

HPTLC : High Performance Thin Layer Chromatography
HPTLC Densitogram

No. 258

Cefpodoxime proxetil

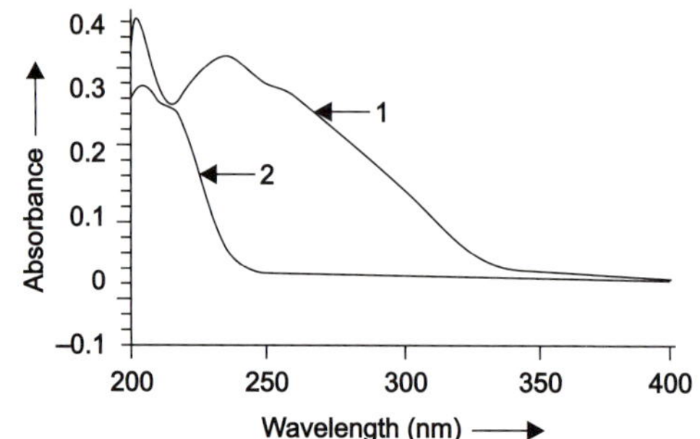

Overlaid UV-spectra of cefpodoxime proxetil (1) and potassium clavulanate (2) for selection of suitable wavelength for densitometric scanning

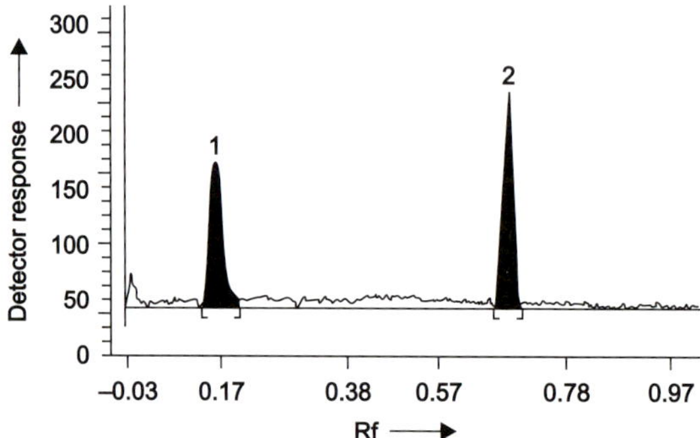

Typical densitogram of the standard containing cefpodoxime proxetil and potassium clavulanate. For detailed experimental and chromatographic condition refer to Protocol No. 258. Peaks identification: 1. Potassium clavulanate; 2. Cefpodoxime proxetil.

PROTOCOL FOR HPTLC ANALYSIS OF PHARMACEUTICAL FORMULATION

Protocol No. 258

Formulation: **Cefpodoxime proxetil, Potassium clavulanate**

Classification: Antibiotics **Dosage form:** Tablets

Standard preparation: Prepare 1 mg/ml solution of each compound separately in methanol. Further dilutions made to get 250 μg/ml of cefpodoxime proxetil and 1000 μg/ml of potassium clavulanate. Apply 2–10 μl of each solution and carry out chromatographic analysis for linearity profile.

Sample preparation: Weigh accurately powdered sample equivalent to 10 mg of cefpodoxime proxetil, suspend in 5 ml of methanol, sonicate for 5 min and dilute to 10 ml with methanol. Filter through Whatman No. 41 filter paper. Dilute 2.5 ml of the filtrate to 10 ml with methanol and apply 4 μl for chromatographic analysis.

Chromatographic equipments:

Sample applicator: Camag Linomat–V

Development chamber: Camag twin–trough glass chamber, 20 × 10 cm

Densitometric scanner: Camag TLC Scanner–III

Chromatographic conditions:

1. Stationary phase: Silica gel $60F_{254}$ pre-coated HPTLC plates, 20 × 10 cm (200 μm) – Merck, pre-washed with methanol and activated at 110°C for 5 min prior to use
2. Mobile phase (MP): Chloroform–methanol–toluene (4 : 3 : 3 v/v)
3. Standard/Sample application:
   Band length: 6 mm Volume applied: 2–10 μl Spacing: 10 mm
4. Chamber saturation: 30 min (MP)
5. RH (%): 55 ± 5
6. Temperature °C: 22 ± 2
7. Separation technique: Ascending
8. Quantity of mobile phase: 20 ml
9. Migration distance: 90 mm
10. Migration time: 30 min

Densitometric evaluation:

Wavelength: UV–215 nm or 315 nm (iso-absorption point)

Scanning mode: Reflectance/Absorbance

HRF: Potassium clavulanate—16; Cefpodoxime proxetil—66

Linearity range (ng band): Cefpodoxime proxetil—500–2500; Potassium clavulanate—2000–10,000

Recovery (%): Cefpodoxime proxetil—99.05–100.25; Potassium clavulanate—97.55–99.25

References: S.V. Gandhi, P.B. Deshpande, U.P. Patel, P.J. Mundhe and P.R. Deshmukh, *Pharma Review*, 148–150, Nov–Dec, 2010.

Comments: The method validated for accuracy, precision, linearity, LOD, LOQ, specificity, robustness and ruggedness.

HPTLC : High Performance Thin Layer Chromatography
HPTLC Densitogram

No. 259

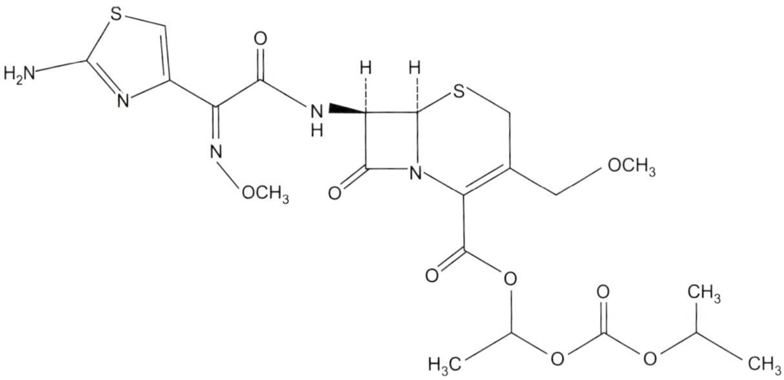

Cefpodoxime proxetil

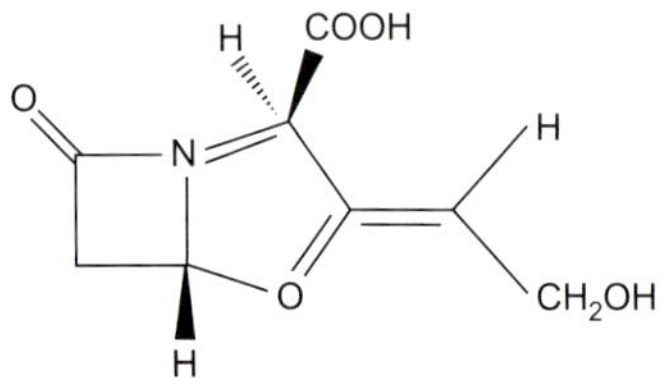

Potassium clavulanate

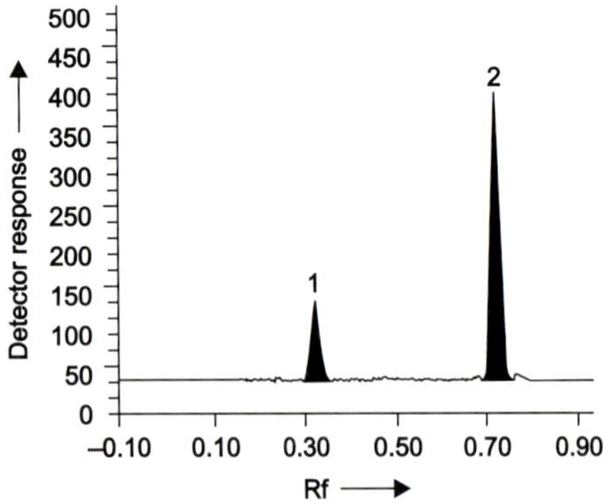

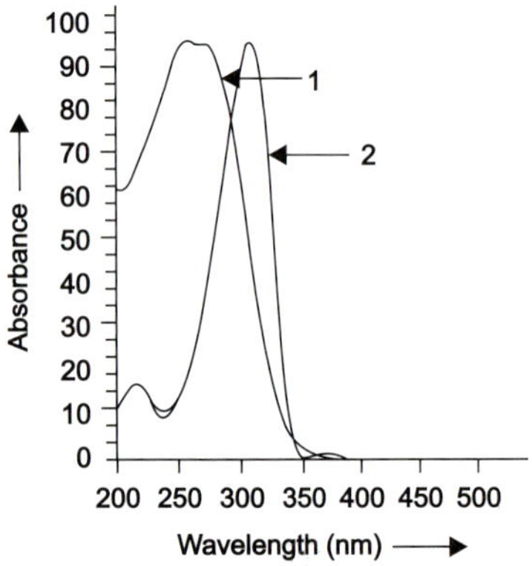

Overlaid UV-spectra of cefpodoxime proxetil (1) and potassium clavulanate (2) for selection of suitable wavelength for densitometric scanning

Typical densitogram of the sample containing cefpodoxime proxetil and potassium clavulanate. For detailed experimental and chromatographic conditions, refer to Protocol No. 259. Peaks identification: 1. Potassium clavulanate; 2. Cefpodoxime proxetil.

PROTOCOL FOR HPTLC ANALYSIS OF PHARMACEUTICAL FORMULATION

Protocol No. 259

Formulation: Cefpodoxime proxetil, Potassium clavulanate
Classification: Antibiotics **Dosage form:** Tablets
Standard preparation: Prepare 1 mg/ml solution of each compound in solvent. Apply varying volumes of standard solution of each compound for chromatographic evaluation after suitable dilution.
Solvent: Methanol–water (60 : 40 v/v).
Sample preparation: Weigh powdered sample equivalent to 100 mg of cefpodoxime proxetil, suspend in 70 ml of solvent, sonicate for 30 min, dilute to 100 ml with the solvent, filter through Whatman filter paper No. 42 and apply 1 μl of the filtrate for chromatographic analysis.
Chromatographic equipments:
Sample applicator: Camag Linomat–IV
Development chamber: Camag twin-trough glass chamber, 10 × 10 cm
Densitometric scanner: Camag TLC Scanner–III
Chromatographic conditions:
1. Stationary phase: Silica gel 60F_{254} pre-coated TLC plates, 10 × 10 cm (250 μm) – Merck, pre-washed with methanol, activated at 110°C for 15 min, prior to use
2. Mobile phase (MP): Toluene–methanol–chloroform–acetonitrile (4 : 3 : 2 : 1.5 v/v)
3. Standard/Sample application:
   Band length: 10 mm Volume applied: 1–10 μl Spacing: 10 mm
4. Chamber saturation: 30 min (MP)
5. RH (%): 55 ± 5
6. Temperature °C: 25 ± 2
7. Separation technique: Ascending
8. Quantity of mobile phase: 10 ml
9. Migration distance: 80 mm
10. Migration time: 20 min

Densitometric evaluation:
Wavelength: UV–278 nm or 315 nm (isobestic point)
Scanning mode: Reflectance/Absorbance
HRF: Potassium clavulanate—33; Cefpodoxime proxetil—72
Linearity (ng/band): Cefpodoxime proxetil—250–3500; Potassium clavulanate—100–4500
Recovery (%): 99.75–100.75 for both the compounds
References: A.B. Thomas, S.B. Dighe, R.K. Nanda, L.P. Kotha Pali, S.N. Jagdale and A.D. Deshpande, *J. Liq. Chromatogr. and Related Tech.*, **33**, 1689–1703, 2010.
Comments:
- The method validated for accuracy, precision, linearity, LOD, LOQ, specificity, robustness and ruggedness.
- The method is stability indicating (acid, base, oxidative, thermal, photolytic). The degradation products were separated from main compounds.

HPTLC : High Performance Thin Layer Chromatography
HPTLC Densitogram

No. 260

Cefuroxime axetil

Potassium clavulanate

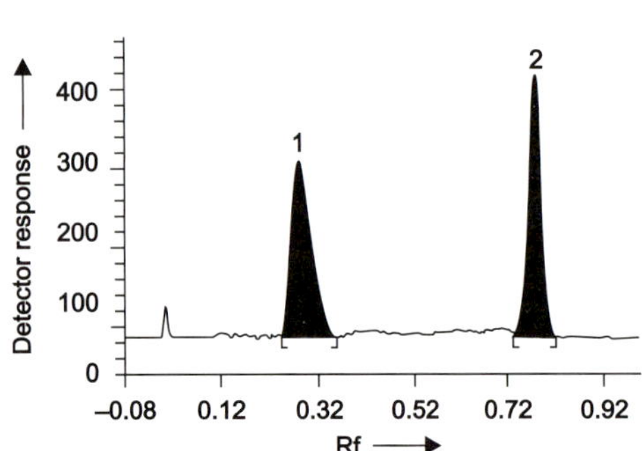

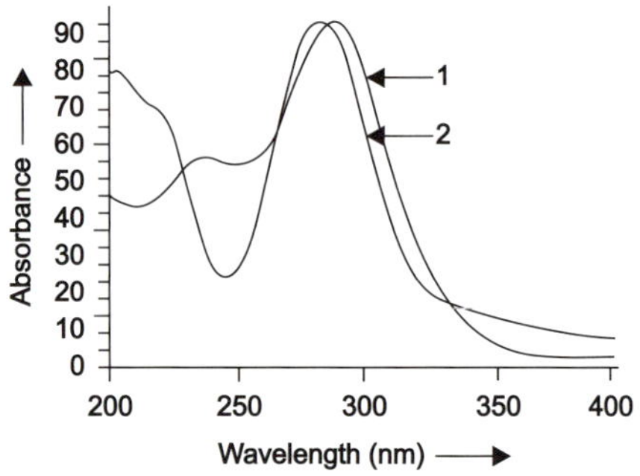

Overlaid UV-spectra of cefuroxime (1) and potassium clavulanate (2) for selection of suitable wavelength for densitometric scanning

Typical densitogram of the standard containing cefuroxime axetil and potassium clavulanate. For detailed experimental and chromatographic conditions, refer to Protocol No. 260. Peaks identification: 1. Potassium clavulanate; 2. Cefuroxime axetil.

PROTOCOL FOR HPTLC ANALYSIS OF PHARMACEUTICAL FORMULATION

Protocol No. 260

Formulation: Cefuroxime axetil, Potassium clavulanate

Classification: Antibiotics **Dosage form:** Tablets

Standard preparation: Prepare 1 mg/ml solution of both the compounds in methanol. Further dilutions are made to get 250 µg/ml of cefuroxime axetil and use solution of potassium clavulanate as such.

Sample preparation: Powdered sample equivalent to 10 mg of cefuroxime axetil suspended in 5 ml of methanol, sonicated for 5 min, diluted to 10 ml with methanol. Further dilutions made suitably and apply 4 µl for assay.

Chromatographic equipments:

Sample applicator: Camag Linomat–V

Development chamber: Camag twin-trough glass chamber, 20 × 10 cm

Densitometric scanner: Camag TLC Scanner–III

Chromatographic conditions:

1. Stationary phase: Silica gel $60F_{254}$ pre-coated HPTLC plates, 20 × 10 cm (200 µm) – Merck, pre-washed with methanol and activated at 110°C for 5 min prior to use
2. Mobile phase (MP): Chloroform–methanol–toluene (4 : 3 : 3 v/v)
3. Standard/Sample application:
   Band length: 6 mm Volume applied: 2–10 µl Spacing: 6.8 mm
4. Chamber saturation: 30 min (MP)
5. RH (%): 55 ± 5
6. Temperature °C: 22 ± 2
7. Separation technique: Ascending
8. Quantity of mobile phase: 20 ml
9. Migration distance: 90 mm
10. Migration time: 30 min

Densitometric evaluation:

Wavelength: UV–225 nm

Scanning mode: Reflectance/Absorbance

HRF: Potassium clavulanate—29; Cefuroxime axetil—77

Linearity (ng/band): Cefuroxime axetil—500–2500; Potassium clavulanate—2000–10,000

Recovery (%): Cefuroxime axetil—98.80–101.48; Potassium clavulanate—99.40–101.26

References: R. Senegar, S.V. Gandhi, U.P. Patil, V.S. Rajmane and K.G. Bothara, *Acta Chromatographica*, **22(1)**, 91–97, 2010.

Comments: The method was validated for accuracy, precision, linearity, LOD and LOQ as per ICH guidelines.

HPTLC : High Performance Thin Layer Chromatography
HPTLC Densitogram

No. 261

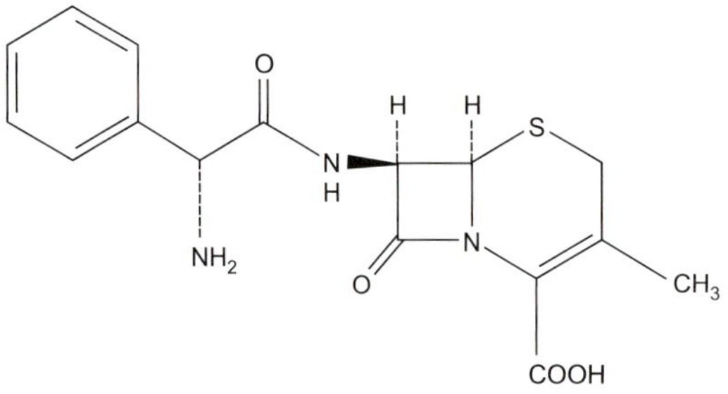

Cephalexin

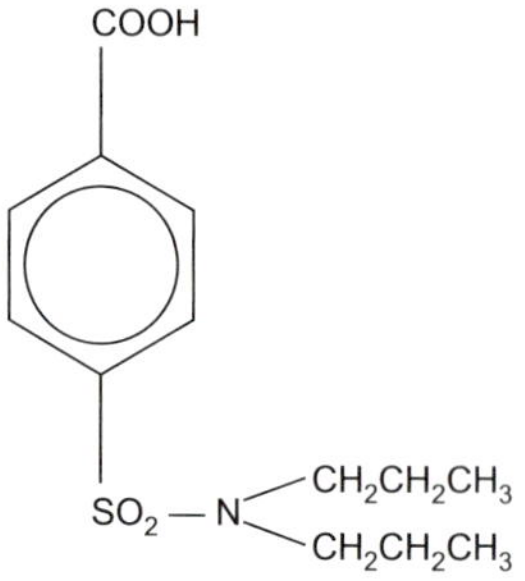

Probenecid

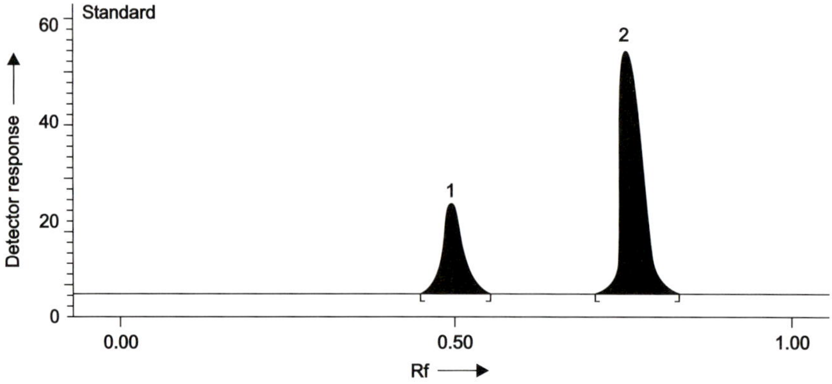

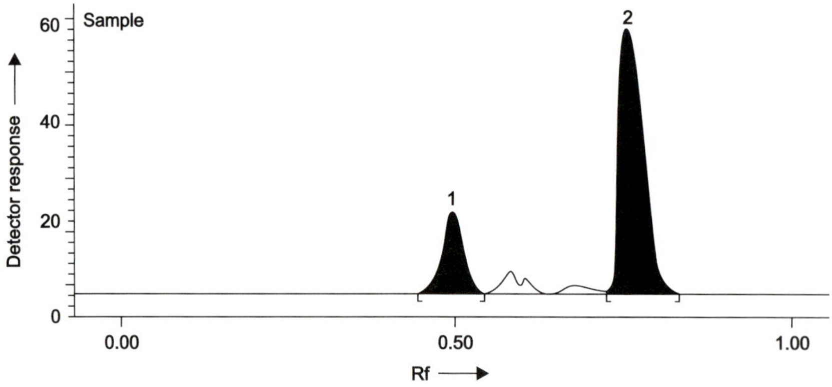

Standard

Sample

Typical densitogram of the standard and sample containing cephalexin and probenecid. For detailed experimental and chromatographic conditions, refer to Protocol No. 261. Peaks identification: 1. Cephalexin; 2. Probenecid.

PROTOCOL FOR HPTLC ANALYSIS OF PHARMACEUTICAL FORMULATION

Protocol No. 261

Formulation: Cephalexin, Probenecid

Classification: Antibiotics **Dosage form:** Capsules, Tablets

Standard preparation: Prepare 500 μg/ml solution of both the compounds in methanol. Further dilute 2.5 ml of each solution to 10 ml with methanol and use for chromatographic analysis.

Sample preparation: Powdered sample equivalent to 125 mg of cephalexin suspended in 30–40 ml of methanol, sonicated for 10 min, diluted to 50 ml. Filter and dilute 0.5 ml to 10 ml with methanol and use for chromatographic evaluation.

Chromatographic equipments:

Sample applicator: Camag Linomat–IV

Development chamber: Camag twin-trough glass chamber, 10 × 10 cm

Densitometric scanner: Camag TLC Scanner–III

Chromatographic conditions:

1. Stationary phase: Silica gel $60F_{254}$ pre-coated HPTLC plates, 10 × 10 cm (200 μm) – Merck
2. Mobile phase (MP): Chloroform–methanol–25% ammonia (7 : 2.5 : 0.7 v/v)
3. Standard/Sample application:
   Band length: 5 mm Volume applied: 5 μl Spacing: 5 mm
4. Chamber saturation: 20 min (MP)
5. RH (%): 55 ± 5
6. Temperature °C: 22 ± 2
7. Separation technique: Ascending
8. Quantity of mobile phase: 10 ml
9. Migration distance: 50 mm
10. Migration time: 22 min

Densitometric evaluation:

Wavelength: UV–260 nm Scanning mode: Reflectance/Absorbance

HRF: Cephalexin—50; Probenecid—75

Linearity: 100–1000 ng/band for both the compounds

Recovery (%): 101.98–102.46 for both the compounds

References: —

Comments:

- The method was optimized and analytical work carried out at **Anchrom's HPTLC Application Laboratory**, Mumbai, India.
- The method was routinely used for estimation of both the compounds in plasma for bio-equivalence studies.

HPTLC : High Performance Thin Layer Chromatography
HPTLC Densitogram

No. 262

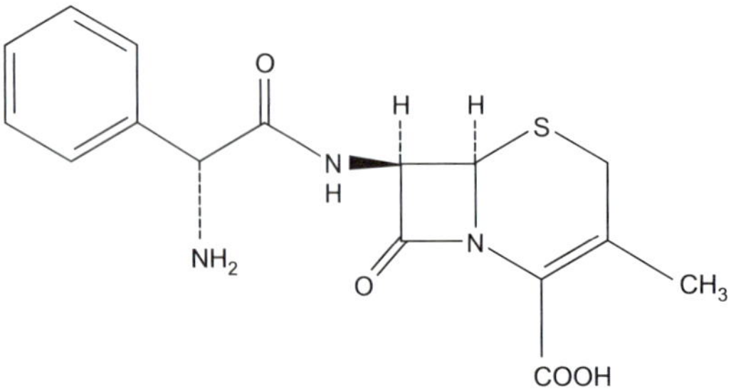

Cephalexin

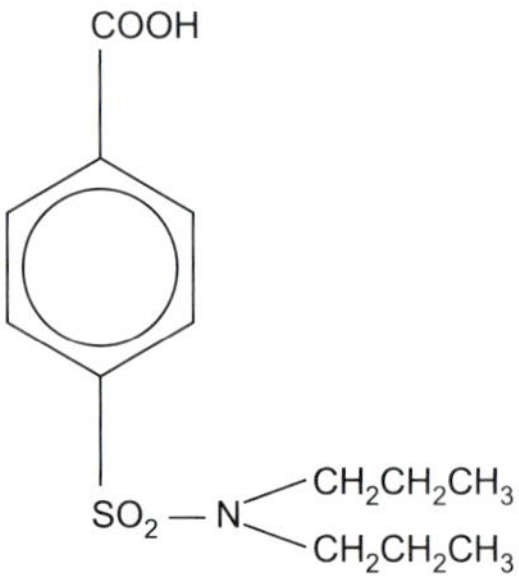

Probenecid

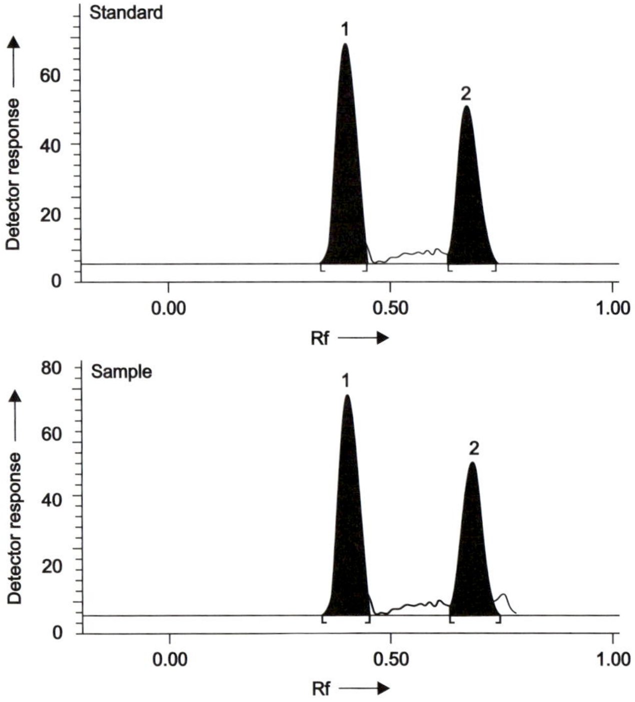

Typical densitogram of the standard and sample containing cephalexin and probenecid. For detailed experimental and chromatographic conditions, refer to Protocol No. 262. Peaks identification: 1. Probenecid; 2. Cephalexin.

PROTOCOL FOR HPTLC ANALYSIS OF PHARMACEUTICAL FORMULATION

Protocol No. 262

Formulation: Cephalexin, Probenecid

Classification: Antibiotics **Dosage form:** Capsules, Tablets

Standard preparation: Prepare 0.5 mg/ml solution of each compound in methanol. Further dilute 2.5 ml of each solution to 10 ml with methanol and use for chromatographic application.

Sample preparation: Powdered sample equivalent to 125 mg of probenecid suspended in 30–40 ml of methanol, sonicated for 5 min, diluted to 50 ml, filtered and 0.5 ml of the filtrate diluted to 10 ml with methanol and used for chromatographic analysis.

Chromatographic equipments:

Sample applicator: Camag Linomat–IV

Development chamber: Camag twin-trough glass chamber, 10 × 10 cm

Densitometric scanner: Camag TLC Scanner–II

Chromatographic conditions:

1. Stationary phase: Silica gel 60 RP–18F$_{254s}$ pre-coated HPTLC plates; 10 × 10 cm (200 μm) – Merck
2. Mobile phase (MP): 0.5 M sodium chloride–methanol–acetonitrile–glacial acetic acid (5 : 2 : 3 : 0.1 v/v)
3. Standard/Sample application:
   Band length: 5 mm Volume applied: 5 μl Spacing: 5 mm
4. Chamber saturation: 20 min (MP)
5. RH (%): 55 ± 5
6. Temperature °C: 22 ± 2
7. Separation technique: Ascending
8. Quantity of mobile phase: 10 ml
9. Migration distance: 50 mm
10. Migration time: 25 min

Densitometric evaluation:

Wavelength: UV–260 nm Scanning mode: Reflectance/Absorbance

HRF: Probenecid—40; Cephalexin—68

Linearity: 100–1000 ng/band

Recovery (%): 101.70–102.93 for both the compounds

References: —

Comments:

- The method was optimized and analytical work carried out at **Anchrom's HPTLC Application Laboratory**, Mumbai, India.
- Reversed-phase chromatography using non-halogen mobile phase resulted in reversal of retention order. When compared to normal-phase chromatography, resolution was better with reversed-phase.

HPTLC : High Performance Thin Layer Chromatography
HPTLC Densitogram

No. 263

Cephalexin

Probenecid

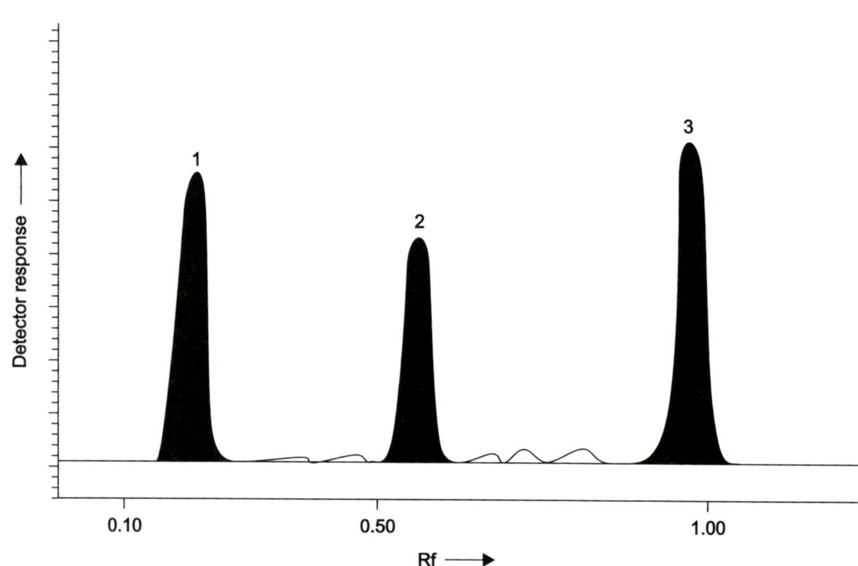

Typical densitogram of the sample containing cephalexin and probenecid. For detailed experimental and chromatographic conditions, refer to Protocol No. 263. Peaks identification: 1. Norfloxacin (IS); 2. Cephalexin; 3. Probenecid.

PROTOCOL FOR HPTLC ANALYSIS OF PHARMACEUTICAL FORMULATION

Protocol No. 263

Formulation: Cephalexin, Probenecid

Classification: Antibiotics **Dosage form:** Tablets

Standard preparation: Prepare 1 mg/ml solution of both the compounds in methanol. Further dilutions made with methanol to get 150–350 μg/ml solution of each. Apply 10 μl of each solution for linearity studies. Internal standard (IS) – 250 μg/ml of norfloxacin in methanol.

Sample preparation: Powdered sample equivalent to 100 mg of cephalexin or probenecid suspended in methanol, sonicated for 10 min, diluted to 100 ml, filtered through 0.45 μm filter. Dilute 2.5 ml of filtrate to 10 ml after adding 1 ml of (IS) solution in methanol. Apply 10 μl of the resulting solution for chromatographic evaluation.

Chromatographic equipments:

Sample applicator: Camag Linomat–IV

Development chamber: Camag twin-trough glass chamber, 10 × 10 cm

Densitometric scanner: Camag TLC Scanner–III

Chromatographic conditions:

1. Stationary phase: Silica gel $60F_{254}$ pre-coated HPTLC plates, 10 × 10 cm (200 μm) – Merck
2. Mobile phase (MP): Chloroform–methanol–25% ammonia (7 : 2.6 : 0.4 v/v)
3. Standard/Sample application:
   Band length: 10 mm Volume applied: 10 μl Spacing: 10 mm
4. Chamber saturation: 15 min (MP)
5. RH (%): 55 ± 5
6. Temperature °C: 22 ± 2
7. Separation technique: Ascending
8. Quantity of mobile phase: 10 ml
9. Migration distance: 70 mm
10. Migration time: 30 min

Densitometric evaluation:

Wavelength: UV–260 nm Scanning mode: Reflectance/Absorbance

HRF: Norfloxacin (IS)—15; Cephalexin—54; Probenecid—95

Linearity (ng/band): 100–1500 for both the compounds

Recovery (%): 100.38–100.68 for both the compounds

References: U.P. Halkar and N.P. Bhandari, *Indian Drugs*, **35(6)**, 382–384, 1998.

Comments: The method was validated for accuracy, precision and linearity.

HPTLC : High Performance Thin Layer Chromatography
HPTLC Densitogram

No. 264

Cephalexin

Cefadroxil

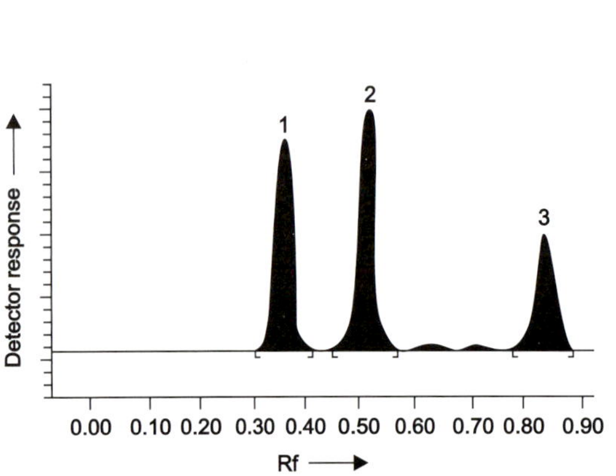

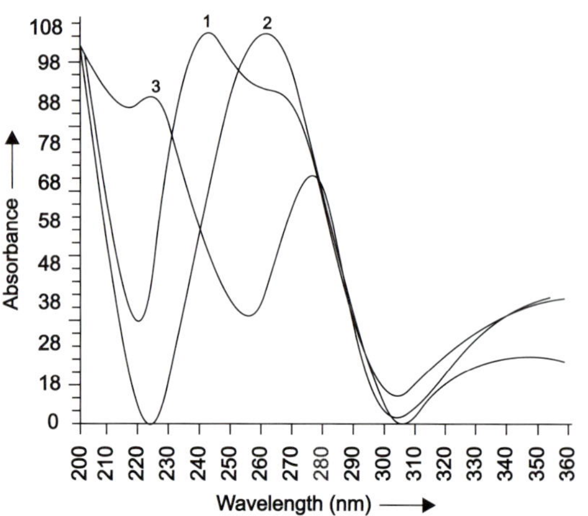

Overlaid UV-spectra of cephalexin (2), cefadroxil (1) and (IS) (3) for selection of suitable wavelength for densitometric scanning

Typical densitogram of the standard containing cephalexin and cefadroxil. For detailed experimental and chromatographic conditions, refer to Protocol No. 264. Peaks identification: 1. Cefadroxil; 2. Cephalexin; 3. p-OH-phenylacetamide (IS).

PROTOCOL FOR HPTLC ANALYSIS OF PHARMACEUTICAL FORMULATION

Protocol No. 264

Formulation: Cephalexin, Cefadroxil

Classification: Antibiotics **Dosage form:** Capsules

Standard preparation: Prepare 2 mg/ml solution of each compound in methanol. Dilute varying volumes (2–10 ml) of the each drug solution to 25 ml with methanol keeping the concentration of (IS) constant. Apply 10 μl of each solution for linearity profile.

Sample preparation: Sample equivalent to 50 mg of cephalexin or cefadroxil suspended in 50–60 ml of methanol, sonicated for 10 min, diluted to 10 ml, filtered and 2 ml of the filtrate diluted to 50 ml after adding 2 ml of (IS) solution (2 mg/ml). Apply 10 μl for chromatographic evaluation.

Chromatographic equipments:

Sample applicator: Camag Linomat–IV

Development chamber: Camag Twin-trough glass chamber, 10 × 10 cm

Densitometric scanner: Camag TLC Scanner–II

Chromatographic conditions:

1. Stationary phase: Silica gel $60F_{254s}$ pre-coated HPTLC plates, 10 × 10 cm (200 μm) – Merck
2. Mobile phase (MP): Chloroform–methanol–acetonitrile–25% ammonia (7.5 : 3.0 : 2.0 : 1.2 v/v)
3. Standard/Sample application:
   Band length: 8 mm Volume applied: 10 μl Spacing: 10 mm
4. Chamber saturation: 20 min (MP)
5. RH (%): 55 ± 5
6. Temperature °C: 22 ± 2
7. Separation technique: Ascending
8. Quantity of mobile phase: 12 ml
9. Migration distance: 90 mm
10. Migration time: 30 min

Densitometric evaluation:

Wavelength: UV–254 nm Scanning mode: Reflectance/Absorbance

HRF: Cefadroxil—36; Cephalexin—51; p-OH-phenylacetamide—(IS)–83

Linearity (ng/band): 200–1000 for both the drugs

Recovery (%): 98.41–99.52 for both the compounds

References: C.V. Shabadi, B.A. Shelar and A.R. Shelar, *Indian Drugs*, **35(12)**, 766–770, 1998.

Comments: —

HPTLC : High Performance Thin Layer Chromatography
HPTLC Densitogram

No. 265

Cefuroxime axetil

Probenecid

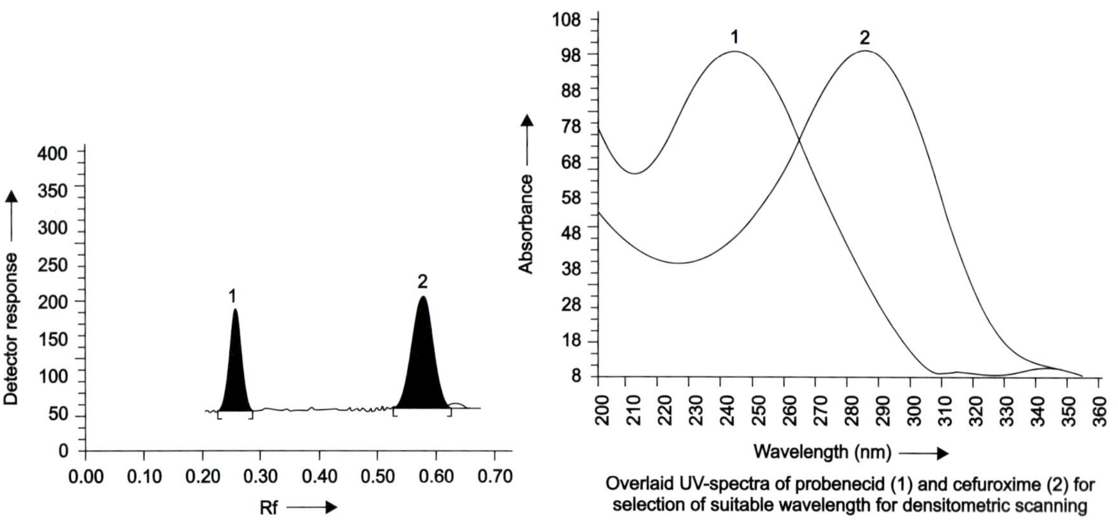

Overlaid UV-spectra of probenecid (1) and cefuroxime (2) for selection of suitable wavelength for densitometric scanning

Typical densitogram of the standard containing probenecid and cefuroxime axetil. For detailed experimental and chromatographic conditions, refer to Protocol No. 265. Peaks identification: 1. Probenecid; 2. Cefuroxime axetil.

PROTOCOL FOR HPTLC ANALYSIS OF PHARMACEUTICAL FORMULATION

Protocol No. 265

Formulation: **Probenecid, Cefuroxime axetil**

Classification: Antibiotics **Dosage form:** Capsules

Standard preparation: Prepare 100 µg/ml solution of each compound in methanol. Apply 1–6 µl of each solution for linearity profile.

Sample preparation: Sample equivalent to 100 mg of probenecid or cefuroxime suspended in 70–80 ml of methanol, sonicated for 15 min, diluted to 100 ml, filtered through Whatman No. 41 filter paper and further dilutions made to get solution of 100 µg/ml and used for chromatographic application.

Chromatographic equipments:

Sample applicator: Camag Linomat–IV

Development chamber: Camag twin-trough glass chamber, 10 × 10 cm

Densitometric scanner: Camag TLC Scanner–III

Chromatographic conditions:

1. Stationary phase: Silica gel 60F_{254} pre-coated HPTLC plates; 10 × 10 cm (200 µm) – Merck pre-washed with methanol, activated at 50°C for 5 min, prior to use
2. Mobile phase (MP): Chloroform–acetonitrile–toluene–acetate buffer, pH 6.0 (5 : 4 : 1 : 0.3 v/v)
3. Standard/Sample application:
   Band length: 10 mm Volume applied: 10 µl Spacing: 10 mm
4. Chamber saturation: 30 min (MP)
5. RH (%): 55 ± 5
6. Temperature °C: 22 ± 2
7. Separation technique: Ascending
8. Quantity of mobile phase: 10 ml
9. Migration distance: 75 mm
10. Migration time: 15 min

Densitometric evaluation:

Wavelength: UV–260 nm Scanning mode: Reflectance/Absorbance

HRF: Probenecid—28; Cefuroxime—58

Linearity: 100–500 ng/band for both the compounds

Recovery (%): 99.2—99.9 for both the compounds

References: K.R. Sireesha et al., *Ind. J. Pharm Sci.*, **66(3)**, 278–282, 2004.

Comments:

- The method validated for accuracy, precision, linearity, specificity, LOD and LOQ.
- Since cephalosporins are likely to undergo degradation on silica gel layers, active polar surface, stability was tested at different times prior to densitometric scanning.
- No decomposition observed during development. No decomposition observed when the drop was spotted and left upto 3 hrs. Decomposition observed 3 hrs. after development of the plate.

HPTLC : High Performance Thin Layer Chromatography
HPTLC Densitogram

No. 266

Ceftriaxone

Cefotaxime

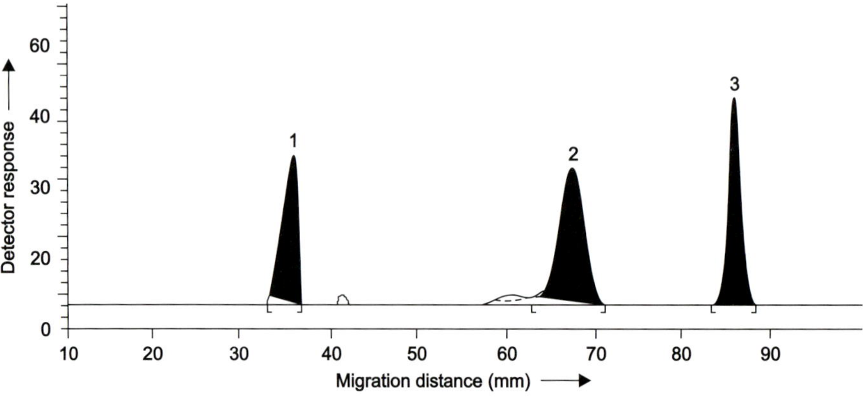

Typical densitogram of the standard containing ceftriaxone, cefixime and cefotaxime. For detailed experimental and chromatographic conditions, refer to Protocol No. 266. Peaks identification: 1. Ceftriaxone; 2. Cefixime; 3. Cefotaxime.

PROTOCOL FOR HPTLC ANALYSIS OF PHARMACEUTICAL FORMULATION

Protocol No. 266

Formulation: Ceftriaxone, Cefixime, Cefotaxime (cephalosporins)

Classification: Antibiotics **Dosage form:** Injections

Standard preparation: Prepare 1 mg/ml solution of each cephalosporin in methanol. Further serial dilutions made for linearity profile. Apply 1 µl of each solution for chromatographic evaluation.

Sample preparation: Appropriate volume of the sample was diluted with methanol to get 250 µg/ml. Apply 1 µl of the resulting solution for assay.

Chromatographic equipments:

Sample applicator: Camag Linomat–III

Development chamber: Camag twin-trough glass chamber, 10 × 10 cm

Densitometric scanner: Camag TLC Scanner–II

Chromatographic conditions:

1. Stationary phase: Silica gel pre-coated plates (2.5 × 10 cm) with concentrating zones – Merck
2. Mobile phase (MP): Ethyl acetate–acetone–methanol–water (5 : 2.5 : 2.5 : 1.5 v/v)
3. Standard/Sample application:
   Band length: — Volume applied: 1 µl Spacing: —
4. Chamber saturation: 20 min (MP)
5. RH (%): 55 ± 5
6. Temperature °C: 22 ± 2
7. Separation technique: Ascending
8. Quantity of mobile phase: 11.5 ml
9. Migration distance: 90 mm
10. Migration time: 20 min

Densitometric evaluation:

Wavelength: UV–270 nm Scanning mode: Reflectance/Absorbance

HRF: See densitogram

Linearity (ng/band): 125–500 for all the three cephalosporins

Recovery (%): 98.1–98.8 for all the three compounds

References: S. Eric-Jovanovic, D. Agbaba, D. Zivanor-Stakic and S. Vladimirov, *J. Pharm. Biomed. Anal.*, **18**, 893–898, 1998

Comments: The method validated for accuracy, precision, linearity, LOD and LOQ.

HPTLC : High Performance Thin Layer Chromatography
HPTLC Densitogram

No. 267

Compound	λ_{max} (nm)	*Rf*	Linearity (ng/band)
Cefadroxil	270	0.20	180–480
Cefaclor	274	0.23	80–800
Cefazolin	280	0.30	40–1200
Cephalexin	268	0.35	40–400
Cefotaxime	270	0.39	150–1200
Ceftriaxone	280	0.51	170–1000
Cefuroxime	275	0.53	50–500
Cefuroxime axetil	284	0.94	50–500

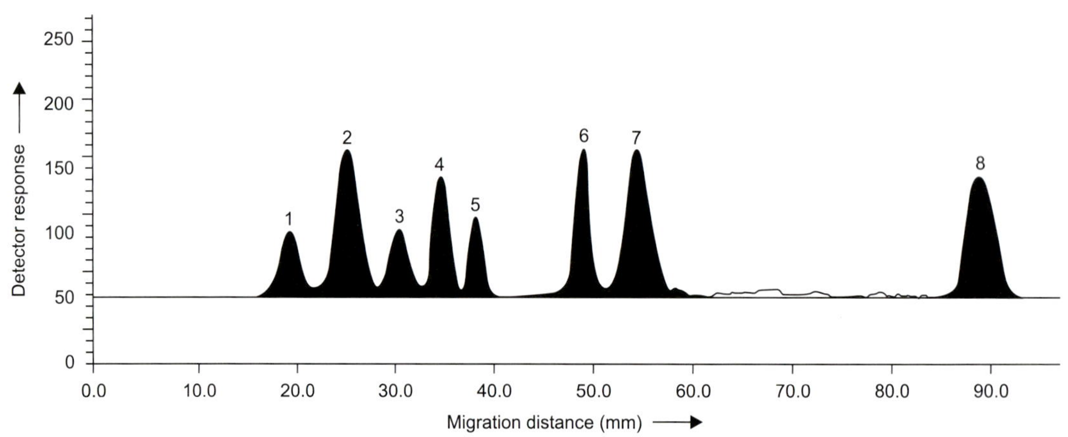

Typical densitogram of the standard containing different cephalosporins. For detailed experimental and chromatographic conditions, refer to Protocol No. 267. Peaks identification: 1. Cefadroxil; 2. Cefaclor; 3. Cefazolin; 4. Cephalexin; 5. Cefotaxime; 6. Ceftriaxone; 7. Cefuroxime; 8. Cefuroxime axetil.

PROTOCOL FOR HPTLC ANALYSIS OF PHARMACEUTICAL FORMULATION

Protocol No. 267

Formulation: **Cephalosporins (First generation: Cephalexin, Cefadroxil and Cefazolin; Second generation: Cefaclor, Cefuroxime and Cefuroxime axetil; Third generation: Ceftriaxone, Cefotaxime)**

Classification: Antibiotics

Dosage form: Capsules and powder for injection

Standard preparation: Standard solution of each drug was prepared in solvent to get 10 μg/ml. Further serial dilutions made for linearity studies. Apply 10 μl of each solution for chromatographic analysis.

Solvent: Methanol–water (1 : 1 v/v).

Sample preparation: Contents of the capsules or powder for injection were dissolved in solvent to get 10 μg/ml. Filter and dilute the filtrate suitably for assay.

Chromatographic equipments:

Sample applicator: Camag Linomat–IV

Development chamber: Sigma–Aldrich glass chamber, 18 × 9 × 18 cm

Densitometric scanner: Camag TLC Scanner–III

Chromatographic conditions:

1. Stationary phase: Silica gel $60F_{254}$ pre-coated TLC plates, 15 × 10 cm (250 μm) – Merck
2. Mobile phase (MP): Chloroform–ethyl acetate–glacial acetic acid–water (4 : 4 : 4 : 1 v/v)
3. Standard/Sample application:
   Band length: 10 mm Volume applied: 10 μl Spacing: 8 mm
4. Chamber saturation: 30 min (MP)
5. RH (%): —
6. Temperature °C: 22 ± 1
7. Separation technique: Ascending
8. Quantity of mobile phase: 26 ml
9. Migration distance: 95 mm
10. Migration time: —

Densitometric evaluation:

Wavelength: See table, preferable at 275 nm

Scanning mode: Reflectance/Absorbance

HRF: See densitogram

Linearity (ng/band): See table

Recovery (%): 98.30–100.85 for all the drugs

References: Monika Dabrowska, Malgorzata Starck and Sabina Pikulska, *J. Planar Chromatogr.*, **24(1)**, 23–29, 2011.

Comments: The method validated for accuracy, precision, linearity, LOD, LOQ, specificity, robustness and ruggedness.

Cefaclor

Cefadroxil

Cefuroxime

Cefazolin

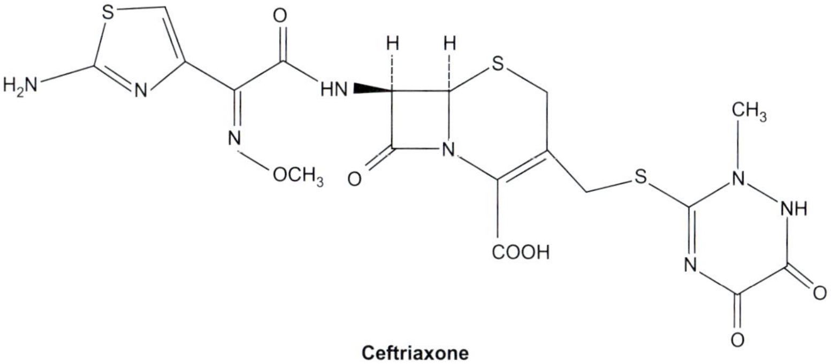

Ceftriaxone

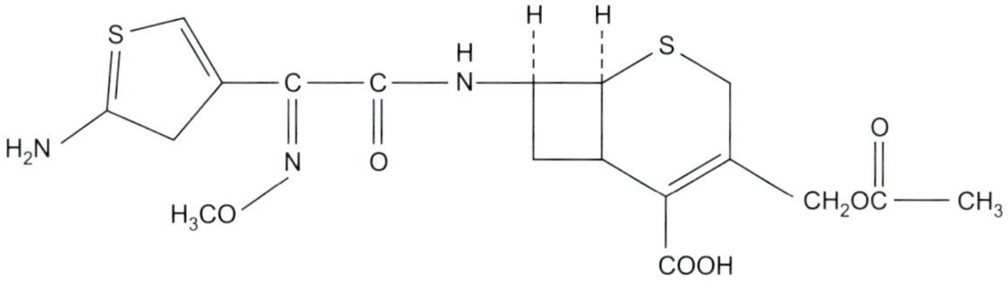

Cefotaxime

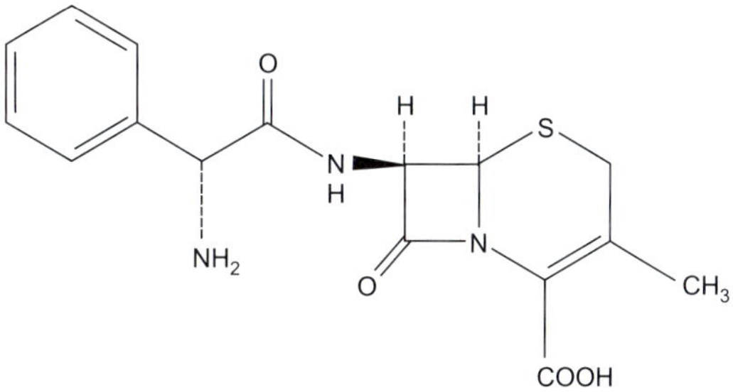

Cephalexin

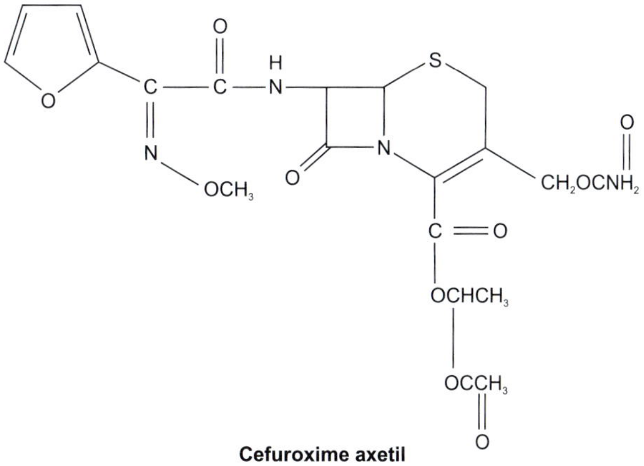

Cefuroxime axetil

HPTLC : High Performance Thin Layer Chromatography
HPTLC Densitogram

No. 268

Amikacin

Kanamycin

Neomycin B: $R_1 = -CH_2NH_2$
$R_2 = -H$
Neomycin C: $R_1 = -H$
$R_2 = -CH_2NH_2$

Neomycin

Tobramycin

Netilmicin

Typical densitogram of the standard solution containing six different antibiotics. For detailed experimental and chromatographic conditions, refer to Protocol No. 268. Peaks identification: 1. Neomycin; 2. Kanamycin; 3. Tobramycin; 4. Gentamicin (G1); 5. Gentamicin (G2); 6. Netilmicin.

PROTOCOL FOR HPTLC ANALYSIS OF PHARMACEUTICAL FORMULATION

Protocol No. 268

Formulation: **Gentamicin, Neomycin, Amikacin, Kanamycin, Netilmicin, Tobramycin**
Classification: Antibiotics **Dosage form:** Injections, tablets, eye drops
Standard preparation: Tobramycin, amikacin and netilmicin—250 μg/ml in water; gentamicin, kanamycin and neomycin, prepare 1 mg/ml solution in methanol. Further dilute with methanol–water (1 : 1) to get 500 μg/ml to carry out the chromatographic analysis.
Sample preparation: Sample of each antibiotic was processed as under standard preparation and used for analysis.
Chromatographic equipments:
Sample applicator: Camag Linomat–IV
Development chamber: Sigma-Aldrich glass chamber, 16 × 9 × 18 cm
Densitometric scanner: Camag TLC Scanner–III
Chromatographic conditions:
1. Stationary phase: Silica gel $60F_{254}$ pre-coated HPTLC plates; 11 × 10 cm (200 μm) – Merck
2. Mobile phase (MP): Methanol–chloroform–25% ammonia (3 : 1 : 2 v/v)
3. Standard/Sample application:
Band length: 8 mm Volume applied: 5 μl Spacing: 8 mm
4. Chamber saturation: 20 min (MP)
5. RH (%): 55 ± 5
6. Temperature °C: 22 ± 2
7. Separation technique: Ascending
8. Quantity of mobile phase: 18 ml
9. Migration distance: 90 mm
10. Migration time: 30 min

Densitometric evaluation:
Wavelength: UV–Vis 500 nm Scanning mode: Reflectance/Absorbance
HRF: See densitogram
Linearity (μg/band): Amikacin and Netilmicin—0.75–6.25; Gentamicin, Kanamycin, Neomycin and Tobramycin—1.5–12.5
Recovery (%): 100.23–101.01 for all the compounds
References: Urszula Hubicka, Jan Krzek, Hanna Woltynska and Bozena Stachaz, *J. AOAC Int.*, **92(4)**, 1068–1075, 2009.
Comments:
- The method validated for accuracy, precision, linearity, LOD, LOQ, specificity and robustness.
- The developed and dried plate immersed in 0.2% ethanolic ninhydrin solution (15 s), heated for 5 min (100°C) and scanned at 500 nm.
- As observed by the authors, the use of HPTLC plate led to increased development time. TLC pre-coated plates may be used for chromatographic quantification.

HPTLC : High Performance Thin Layer Chromatography
HPTLC Densitogram

No. 269

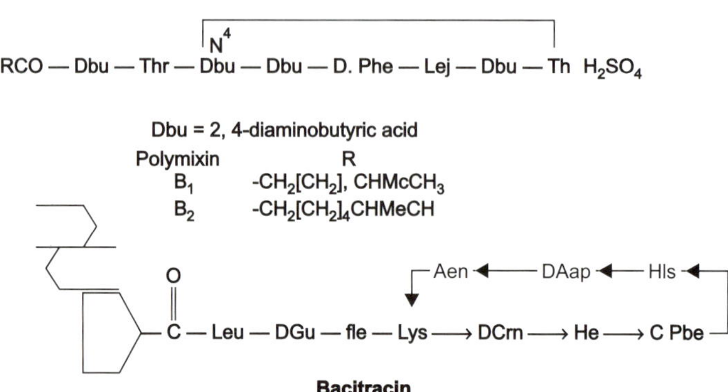

Application scheme		
	Standard	**Sample**
Neomycin	6 µl	20 µl
Polymixin B	2 µl	40 µl
Bacitracin	6 µl	10 µl
Preservatives	3 µl	3 µl

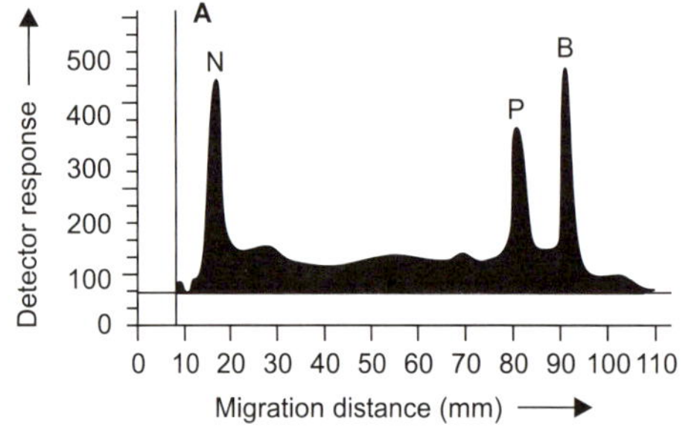

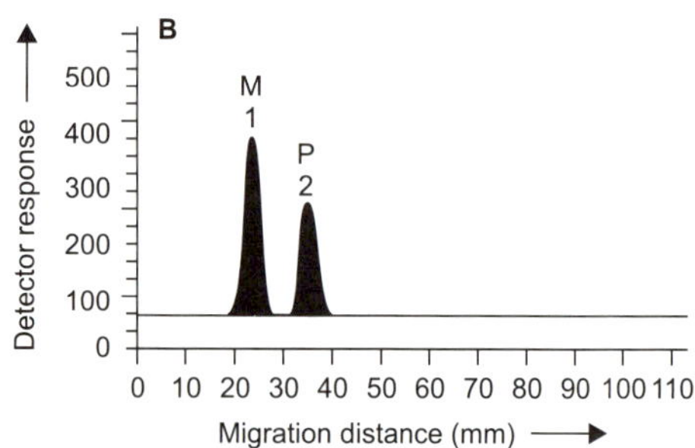

Typical densitogram of the sample containing three antibiotics and two preservatives. For detailed experimental and chromatographic conditions, refer to Protocol No. 269. Peaks identification: A—1. Neomycin (N); 2. Polymixin (P); 3. Bacitracin (B). B—1. Methylparaben (M); 2. Propylparaben (P).

PROTOCOL FOR HPTLC ANALYSIS OF PHARMACEUTICAL FORMULATION

Protocol No. 269

Formulation: **Neomycin sulphate, Polymixin B. sulphate, Zinc bacitracin, Methyl paraben, Propylparaben**

Classification: Antibiotics **Dosage form:** Ointment

Standard preparation: Antibiotic—700 μg/ml obtained by dissolving in small volume of water, dilutions with methanol, preservatives—40 μg/ml of each in methanol. Apply different volumes for analysis.

Sample preparation: Antibiotics: 2 g of the sample suspended in 30 ml of diethylether, extracted with 3 × 10 ml water to ensure complete extraction of antibitocis into aq. layer, dilute to 50 ml with water and use for applicaltion. Preservatives: 1.5 g of sample suspended in 40 ml methanol, heated in water-bath for 30 min, cooled, filtered and diluted to 50 ml with methanol and used for analysis.

Chromatographic equipments:

Sample applicator: Camag Linomat–IV

Development chamber: Sigma-Aldrich, TLC chamber

Densitometric scanner: Camag TLC Scanner–III

Chromatographic conditions:

1. Stationary phase: Silica gel F_{254} pre-coated HPTLC plates, 10 × 10 cm (200 μm) – Merck
2. Mobile phase (MP): (A) Methanol–n-butanol–25% ammonia–chloroform (14 : 4 : 9 : 12 v/v) for antibiotics; n-pentane–glacial acetic acid (66 : 9 v/v) for preservatives
3. Standard/Sample application: See application scheme
   Band length: 10 mm Volume applied: 5 μl Spacing: 10 mm
4. Chamber saturation:
5. RH (%): 55 ± 5
6. Temperature °C: 22 ± 2
7. Separation technique: Ascending
8. Quantity of mobile phase: 39 ml, 38 ml
9. Migration distance: 110 mm
10. Migration time: 90 min (A); 60 min (B)

Densitometric evaluation:

Wavelength: UV–260 nm (preservatives); 550 nm (antibiotics)

Scanning mode: Reflectance/Absorbance

HRF: —

Linearity range (ng/band): Neomycin—0.03–0.09; Polymixin B—0.045–0.085; Bacitracin—0.03–0.095; Methylparaben—0.0025–0.0175; Propylparaben—0.0015–0.010

Recovery (%): Antibiotics—103.76–104.95; Preservatives—98.08–101.53

References: Jan Krzek, Malgorzata Starck, Anna Kwiecien and Wlodzimierz Rzesutko, *J. Pharm. and Biomed. Analysis*, **24**, 629–636, 2001.

Comments:

- The method validated for accuracy, precision, linearity, robustness, LOD and LOQ.
- Visualization of the developed plate was done by immersing in 0.2% ethanolic ninhydrin solution, heating at 100°C for 5 min; preservative scanned at 550 nm.

HPTLC : High Performance Thin Layer Chromatography
HPTLC Densitogram

No. 270

Pyrantel pamoate

Mebendazole

Typical densitogram of the sample containing mebendazole and pyrantel pamoate. For detailed experimental and chromatographic condition refer to Protocol No. 270. Peaks identification: 1. Pyrantel pamoate; 2. Mebendazole; 3. (IS).

PROTOCOL FOR HPTLC ANALYSIS OF PHARMACEUTICAL FORMULATION

Protocol No. 270

Formulation: Mebendazole, Pyrantel pamoate

Classification: Antibiotics **Dosage form:** Ointment

Standard preparation: Dissolve 100 mg of pyrantel pamoate and 150 mg of mebendazole separately in minimum volume of DMF, dilute to 100 ml with methanol. Further dilutions made with methanol for linearity studies. Each solution contained 20 μg/ml of 2-methylmercaptothiadiazole as (IS).

Sample preparation: Powdered sample equivalent to 100 mg of pyrantel pamoate or 150 mg of mebendazole dissolved in minimum volume of DMF, dilute to 100 ml with methanol, filter through Whatman No. 1 filter paper. 20 ml of the filtrate diluted to 50 ml after adding 5 ml of (IS) solution (4 mg/ml in methanol) and used for chromatographic application.

Chromatographic equipments:

Sample applicator: Camag Linomat–IV

Development chamber: Camag twin-trough glass chamber, 10 × 10 cm

Densitometric scanner: Camag TLC Scanner–III

Chromatographic conditions:

1. Stationary phase: Silica gel $60F_{254}$ pre-coated HPTLC plates, 10 × 10 cm (200 μm) – Merck
2. Mobile phase (MP): Toluene–ethyl acetate–acetic acid (5 : 5 : 0.2 v/v)
3. Standard/Sample application: —
   Band length: 5 mm Volume applied: 4 μl Spacing: 5 mm
4. Chamber saturation: 20 min (MP)
5. RH (%): 55 ± 5
6. Temperature °C: 22 ± 2
7. Separation technique: Ascending
8. Quantity of mobile phase: 10 ml
9. Migration distance: 75 mm
10. Migration time: 20 min

Densitometric evaluation:

Wavelength: UV–265 nm Scanning mode: Reflectance/Absorbance

HRF: Pyrantel pamoate—21; Mebendazole—63; IS—84

Linearity range (ng/band): Pyrantel pamoate—50–400; Mebendazole—75–600

Recovery (%): 100.05–100.08 for both the compounds

References: SS Zarapkar, SS Kolte and S.H. Rane, *Indian Drugs*, **35(1)**, 49–51, 1998.

Comments: The method validated for accuracy, precision, linearity, LOD and LOQ.

HPTLC : High Performance Thin Layer Chromatography
HPTLC Densitogram

No. 271

Pyrantel pamoate

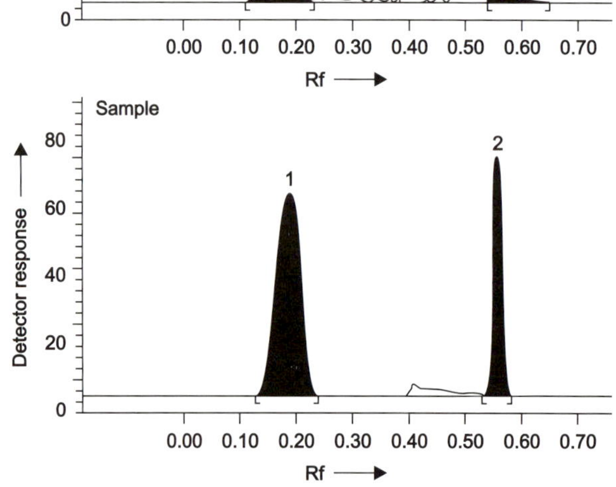

Typical densitogram of the standard and the sample containing mebendazole and pyrantel pamoate. For detailed experimental and chromatographic condition refer to Protocol No. 271. Peaks identification: 1. Pyrantel pamoate; 2. Mebendazole.

PROTOCOL FOR HPTLC ANALYSIS OF PHARMACEUTICAL FORMULATION

Protocol No. 271

Formulation: Mebendazole, Pyrantel pamoate

Classification: Antibiotics **Dosage form:** Ointment

Standard preparation: (a) Prepare 1 mg/ml solution of pyrantel pamoate (base) in 'DMF'. (b) Prepare 1.5 mg of mebendazole solution in DMF. Mix 0.4 ml of solution (a) and (b) and dilute to 10 ml for application.

Sample preparation: Suspend powdered sample equivalent to 150 mg of mebendazole in 60 ml of DMF, sonicate for 10 min, dilute to 100 ml with methanol, filter and dilute 0.4 ml of filtrate to 10 ml with methanol and use for chromatographic evaluation.

Chromatographic equipments:

Sample applicator: Camag Linomat–IV

Development chamber: Camag twin-trough glass chamber, 10 × 10 cm

Densitometric scanner: Camag TLC Scanner–III

Chromatographic conditions:

1. Stationary phase: Silica gel 60F_{254} pre-coated HPTLC plates, 10 × 10 cm (200 μm) – Merck
2. Mobile phase (MP): Xylene–ethyl acetate–glacial acetic acid (5 : 5 : 0.2 v/v)
3. Standard/Sample application: —
   Band length: 5 mm Volume applied: 5 μl Spacing: 5 mm
4. Chamber saturation: 10 min (MP)
5. RH (%): 55 ± 5
6. Temperature °C: 22 ± 2
7. Separation technique: Ascending
8. Quantity of mobile phase: 10 ml
9. Migration distance: 50 mm
10. Migration time: 25 min

Densitometric evaluation:

Wavelength: UV–254 nm Scanning mode: Reflectance/Absorbance

HRF: Pyrantel pamoate—18; Mebendazole—58

Linearity range (%): 100–500 ng/band for both the compounds

Recovery (%): 98.37–102.35 for both the compounds

References: —

Comments:

- The method was optimized and analytical work carried out at **Anchrom's HPTLC Application Laboratory**, Mumbai, India.
- Several market samples of similar composition were analysed by the proposed method and found to give reproducible results.

HPTLC : High Performance Thin Layer Chromatography
HPTLC Densitogram

No. 272

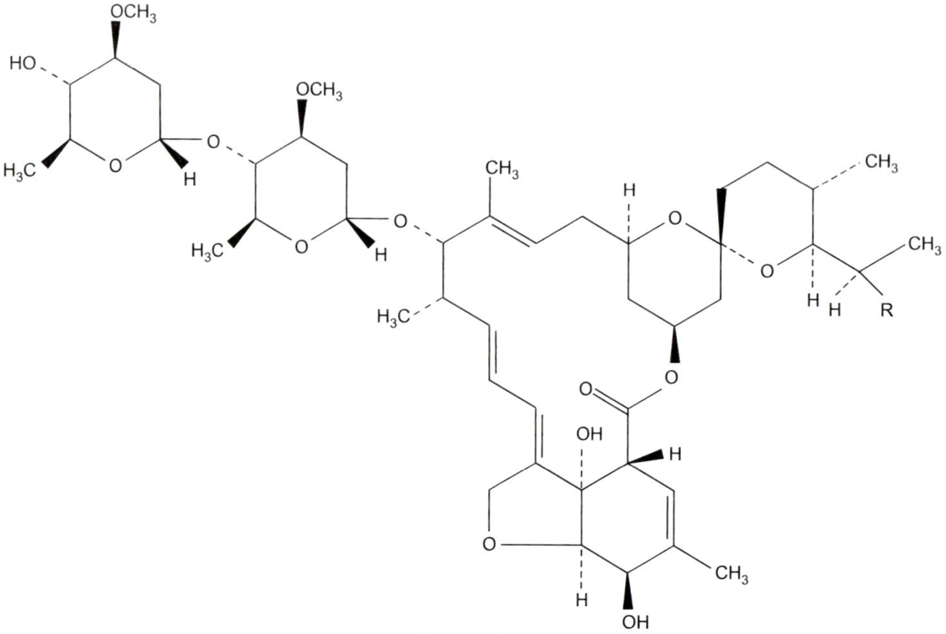

Ivermectin

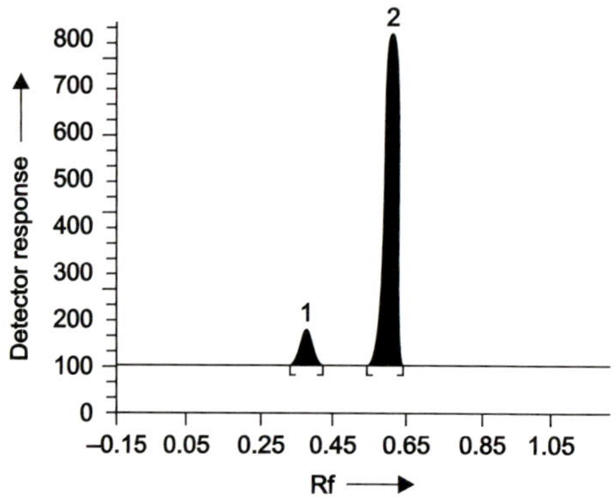

Typical densitogram of the standard containing ivermectin and albendazole. For detailed experimental and chromatographic condition refer to Protocol No. 272. Peaks identification: 1. Ivermectin; 2. Albendazole.

PROTOCOL FOR HPTLC ANALYSIS OF PHARMACEUTICAL FORMULATION

Protocol No. 272

Formulation: **Ivermectin, Albendazole**

Classification: Antibiotics **Dosage form:** Tablets

Standard preparation: Dissolve 6 mg of ivermectin in 5 ml of formic acid and dilute to 100 ml with methanol (60 μg/ml). Prepare 4000 μg/ml solution of albendazole by first dissolving pure drug in 5 ml of formic acid and then diluting to 100 ml with methanol. Apply 2–9 μl of each solution for linearity profile.

Sample preparation: Powdered sample equivalent to 6 mg of ivermectin and 400 mg of albendazole transferred to a 100 ml volumetric flask containing 5 ml of formic acid and 50 ml of methanol, shake for 10 min, dilute to volume with methanol and use for chromatographic analysis.

Chromatographic equipments:

Sample applicator: Camag Linomat–V

Development chamber: Camag twin-trough glass chamber, 10 × 10 cm

Densitometric scanner: Camag TLC Scanner–III

Chromatographic conditions:

1. Stationary phase: Silica gel $60F_{254}$ pre-coated TLC plates, 10 × 10 cm (250 μm) – Merck
2. Mobile phase (MP): Toluene–ethyl acetate–glacial acetic acid (6 : 4 : 0.5 v/v)
3. Standard/Sample application: —
   Band length: 10 mm Volume applied: 2–9 μl Spacing: 10 mm
4. Chamber saturation: 30 min (MP)
5. RH (%): 55 ± 5
6. Temperature °C: Ambient
7. Separation technique: Ascending
8. Quantity of mobile phase: 10 ml
9. Migration distance: 80 mm
10. Migration time: 20 min

Densitometric evaluation:

Wavelength: UV–247 nm Scanning mode: Reflectance/Absorbance

HRF: Ivermectin—39; Albendazole—62

Linearity (μg/band): Ivermectin—0.12–0.54; Albendazole—8–36

Recovery (%): 98.0–101.0 for both the compounds

References: Susheel John Varghese, P. Vasanthi, T.K. Ravi, *J. Planar Chromatogr.*, **24(4)**, 344–347, 2011.

Comments: Several market samples of similar composition were analysed by the proposed method with reproducible results.

HPTLC : High Performance Thin Layer Chromatography
HPTLC Densitogram

No. 273

H_2N N NH_2 HCl N : NC = H_5

Phenazopyridine hydrochloride

NO_2 O C=N N O NH O

Nitrofurantoin

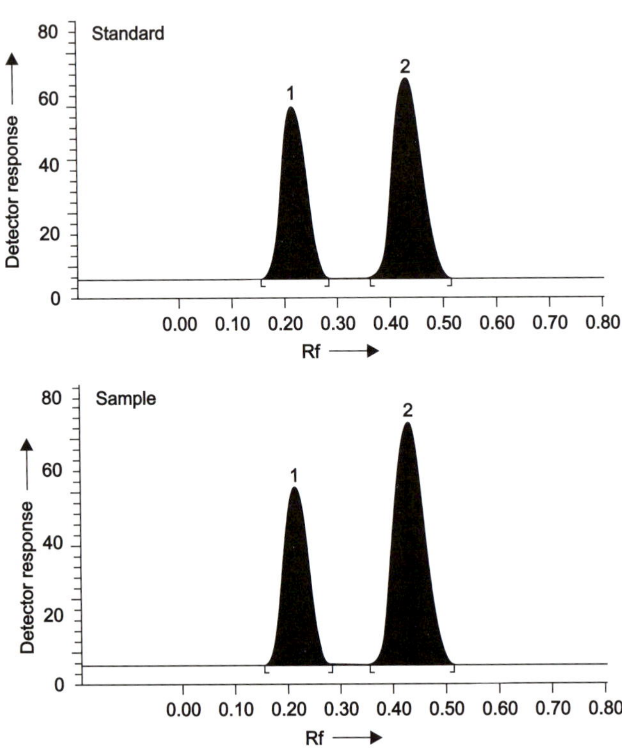

Typical densitogram of the standard and the sample containing phenazopyridine HCl and nitrofurantoin. For detailed experimental and chromatographic condition refer to Protocol No. 273. Peaks identification: 1. Nitrofurantoin; 2. Phenazopyridine HCl.

PROTOCOL FOR HPTLC ANALYSIS OF PHARMACEUTICAL FORMULATION

Protocol No. 273

Formulation: Phenazopyridine hydrochloride, Nitrofurantoin

Classification: Antibiotics **Dosage form:** Ointment

Standard preparation: (i) Weigh accurately 15 mg of phenazopyridine (P), add 2 ml of DMF and dilute to 10 ml with methanol (2). Weigh accurately about 10 mg of nitrofurantoin (N), add 2 ml of DMF and dilute to 10 ml with methanol (1). Mix 0.2 ml of solution (1) and 0.1 ml of solution (2) and dilute to 10 ml with methanol and use for chromatographic analysis.

Sample preparation: Weigh accurately sample equivalent to 20 mg of nitrofurantoin, add 50 ml of DMF, vortex for 10 min, dilute to 100 ml with methanol, filter and dilute 1 ml to 10 ml with methanol and use for chromatographic analysis.

Chromatographic equipments:

Sample applicator: Camag Linomat–IV

Development chamber: Camag twin-trough glass chamber, 10 × 10 cm

Densitometric scanner: Camag TLC Scanner–III

Chromatographic conditions:

1. Stationary phase: Silica gel $60F_{254}$ pre-coated HPTLC plates, 10 × 10 cm (200 μm) – Merck
2. Mobile phase (MP): n-hexane–ethyl acetate–glacial acetic acid (5 : 5 : 0.1 v/v)
3. Standard/Sample application: —
   Band length: 10 mm Volume applied: 10 μl Spacing: 10 mm
4. Chamber saturation: 10 min (MP)
5. RH (%): 55 ± 5
6. Temperature °C: 22 ± 2
7. Separation technique: Ascending
8. Quantity of mobile phase: 10 ml
9. Migration distance: 50 mm
10. Migration time: 25 min

Densitometric evaluation:

Wavelength: UV–361 nm Scanning mode: Reflectance/Absorbance

HRF: Nitrofuranton—21; Phenazopyridine HCl—42

Linearity range (ng/band): Nitrofuranton—25–250; Phenazopyridine HCl—100–750

Recovery (%): 98.6–100.7 for both the compounds

References: —

Comments:

- The method was optimized and analytical work carried out at **Anchrom's HPTLC Application Laboratory**, Mumbai, India.
- Several market samples of similar composition were analysed by the proposed method and found to give reproducible results.

HPTLC : High Performance Thin Layer Chromatography
HPTLC Densitogram

No. 274

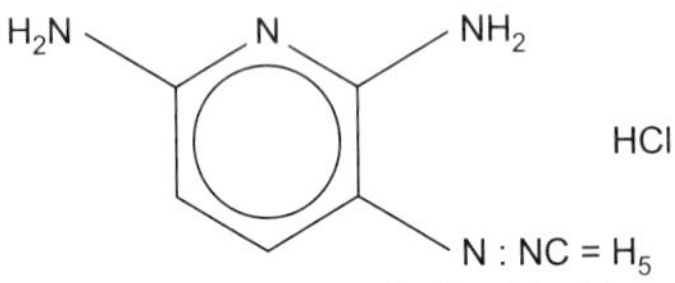

HCl

Phenazopyridine hydrochloride

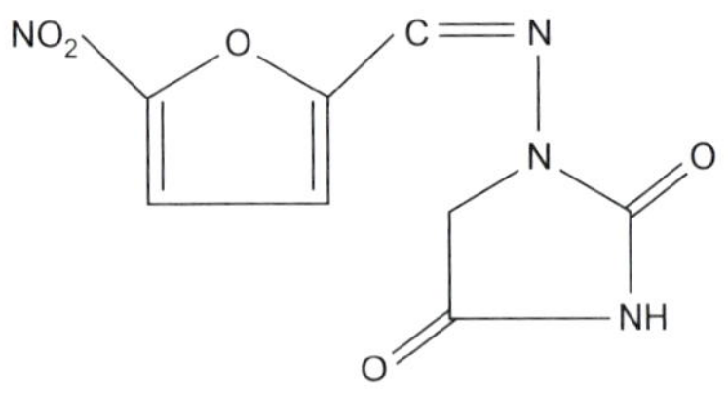

Nitrofurantoin

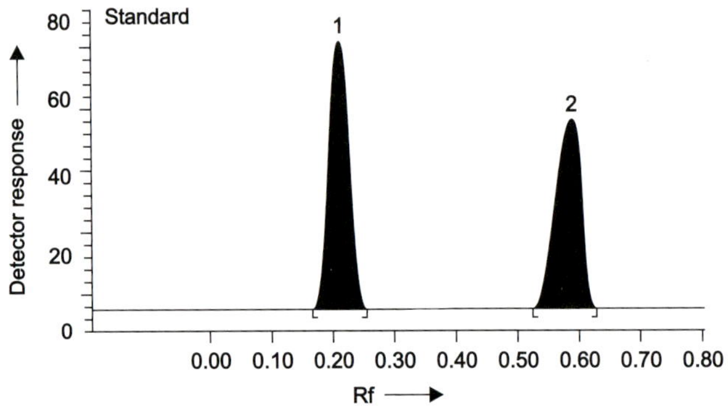

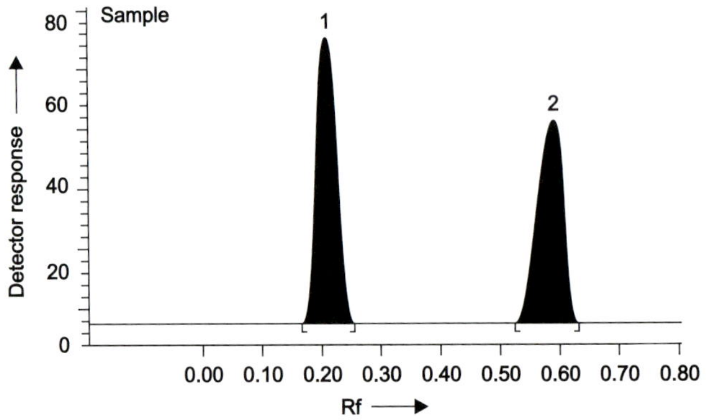

Typical densitogram of the standard and the sample containing phenazopyridine HCl and nitrofurantoin. For detailed experimental and chromatographic condition refer to Protocol No. 274. Peaks identification: 1. Phenazopyridine HCl; 2. Nitrofurantoin.

PROTOCOL FOR HPTLC ANALYSIS OF PHARMACEUTICAL FORMULATION

Protocol No. 274

Formulation: Phenazopyridine hydrochloride, Nitrofurantoin

Classification: Antibiotics **Dosage form:** Ointment

Standard preparation: (i) Weigh accurately 15 mg of phenazopyridine (P), add 2 ml of DMF and dilute to 10 ml with methanol (2). Weigh accurately about 10 mg of nitrofurantoin (N), add 2 ml of DMF and dilute to 10 ml with methanol (1). Mix 0.2 ml of solution (1) and 0.1 ml of solution (2) and dilute to 10 ml with methanol and use for chromatographic analysis.

Sample preparation: Weigh accurately sample equivalent to 20 mg of nitrofurantoin, add 50 ml of DMF, vortex for 10 min, dilute to 100 ml with methanol, filter and dilute 1 ml to 10 ml with methanol and use for chromatographic analysis.

Chromatographic equipments:

Sample applicator: Camag Linomat–IV

Development chamber: Camag twin-trough glass chamber, 10 × 10 cm

Densitometric scanner: Camag TLC Scanner–III

Chromatographic conditions:

1. Stationary phase: Silica gel 60 RP–18F_{254s} pre-coated HPTLC plates, 10 × 10 cm (200 μm) – Merck
2. Mobile phase (MP): 0.5 M sodium chloride–methanol–glacial acetic acid (2 : 8 : 0.01 v/v)
3. Standard/Sample application: —
   Band length: 10 mm Volume applied: 10 μl Spacing: 10 mm
4. Chamber saturation: 30 min (MP)
5. RH (%): 55 ± 5
6. Temperature °C: 22 ± 2
7. Separation technique: Ascending
8. Quantity of mobile phase: 20 ml
9. Migration distance: 50 mm
10. Migration time: 35 min

Densitometric evaluation:

Wavelength: UV–361 nm Scanning mode: Reflectance/Absorbance

HRF: Phenazopyridine HCl—20; Nitrofuranton—58

Linearity range (ng/band): Phenazopyridine HCl—100–750; Nitrofuranton—25–250

Recovery: 99.25–101.10 for both the compounds

References: —

Comments:

- The method was optimized and analytical work carried out at **Anchrom's HPTLC Application Laboratory**, Mumbai, India.
- Reversed-phase chromatography resulted in reversal of retention order as compared to normal-phase chromatography.
- The separation was superior in RP–chromatography.

HPTLC : High Performance Thin Layer Chromatography
HPTLC Densitogram

No. 275

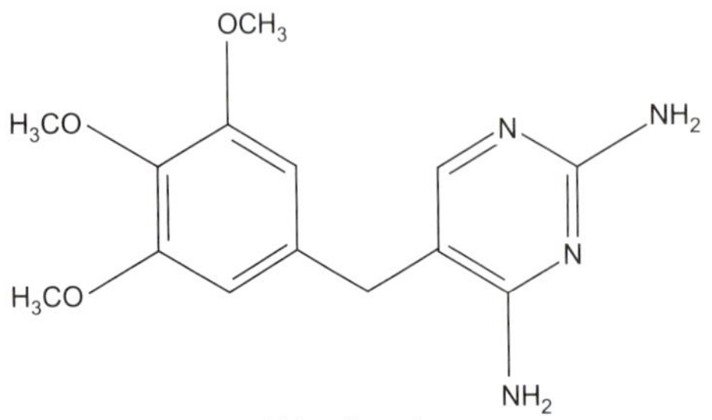

Trimethoprim

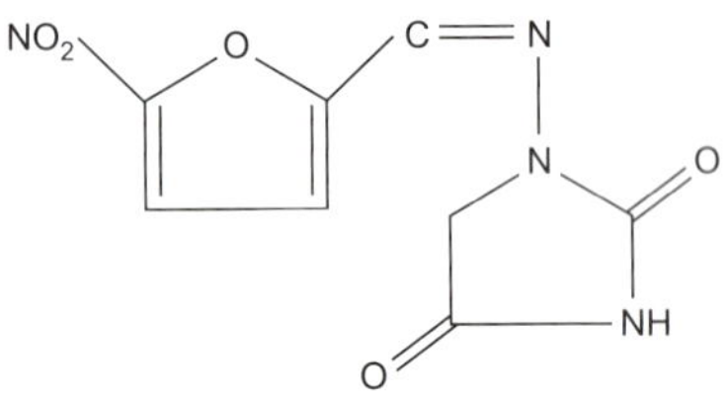

Nitrofurantoin

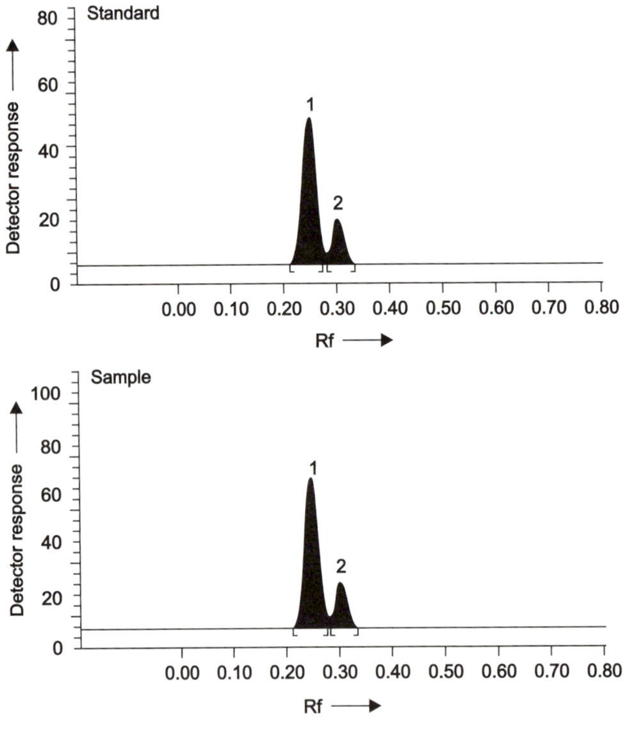

Standard

Sample

Typical densitogram of the standard and the sample containing trimethoprim and nitrofurantoin. For detailed experimental and chromatographic condition refer to Protocol No. 275. Peaks identification: 1. Trimethoprim; 2. Nitrofurantoin.

PROTOCOL FOR HPTLC ANALYSIS OF PHARMACEUTICAL FORMULATION

Protocol No. 275

Formulation: Trimethoprim, Nitrofurantoin

Classification: Antibiotics **Dosage form:** Tablets, Capsules

Standard preparation: (a) Weigh10 mg of nitrofurantoin, dissolve in 2 ml of DMF, dilute to 20 ml with methanol. (b) Dissolve 10 mg of trimethoprim in methanol to produce 20 ml. Mix 0.5 ml of solution (a) and 0.4 ml of solution (b) and dilute to 10 ml with methanol to use for application.

Sample preparation: Powdered sample equivalent to 20 mg of trimethoprim suspended in 70–80 ml methanol, sonicated for 10 min, diluted to 100 ml, filtered and 1 ml of the filtrate diluted to 10 ml with methanol for chromatographic evaluation.

Chromatographic equipments:

Sample applicator: Camag Linomat–IV

Development chamber: Camag twin-trough glass chamber, 10 × 10 cm

Densitometric scanner: Camag TLC Scanner–III

Chromatographic conditions:

1. Stationary phase: Silica gel $60F_{254}$ pre-coated HPTLC plates, 10 × 10 cm (200 μm) – Merck
2. Mobile phase (MP): Chloroform–methanol (9.5 : 0.5 v/v)
3. Standard/Sample application: —
   Band length: 5 mm Volume applied: 4 μl Spacing: 5 mm
4. Chamber saturation: 20 min (MP)
5. RH (%): 55 ± 5
6. Temperature °C: 22 ± 2
7. Separation technique: Ascending
8. Quantity of mobile phase: 10 ml
9. Migration distance: 50 mm
10. Migration time: 18 min

Densitometric evaluation:

Wavelength: UV–278 nm or 361 nm Scanning mode: Reflectance/Absorbance

HRF: Trimethoprim—25; Nitrofurantoin—32

Linearity range (%): 25–250 ng/band for both the compounds

Recovery (%): 100.34–102.21 for both the compounds

References: —

Comments:

- The method was optimized and analytical work carried out at **Anchrom's HPTLC Application Laboratory**, Mumbai, India.
- Several market samples of similar composition were analysed by the proposed method and found to give reproducible results.

HPTLC : High Performance Thin Layer Chromatography
HPTLC Densitogram

No. 276

OCH_3 H_3CO H_3CO N NH_2 N NH_2

Trimethoprim

NO_2 O C ═ N N O NH O

Nitrofurantoin

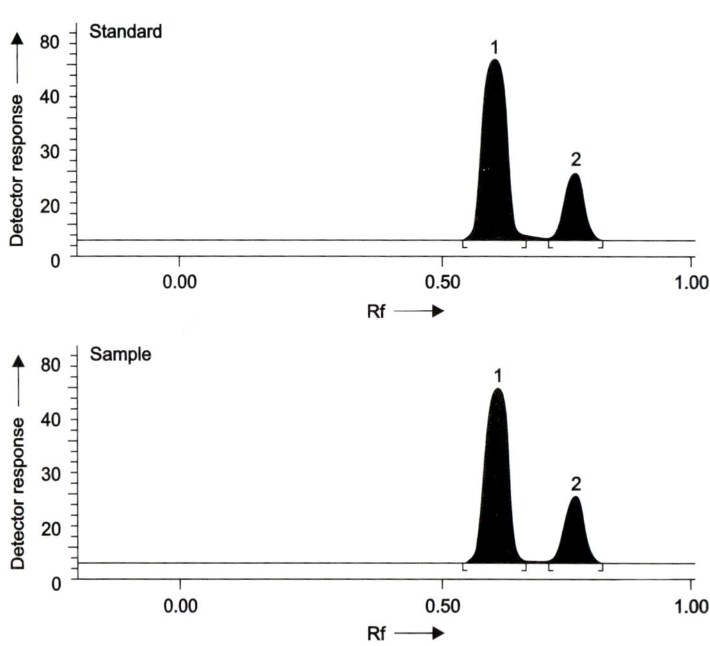

Typical densitogram of the standard and the sample containing trimethoprim and nitrofurantoin. For detailed experimental and chromatographic condition refer to Protocol No. 276. Peaks identification: 1. Trimethoprim; 2. Nitrofurantoin.

PROTOCOL FOR HPTLC ANALYSIS OF PHARMACEUTICAL FORMULATION

Protocol No. 276

Formulation: Trimethoprim, Nitrofurantoin

Classification: Antibiotics **Dosage form:** Tablets, Capsules

Standard preparation: (a) Weigh10 mg of nitrofurantoin, dissolve in 2 ml of DMF, dilute to 20 ml with methanol. (b) Dissolve 10 mg of trimethoprim in methanol to produce 20 ml. Mix 0.5 ml of solution (a) and 0.4 ml of solution (b) and dilute to 10 ml with methanol to use for application.

Sample preparation: Powdered sample equivalent to 20 mg of trimethoprim suspended in 70–80 ml methanol, sonicated for 10 min, diluted to 100 ml, filtered and 1 ml of the filtrate diluted to 10 ml with methanol for chromatographic evaluation.

Chromatographic equipments:

Sample applicator: Camag Linomat–IV

Development chamber: Camag twin-trough glass chamber, 10 × 10 cm

Densitometric scanner: Camag TLC Scanner–III

Chromatographic conditions:

1. Stationary phase: Silica gel 60 RP–18F_{254s} pre-coated HPTLC plates; 10 × 10 cm (200 μm) – Merck
2. Mobile phase (MP): 0.5 M sodium chloride–methanol–glacial acetic acid (12 : 8 : 0.1 v/v)
3. Standard/Sample application: —
   Band length: 5 mm Volume applied: 5 μl Spacing: 5 mm
4. Chamber saturation: 30 min (MP)
5. RH (%): 55 ± 5
6. Temperature °C: 22 ± 2
7. Separation technique: Ascending
8. Quantity of mobile phase: 20 ml
9. Migration distance: 50 mm
10. Migration time: 30 min

Densitometric evaluation:

Wavelength: UV–278 nm or 361 nm Scanning mode: Reflectance/Absorbance

HRF: Trimethoprim—60; Nitrofurantoin—75

Linearity range: 25–500 ng/band for both the compounds

Recovery (%): 98.75–100.75 for both the compounds

References: —

Comments:

- The method was optimized and analytical work carried out at **Anchrom's HPTLC Application Laboratory**, Mumbai, India.
- No change in retention order was observed in RP-chromatography as compared to NP chromatography. RP phase gave better separation.

HPTLC : High Performance Thin Layer Chromatography
HPTLC Densitogram

No. 277

Metronidazole

Nalidixic acid

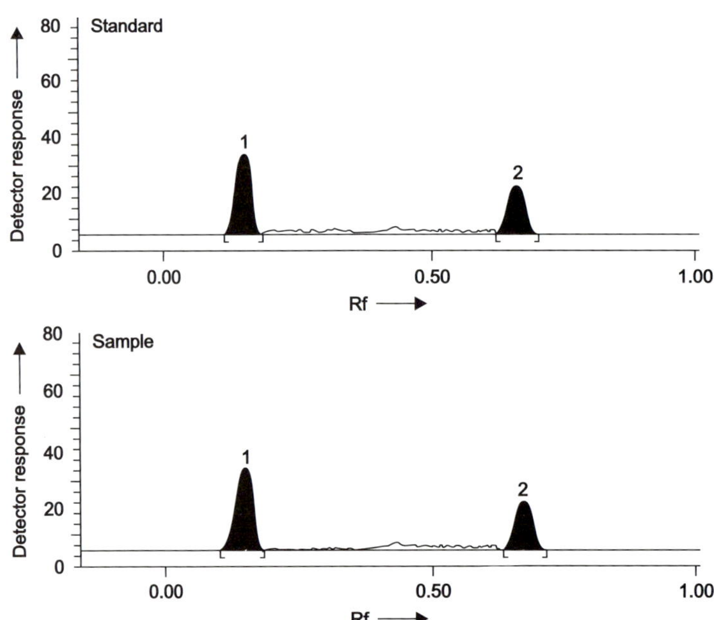

Typical densitogram of the standard and the sample containing metronidazole and nalidixic acid. For detailed experimental and chromatographic condition refer to Protocol No. 277. Peaks identification: 1. Nalidixic acid; 2. Metronidazole.

PROTOCOL FOR HPTLC ANALYSIS OF PHARMACEUTICAL FORMULATION

Protocol No. 277

Formulation: Metronidazole, Nalidixic acid

Classification: Antibiotics **Dosage form:** Tablets, Capsules

Standard preparation: Take 20 mg of metronidazole (M) and 30 mg of nalidixic acid (NA), dissolve in methanol to make 100 ml. Further dilute 2.5 ml to 25 ml for analysis.

Sample preparation: Weigh accurately quantity of the sample equivalent to 200 mg of metronidazole, add 60 ml of methanol, sonicate for 50 min, dilute to 100 ml, filter and dilute 0.1 ml of filtrate to 10 ml with methanol and use for analysis.

Chromatographic equipments:

Sample applicator: Camag Linomat–IV

Development chamber: Camag twin-trough glass chamber, 10 × 10 cm

Densitometric scanner: Camag TLC Scanner–III

Chromatographic conditions:

1. Stationary phase: Silica gel $60F_{254}$ pre-coated HPTLC plates, 10 × 10 cm (200 μm) – Merck
2. Mobile phase (MP): Ethyl acetate–chloroform–methanol–25% ammonia (2.5 : 2.5 : 1.5 : 0.5 v/v)
3. Standard/Sample application: —
   Band length: 5 mm Volume applied: 2 μl Spacing: 5 mm
4. Chamber saturation: 20 min (MP)
5. RH (%): 55 ± 5
6. Temperature °C: 22 ± 2
7. Separation technique: Ascending
8. Quantity of mobile phase: 14 ml
9. Migration distance: 50 mm
10. Migration time: 14 min

Densitometric evaluation:

Wavelength: UV–320 nm Scanning mode: Reflectance/Absorbance

HRF: Nalidixic acid—15; Metronidazole—67

Linearity range (ng/band): Nalidixic acid—10–100; Metronidazole—20–200

Recovery (%): 98.22–101.41 for both the compounds

References: A.P. Argekar, S.V. Raj and S.U. Kapadia, *Indian Drugs*, **33**, 167–170, 1996.

Comments: The method was validated for accuracy, precision, linearity, LOD and LOQ.

HPTLC : High Performance Thin Layer Chromatography
HPTLC Densitogram

No. 278

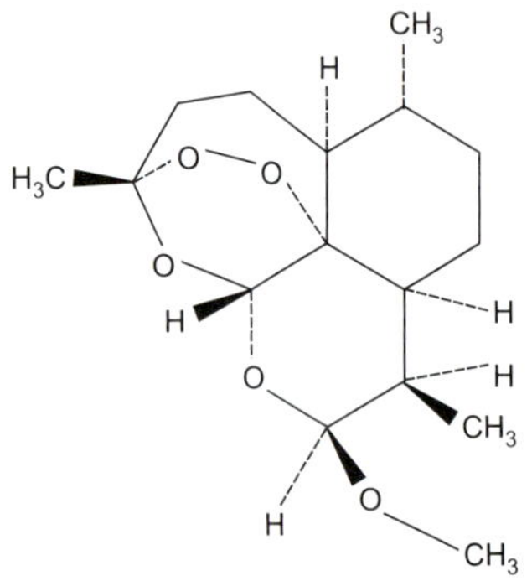

Artemether

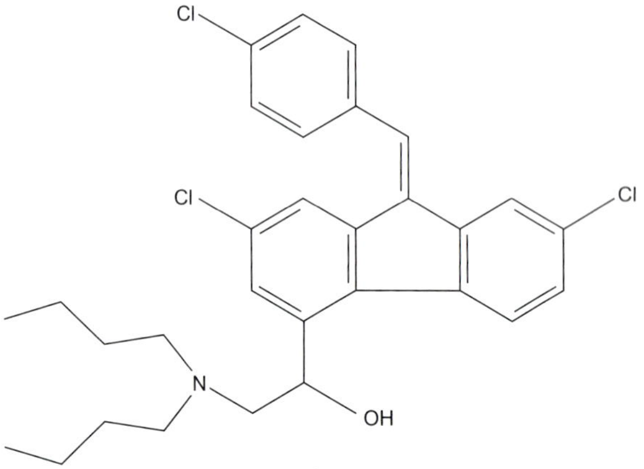

Lumefantrine

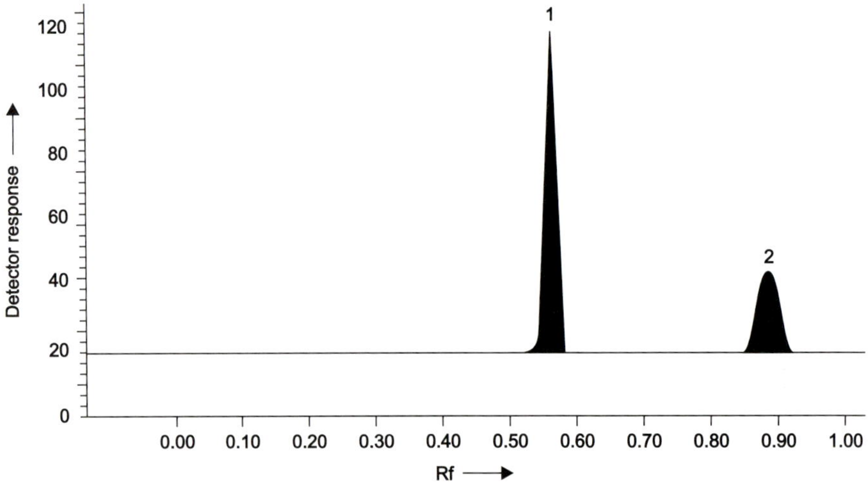

Typical densitogram of the standard containing lumefantrine and artemether. For detailed experimental and chromatographic condition refer to Protocol No. 278. Peaks identification: 1. Lumefantrine; 2. Artemether.

PROTOCOL FOR HPTLC ANALYSIS OF PHARMACEUTICAL FORMULATION

Protocol No. 278

Formulation: Artemether, Lumefantrine

Classification: Antibiotics **Dosage form:** Tablets

Standard preparation: Prepare standard solution of both the compounds in ethyl acetate to get 1 mg/ml of lumefantrine and 100 μg/ml of artemether. Apply varying volumes of each solution (2–10 μl) for linearity profile.

Sample preparation: Powdered sample equivalent to 10 mg of LUMI suspended in 6 ml of ethyl acetate, sonicated for 10 min, diluted to 10 ml, filtered through Whatman No. 41 filter paper and used for application and chromatographic evaluation.

Chromatographic equipments:

Sample applicator: Camag Linomat–V
Development chamber: Camag twin-trough glass chamber, 10 × 10 cm
Densitometric scanner: Camag TLC Scanner–III

Chromatographic conditions:

1. Stationary phase: Silica gel $60F_{254}$ pre-coated HPTLC plates, 10 × 10 cm (200 μm) – Merck, pre-washed with methanol and dried (5 min) prior to use
2. Mobile phase (MP): Toluene–ethyl acetate–formic acid (6 : 6 : 0.7 v/v)
3. Standard/Sample application: —
   Band length: 10 mm Volume applied: 2–10 μl Spacing: 10 mm
4. Chamber saturation: 15 min (MP)
5. RH (%): 55 ± 5
6. Temperature °C: 22 ± 2
7. Separation technique: Ascending
8. Quantity of mobile phase: 12 ml
9. Migration distance: 80 mm
10. Migration time: 35 min

Densitometric evaluation:

Wavelength: UV-267 nm (LUMi); Vis-567 nm (ART)
Scanning mode: Reflectance/Absorbance
HRF: Lumefantrine—54; Artemether—89
Linearity range (ng/band): Artemether—200–1000; Lumefantrine—1200–6000
Recovery (%): 98–102 for both the compounds

References: Vora Asfaq, Darekar Rahul, Mahendra Ratnakar and Damle Mrinalini, *J. Pharm. Res.*, **7(4)**, 229–232, 2008.

Comments:

- The method was validated for accuracy, precision, linearity, LOD, LOQ, specificity and robustness.
- After sanning the plate at 267 nm for lumefantrine, the plate was treated with anisaldehyde–sulphunic acid reagent, heated at 110°C for 12 min and then scanned at 567 nm for 'ART' estimation.

HPTLC : High Performance Thin Layer Chromatography
HPTLC Densitogram

No. 279

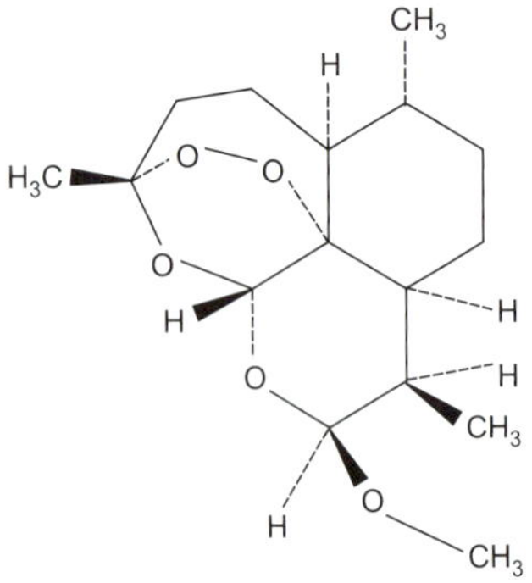

Artemether

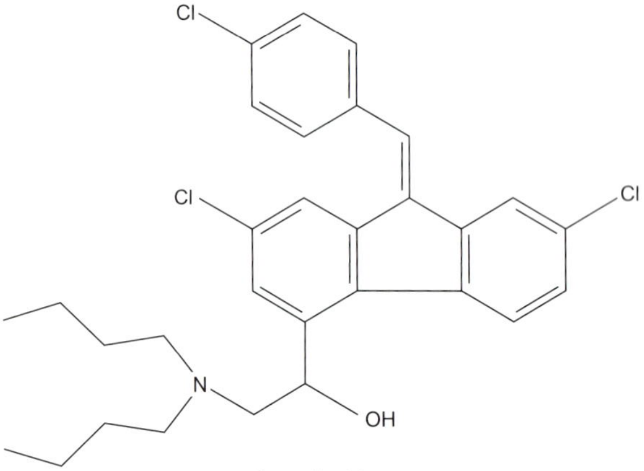

Lumefantrine

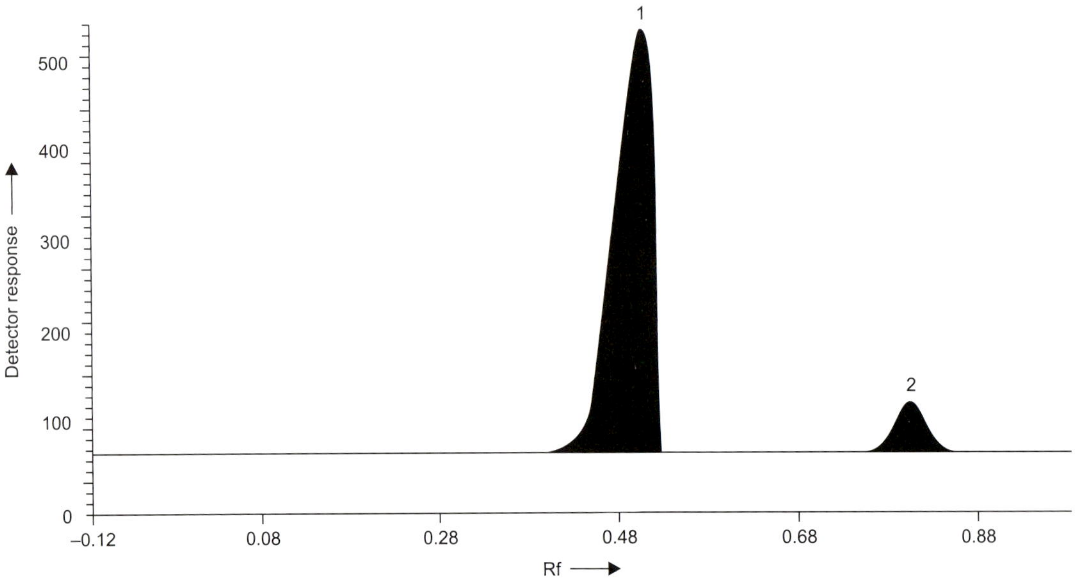

Typical densitogram of the standard containing lumefantrine and artemether. For detailed experimental and chromatographic condition refer to Protocol No. 279. Peaks identification: 1. Lumefantrine; 2. Artemether.

PROTOCOL FOR HPTLC ANALYSIS OF PHARMACEUTICAL FORMULATION

Protocol No. 279

Formulation: Artemether, Lumefantrine

Classification: Antibiotics **Dosage form:** Tablets

Standard preparation: 10 mg of artemether and 60 mg of lumefantrine accurately weighed, dissolved in dichloromethane to get final concentration of 40 µg/ml of artemether and 240 µg/ml of lumefantrine. Apply 2–10 µl of each solution for linearity and chromatographic analysis.

Sample preparation: Powdered sample equivalent to 20 mg of artemether suspended in dichloromethane, sonicated for 2 min, filtered through Whatman No. 42 filter paper, suitably diluted to get 160 ng of artemether and 960 ng of lumefantrine per 10 µl of the final solution. Apply 10 µl for assay.

Chromatographic equipments:

Sample applicator: Camag Linomat–V sample applicator
Development chamber: Camag twin-trough glass chamber
Densitometric scanner: Camag TLC Scanner–III

Chromatographic conditions:

1. Stationary phase: Silica gel $60F_{254}$ pre-coated HPTLC plates, 10 × 10 cm (200 µm) – Merck
2. Mobile phase (MP): n-hexane–ethyl acetate (8 : 2 v/v)
3. Standard/Sample application: —
   Band length: 6 mm Volume applied: 2–10 µl Spacing: 10 mm
4. Chamber saturation: 15 min (MP)
5. RH (%): 55 ± 5
6. Temperature °C: 22 ± 2
7. Separation technique: Ascending
8. Quantity of mobile phase: 10 ml
9. Migration distance: 90 mm
10. Migration time: 20 min

Densitometric evaluation:

Wavelength: UV–357 nm Scanning mode: Reflectance/Absorbance
HRF: Lumefantrine—51; Artemether—83
Linearity range (ng/band): Artemether—80–480; Lumefantrine—480–2880
Recovery (%): Artemether—100.31–100.69; Lumefantrine—99.38–99.68

References: Pawan K. Saini, Raman M. Singh, Satish C. Mathur, Gyanendra N. Singh, Chhoten L. Jain, Roop K. Khar and Abdul Hafeez, *J. Planar Chromatography*, **23(2)**, 119–122, 2010.

Comments:

- The method was validated as per ICH guidelines.
- The method was stability, indicating (acid, base, oxidative).
- MP consisting of toluene-ethylacetatic-glacial acetic acid (9 : 2 : 1 v/v) gave excellant separation of both the compounds with HRF values of Lamefantrine—16; Artemether—56 (GPHF-Minilab, 415 supplement to Vol. II TLC, p. 10–13).

HPTLC : High Performance Thin Layer Chromatography
HPTLC Densitogram

No. 280

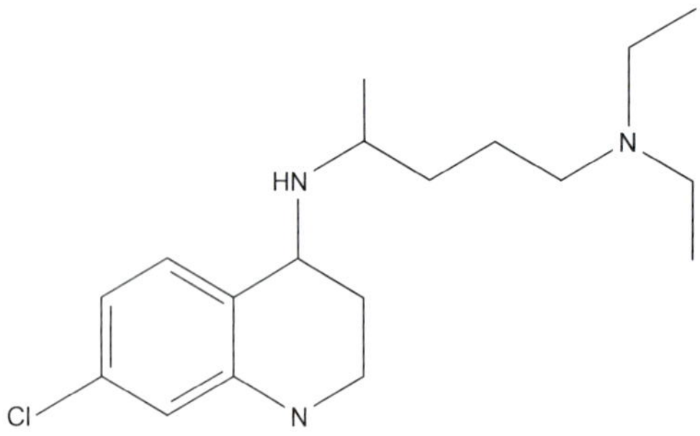

Chloroquine

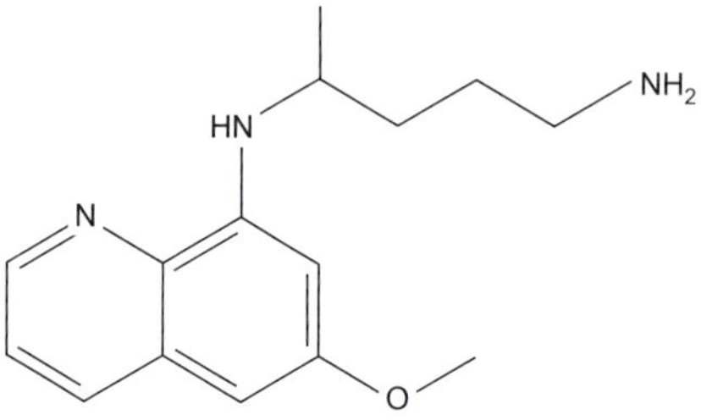

Primaquine

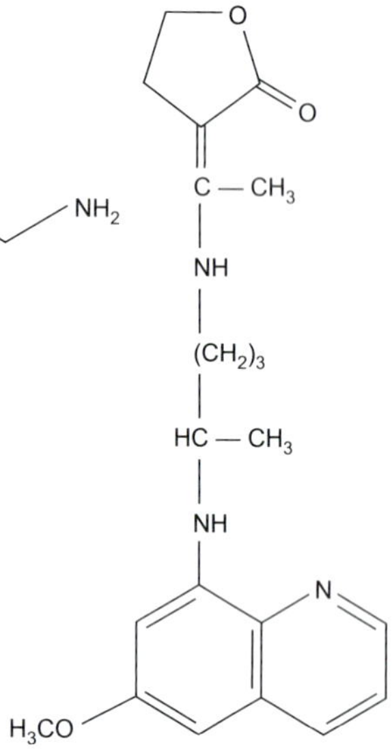

Bulaquine

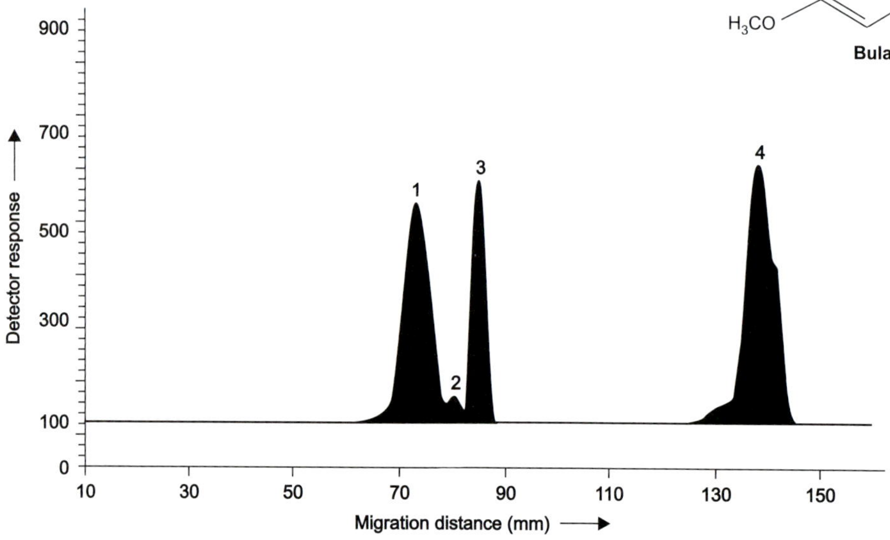

Typical densitogram of the standard containing chloroquine, primaquine and bulaquine. For detailed experimental and chromatographic condition refer to Protocol No. 280. Peaks identification: 1. Primaquine; 2. Dimethyloctylamine (stablizer for bulaquine); 3. Chloroquine; 4. Bulaquine.

PROTOCOL FOR HPTLC ANALYSIS OF PHARMACEUTICAL FORMULATION

Protocol No. 280

Formulation: **Chloroquine, Primaquine, Bulaquine**

Classification: Antibiotics **Dosage form:** Tablets

Standard preparation: Dissolve 25 mg of each chloroquine phosphate and primaquine in water containing 50 mg of K_2CO_3, dilute to 50 ml with methanol. Dissolve 25 mg of bulaquine in methanol containing 0.1% dimethyloctylamine. Further dilutions of above solutions are made with methanol to get 0.5–35 μg/ml (bulaquine); 1.5–50 μg/ml (chloroquine) and 0.5–35 μg/ml (primaquine). Apply 5 μl for analysis.

Sample preparation: Powdered sample suspended in methanol, sonicated, centrifuged and clear supernatant liquid suitably diluted. Apply 5 μl for assay.

Chromatographic equipments:

Sample applicator: Camag Nanomat–III

Development chamber: Camag twin-trough glass chamber, 20 × 20 cm

Densitometric scanner: Camag TLC Scanner–III

Chromatographic conditions:

1. Stationary phase: Silica gel $60F_{254}$ pre-coated HPTLC plates, 20 × 20 cm (200 μm) – Merck
2. Mobile phase (MP): N-hexane–diethylether–methanol–diethylamine (37.5 : 37.5 : 25 : 0.5 v/v)
3. Standard/Sample application: —
   Band length: 5 mm Volume applied: 5 μl Spacing: 10 mm
4. Chamber saturation: 15 min (MP)
5. RH (%): 55 ± 2
6. Temperature °C: 27 ± 3
7. Separation technique: Ascending
8. Quantity of mobile phase: 20 ml
9. Migration distance: 150 mm
10. Migration time: 60 min

Densitometric evaluation:

Wavelength: UV–254 nm Scanning mode: Reflectance/Absorbance

HRF: Primaquine—28; Chloroquine—39; Bulaquine—88

Linearity range (ng band): Primaquine and chloroquine—1–25; Bulaquine—0.5–20

Recovery (%): 98.75–101.25 for all the three compounds

References: A.K. Dwidi, D. Saxena and S. Singh, *J. Pharm. Biomed. Anal.*, **26**, 851–858, 2003.

Comments:

- The method validated for accuracy, precision, linearity, LOD, LOQ, specificity, robustness and ruggedness.
- The author reported simultaneously estimation by HPLC with comparable results.

HPTLC : High Performance Thin Layer Chromatography
HPTLC Densitogram

No. 281

Cefaclor

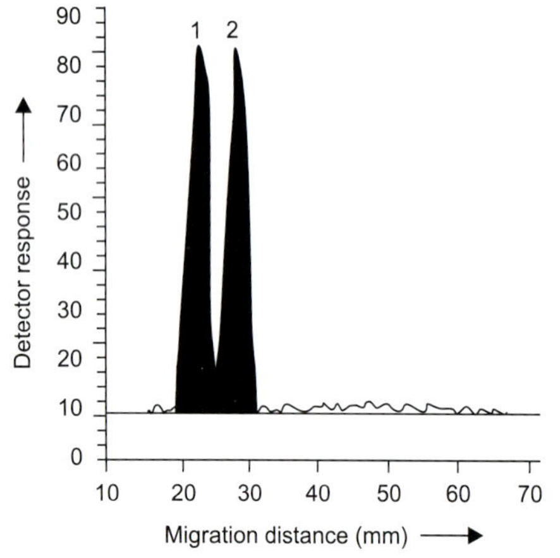

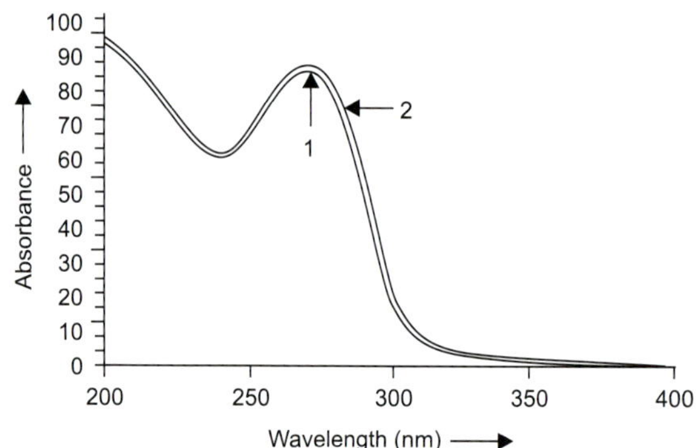

UV-absorption spectra of epimer-1 (1) and epimer-2 (2) for selection of suitable wavelength (274 nm) for densitometric scanning (both epimers have similar UV-spectra)

Typical densitogram of the standard containing cefaclor. For detailed experimental and chromatographic condition refer to Protocol No. 281. Peaks identification: 1. Epimer-1; 2. Epimer-2.

PROTOCOL FOR HPTLC ANALYSIS OF PHARMACEUTICAL FORMULATION

Protocol No. 281

Formulation: **Cefaclor (Epimers)**

Classification: Antibiotics **Dosage form:** Capsules

Standard preparation: Prepare 200 μg/ml solution of cefaclor in the solvent. Apply 5–30 μl for linearity assessment.

Solvent: 1.5% aq. β-cyclodextrin solution–methanol (1 : 1 v/v).

Sample preparation: The sample was shaken with the solvent for 10 min, filtered and suitably diluted with the solvent and used for chromatographic separation and analysis.

Chromatographic equipments:

Sample applicator: Camag Linomat–V

Development chamber: Sigma-Aldrich glass TLC chamber, 18 cm × 9 cm × 18 cm

Densitometric scanner: Camag TLC Scanner–III

Chromatographic conditions:

1. Stationary phase: Silica gel 60F_{254} pre-coated HPTLC plates; 5 × 10 cm (200 μm) – Merck, impregnated with β-cyclodextrin solution, dried in open air, then activated at 60° for 24 h.
2. Mobile phase (MP): Chloroform–methyl acetate–glacial acetic acid–water (4 : 4 : 4 : 1 v/v)
3. Standard/Sample application: —
   Band length: 10 mm Volume applied: 1–35 μl Spacing: 8 mm
4. Chamber saturation: 30 min (MP)
5. RH (%): —
6. Temperature °C: 5 ± 0.1
7. Separation technique: Ascending
8. Quantity of mobile phase: 13 ml
9. Migration distance: 95 mm
10. Migration time: 25 min

Densitometric evaluation:

Wavelength: UV–274 nm Scanning mode: Reflectance/Absorbance

HRF: Epimer-1—26; Epimer-2—30

Linearity range: 1.26–4.25 μg/band for both the epimers

Recovery (%): 100.03–100.81 for both the epimers

References: Monika Dabrowska and Jan Krzek, *J. Planar Chromatogr.*, **23(4)**, 265–269, 2010.

Comments:

- Solution of chiral selector: 1.5% w/v solution of β-cyclodextrin in water.
- Impregnating solution: β-cyclodextrin solution–methanol (9 : 1 v/v).
- Preparation of impregnated TLC plates: Pre-coated TLC plate (5 × 10 cm) was developed with impregnating solution prior to use for analysis.
- The method validated for accuracy, precision, linearity, LOD, LOQ, specificity, robustness and ruggedness.
- At room temperature peaks were not well separated; at 5°C good separation was obtained. Ratio of epimer-1 and 2 was close (1 : 1 v/v).

HPTLC : High Performance Thin Layer Chromatography
HPTLC Densitogram

No. 282

Cefuroxime axetil

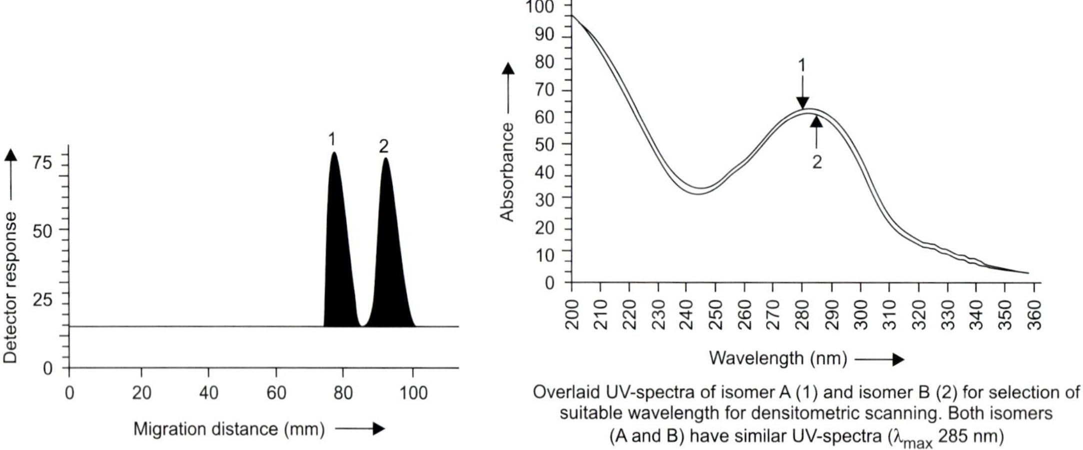

Overlaid UV-spectra of isomer A (1) and isomer B (2) for selection of suitable wavelength for densitometric scanning. Both isomers (A and B) have similar UV-spectra (λ_{max} 285 nm)

Typical densitogram of the sample containing cefuroxime axetil. For detailed experimental and chromatographic condition refer to Protocol No. 282. Peaks identification: 1. Isomer-A(S); 2. Isomer-B(R).

PROTOCOL FOR HPTLC ANALYSIS OF PHARMACEUTICAL FORMULATION

Protocol No. 282

Formulation: **Cefuroxime axetil, Isomers – A(S) and B(R)**

Classification: Antibiotics **Dosage form:** Tablets

Standard preparation: Prepare 10 μg/ml solution of the substance by dissolving in hot (60°C) aqueous ammonium dihydrogen phosphate–methanol (31 : 19 v/v). Apply 10 μl for chromatographic analysis.

Sample preparation: Powdered sample extracted with hot (60°C) solution of $NH_4H_2PO_4$–methanol (31 : 19 v/v) by shaking for 10 min, filtered and the filtrate suitably diluted with above solvent to get 10 μg/ml solution and used for analysis.

Chromatographic equipments:

Sample applicator: Camag Linomat–V

Development chamber: Sigma-Aldrich glass TLC chamber, 18 × 9 × 18 cm

Densitometric scanner: Camag TLC Scanner–III

Chromatographic conditions:

1. Stationary phase: Cellulose coated HPTLC plates, 5 × 10 cm (200 μm) – Merck, activated at 60°C for 24 h
2. Mobile phase (MP): 1% aqueous β-cyclodextrin–methanol (15 : 1 v/v) – chiral mobile phase
3. Standard/Sample application: —

   Band length: 10 mm Volume applied: 30 μl Spacing: 10 mm
4. Chamber saturation: 30 min (MP)
5. RH (%): —
6. Temperature °C: 22 ± 2
7. Separation technique: Ascending
8. Quantity of mobile phase: 16 ml
9. Migration distance: 95 mm
10. Migration time: —

Densitometric evaluation:

Wavelength: UV–285 nm Scanning mode: Reflectance/Absorbance

HRF: Isomer-A—80; Isomer-B—93

Linearity range: 100–450 ng/band for both the isomers

Recovery (%): 96.63–104.16 for both the isomers

References: Monika Dabrowska and Jan Krzek, *J. AOAC. Int.*, **93(3)**, 771–777, 2010.

Comments: The method validated for accuracy, precision, linearity, LOD, LOQ, specificity, robustness and ruggedness.

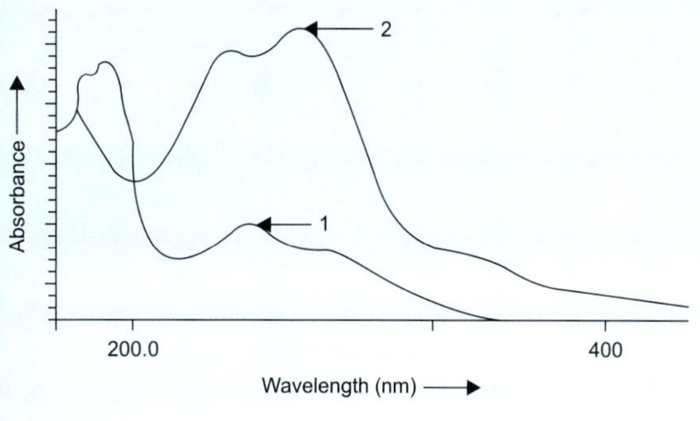

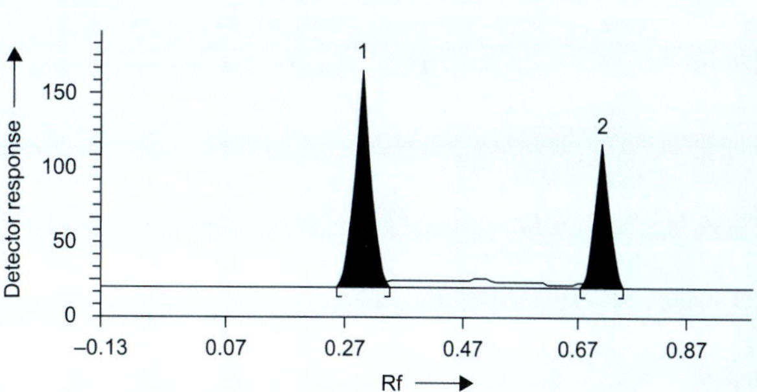

Respiratory System and Anti-Allergics

- Expectorants
- Antitussives and mucolytics
- Bronchodilators (Anti-asthma)
- Anti-allergics

Protocols and Densitograms from 283 to 331

Nothing can be achieved without enthusiasm and dedication.

HPTLC : High Performance Thin Layer Chromatography
HPTLC Densitogram

No. 283

Ephedrine hydrochloride

Triprolidine hydrochloride

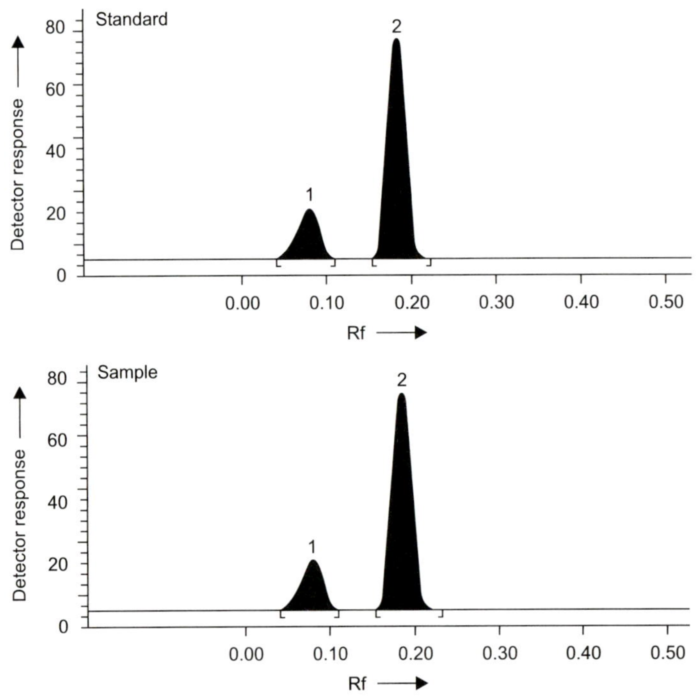

Typical densitogram of the sample and standard containing ephedrine hydrochloride and triprolidine hydrochloride. For detailed experimental and chromatographic conditions, refer to Protocol No. 283. Peaks identification: 1. Ephedrine HCl; 2. Triprolidine HCl.

PROTOCOL FOR HPTLC ANALYSIS OF PHARMACEUTICAL FORMULATION

Protocol No. 283

Formulation: Ephedrine hydrochloride, Triprolidine hydrochloride

Classification: Respiratory System **Dosage form:** Syrup

Standard preparation: Prepare 100 μg/ml solution of each drug in methanol. Mix 6 ml of ephedrine solution and 1 ml of triprolidine solution and dilute to 10 ml with methanol. Apply 10 μl for analysis.

Sample preparation: Dilute 10 ml of the syrup to 25 ml with methanol. Further dilute 0.5 ml to 10 ml with methanol for estimation of the both the compounds.

Chromatographic equipments:

Sample applicator: Camag Linomat–IV

Development chamber: Camag twin-trough glass chamber, 10 × 10 cm

Densitometric scanner: Camag TLC Scanner–II

Chromatographic conditions:

1. Stationary phase: Silica gel $60F_{254}$ pre-coated HPTLC plates, 7 × 10 cm (200 μm) – Merck
2. Mobile phase (MP): Chloroform–methanol–25% ammonia (1 : 0.5 : 0.05 v/v)
3. Standard/Sample application:
   Band length: 10 mm Volume applied: 10 μl Spacing: 10 mm
4. Chamber saturation: 20 min (MP)
5. RH (%): 55 ± 5
6. Temperature °C: 22 ± 2
7. Separation technique: Ascending
8. Quantity of mobile phase: 10 ml
9. Migration distance: 50 mm
10. Migration time: 20 min

Densitometric evaluation:

Wavelength: UV–254 nm (EH and TH); UV–290 nm (TH)

Scanning mode: Reflectance/Absorbance

HRF: Ephedrine HCl (EH)—8; Triprolidine HCl (TH)—18

Linearity (μg/ml): Ephedrine HCl—25–100; Triprolidine HCl—2–20

Recovery (%): 99.60–101.68 for both the drugs

References: —

Comments:

- The method was optimized and analytical work carried out at **Anchrom's HPTLC Application Laboratory**, Mumbai, India.
- Several market samples of similar composition were analysed by the proposed method with reproducible results.

HPTLC : High Performance Thin Layer Chromatography
HPTLC Densitogram

No. 284

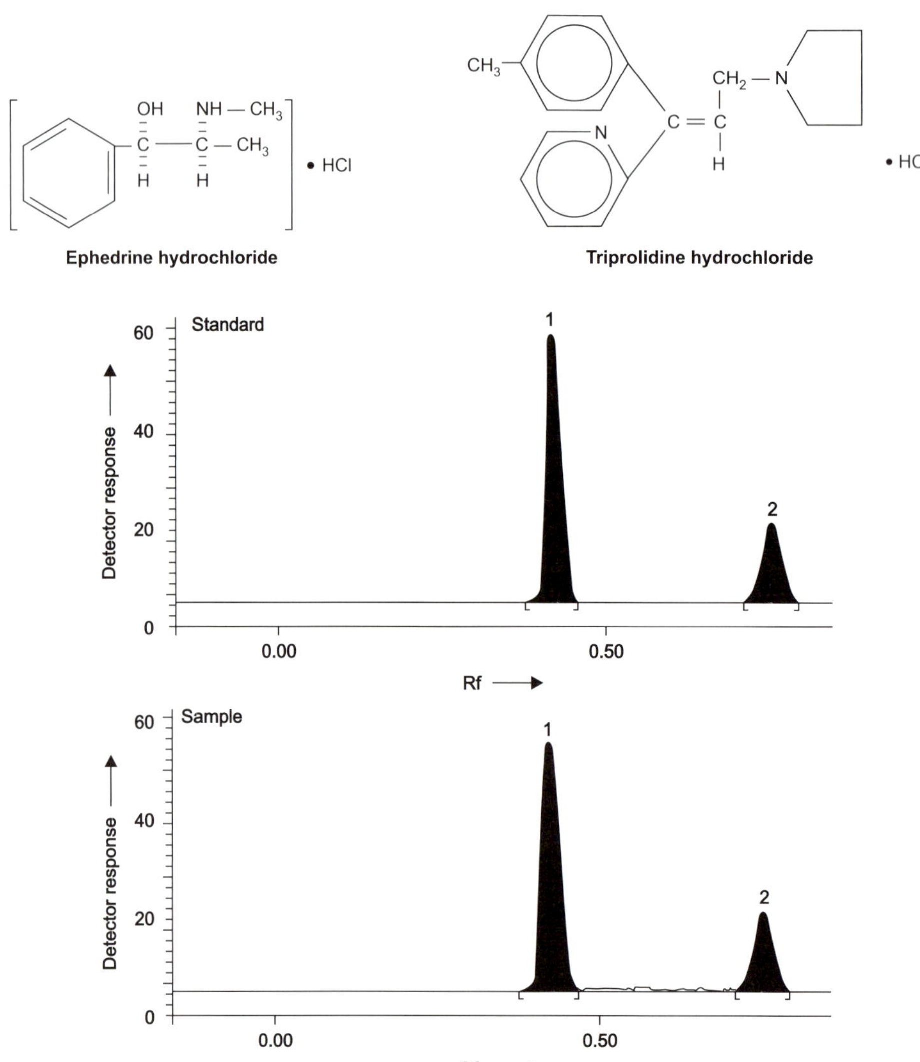

Typical densitogram of the sample and standard containing ephedrine hydrochloride and triprolidine hydrochloride. For detailed experimental and chromatographic conditions, refer to Protocol No. 284. Peaks identification: 1. Triprolidine HCl; 2. Ephedrine HCl.

PROTOCOL FOR HPTLC ANALYSIS OF PHARMACEUTICAL FORMULATION

Protocol No. 284

Formulation: Ephedrine hydrochloride, Triprolidine hydrochloride

Classification: Respiratory System **Dosage form:** Syrup

Standard preparation: Prepare 100 μg/ml solution of each drug in methanol. Mix 6 ml of ephedrine solution with 1 ml of triprolidine solution and dilute to 10 ml with methanol and use for analysis.

Sample preparation: Dilute 10 ml of the sample to 25 ml with methanol. Further dilute 0.5 ml to 10 ml with methanol. Filter and use for analysis.

Chromatographic equipments:

Sample applicator: Camag Linomat–IV

Development chamber: Camag twin-trough glass chamber, 10 × 10 cm

Densitometric scanner: Camag TLC Scanner–II

Chromatographic conditions:

1. Stationary phase: Silica gel RP-18F_{254s} pre-coated HPTLC plates, 10 × 10 cm (200 μm) – Merck
2. Mobile phase (MP): 0.5 M sod. chloride–methanol–acetonitrile–glacial acetic acid (5 : 2 : 3 : 0.1 v/v)
3. Standard/Sample application:
   Band length: 7 mm Volume applied: 10 μl Spacing: 15 mm
4. Chamber saturation: 30 min (MP)
5. RH (%): 55 ± 2
6. Temperature °C: 22 ± 2
7. Separation technique: Ascending
8. Quantity of mobile phase: 10 ml
9. Migration distance: 50 mm
10. Migration time: 25 min

Densitometric evaluation:

Wavelength: UV–254 nm (EH and TH); UV–290 nm (TH)

Scanning mode: Reflectance/Absorbance

HRF: Triprolidine HCl (TH)—40; Ephedrine hydrochloride (EH)—75

Linearity (μg/ml): Ephedrine HCl—25–100; Triprolidine HCl—2–20

Recovery (%): 98.75–103.50 for both the drugs

References: —

Comments:

- The method was optimized and analytical work carried out at **Anchrom's HPTLC Application Laboratory**, Mumbai, India.
- RP-chromatography resulted in reversal of retention order as compared to NP-chromatography.
- RP phase gave better resolution.
- Several market samples of similar composition were analysed by the proposed method with reproducible results.

HPTLC : High Performance Thin Layer Chromatography
HPTLC Densitogram

No. 285

Pseudoephedrine hydrochloride

Triprolidine hydrochloride

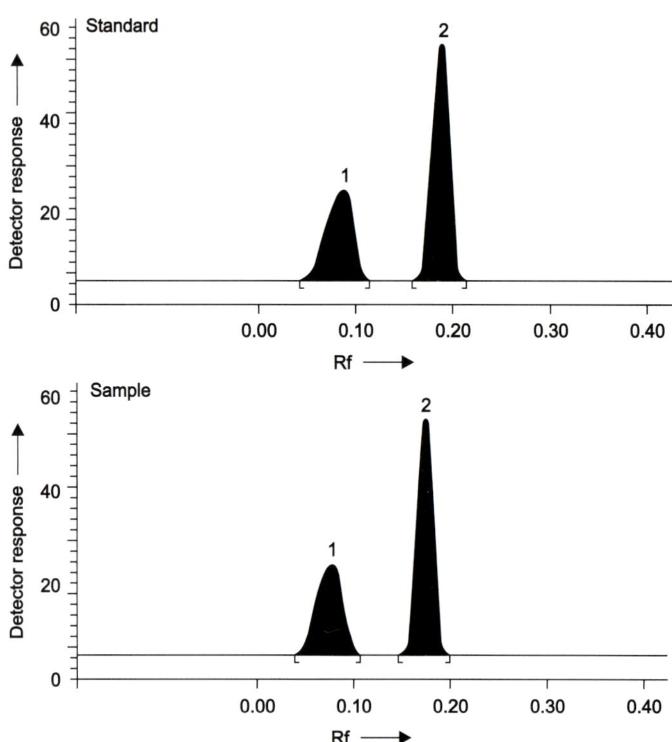

Typical densitogram of the sample and standard containing pseudoephedrine hydrochloride and triprolidine hydrochloride. For detailed experimental and chromatographic conditions, refer to Protocol No. 285. Peaks identification: 1. Pseudoephedrine HCl; 2. Triprolidine HCl.

PROTOCOL FOR HPTLC ANALYSIS OF PHARMACEUTICAL FORMULATION

Protocol No. 285

Formulation: Pseudoephedrine hydrochloride, Triprolidine hydrochloride

Classification: Respiratory System **Dosage form:** Tablets, Syrup

Standard preparation: Prepare 1 mg/ml solution of triprolidine hydrochloride in methanol (1). Weigh 24 mg of pseudoephedrine hydrochloride, add 1 ml of solution (1), vortex for 10 min, dilute to 10 ml with methanol and use for analysis.

Sample preparation: Sample equivalent to 2.5 mg of triprolidine hydrochloride is mixed with 20 ml of methanol, vortex for 10 min, dilute to 25 ml with methanol, filter and use the filtrate for analysis.

Chromatographic equipments:

Sample applicator: Camag Linomat–IV

Development chamber: Camag twin-trough glass chamber, 10 × 10 cm

Densitometric scanner: Camag TLC Scanner–II

Chromatographic conditions:

1. Stationary phase: Silica gel $60F_{254}$ pre-coated HPTLC plates, 10 × 10 cm (200 μm) – Merck
2. Mobile phase (MP): Chloroform–methanol–25% ammonia (10 : 0.5 : 0.05 v/v)
3. Standard/Sample application:
   Band length: 10 mm Volume applied: 5 μl Spacing: 15 mm
4. Chamber saturation: 30 min (MP)
5. RH (%): 55 ± 5
6. Temperature °C: 22 ± 2
7. Separation technique: Ascending
8. Quantity of mobile phase: 10 ml
9. Migration distance: 50 mm
10. Migration time: 20 min

Densitometric evaluation:

Wavelength: UV–254 nm (PH and TH); UV–290 nm (TH)

Scanning mode: Reflectance/Absorbance

HRF: Pseudoephedrine HCl (PH)—9; Triprolidine HCl (TH)—19

Linearity (μg/ml): Triprolidine HCl—50–200; Pseudoephedrine HCl—600–3000

Recovery (%): 98.40–99.63 for both the drugs

References: —

Comments:

- The method was optimized and analytical work carried out at **Anchrom's HPTLC Application Laboratory**, Mumbai, India.
- Several market samples of similar composition were analysed by the proposed method with reproducible results.

HPTLC : High Performance Thin Layer Chromatography
HPTLC Densitogram

No. 286

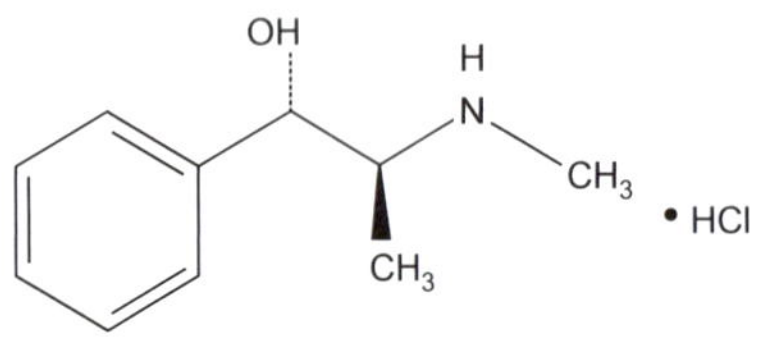

Pseudoephedrine hydrochloride

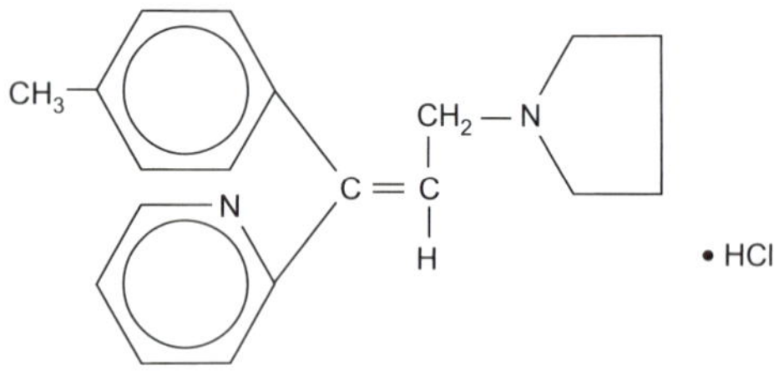

Triprolidine hydrochloride

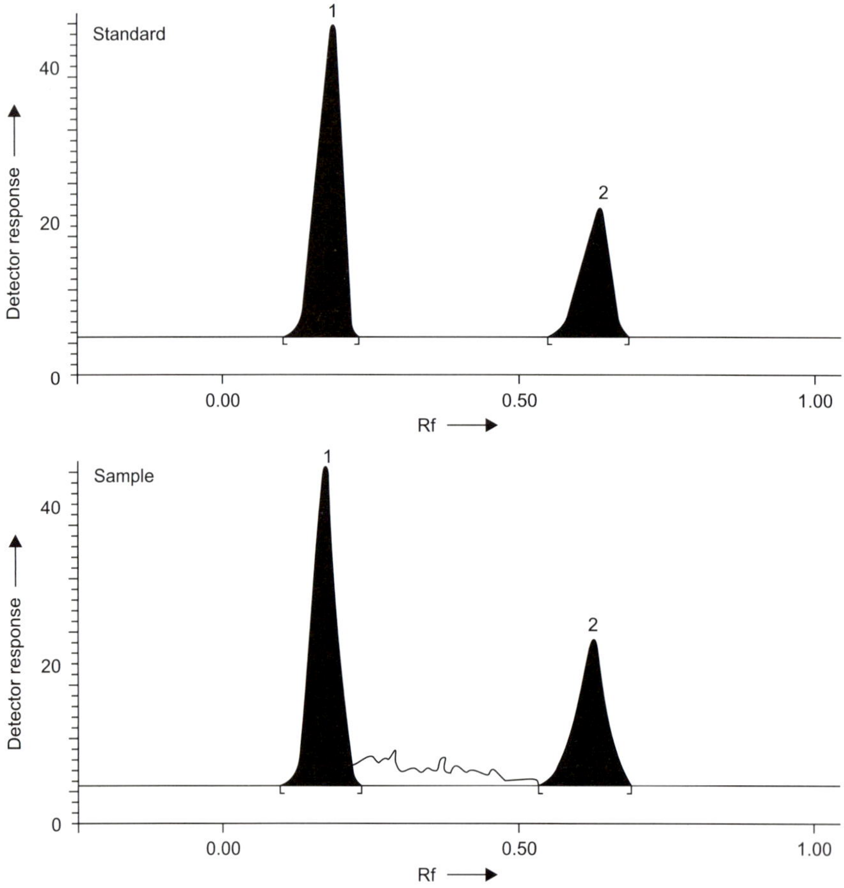

Typical densitogram of the sample and standard containing pseudoephedrine hydrochloride and triprolidine hydrochloride. For detailed experimental and chromatographic conditions, refer to Protocol No. 286. Peaks identification: 1. Triprolidine HCl; 2. Pseudoephedrine HCl.

PROTOCOL FOR HPTLC ANALYSIS OF PHARMACEUTICAL FORMULATION

Protocol No. 286

Formulation: Pseudoephedrine hydrochloride, Triprolidine hydrochloride
Classification: Respiratory System **Dosage form:** Tablets, Syrup
Standard preparation: Prepare 100 μg/ml solution of triprolidine hydrochloride in methanol (1). Weigh 24 mg of pseudoephedrine hydrochloride, add 1 ml of solution (1), dilute to 10 ml with methanol and use for analysis.
Sample preparation: Sample equivalent to 2.5 mg of triprolidine hydrochloride suspended in 20 ml of methanol, vortexed for 10 min, diluted to 25 ml, filtered and the filtrate used for assay.
Chromatographic equipments:
Sample applicator: Camag Linomat–IV
Development chamber: Camag twin-trough glass chamber, 10 × 10 cm
Densitometric scanner: Camag TLC Scanner–II
Chromatographic conditions:

1. Stationary phase: Silica gel 60 RP-18 F_{254s} pre-coated HPTLC plates, 10 × 10 cm (200 μm) – Merck
2. Mobile phase (MP): 0.5 M sod. chloride–methanol–acetonitrile–glacial acetic acid (5 : 2 : 3 : 0.1 v/v)
3. Standard/Sample application:
   Band length: 5 mm Volume applied: 5 μl Spacing: 20 mm
4. Chamber saturation: 30 min (MP)
5. RH (%): 55 ± 5
6. Temperature °C: 22 ± 2
7. Separation technique: Ascending
8. Quantity of mobile phase: 10 ml
9. Migration distance: 50 mm
10. Migration time: 25 min

Densitometric evaluation:
Wavelength: UV–254 nm (TH and PH); UV–290 nm (TH)
Scanning mode: Reflectance/Absorbance
HRF: Triprolidine HCl—17; Pseudoephedrine HCl—63
Linearity (μg/ml): Triprolidine HCl (TH)—50–200; Pseudoephedrine HCl (PH)—600–3000
Recovery (%): 98.75–99.60 for both the drugs
References: —
Comments:

- The method was optimized and analytical work carried out at **Anchrom's HPTLC Application Laboratory**, Mumbai, India.
- Reversed-phase chromatography resulted in reversal of retention order as compared to NP-chromatography.
- The resolution was better with RP-system.
- Several market samples of similar composition were analysed by the proposed method with reproducible results.

HPTLC : High Performance Thin Layer Chromatography
HPTLC Densitogram

No. 287

Pseudoephedrine hydrochloride

Cetirizine

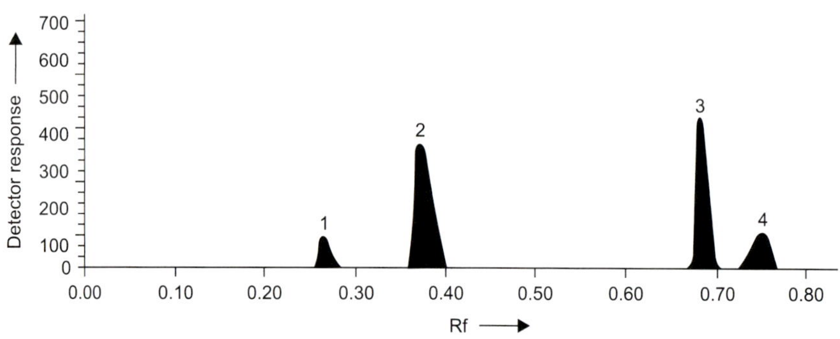

Typical densitogram of the sample containing pseudoephedrine hydrochloride and cetirizine treated with H_2O_2. For detailed experimental and chromatographic conditions, refer to Protocol No. 287. Peaks identification: 1. Decomposition product of cetirizine; 2. Cetirizine; 3. Pseudoephedrine HCl; 4. Decomposition product of pseudoephedrine hydrochloride.

PROTOCOL FOR HPTLC ANALYSIS OF PHARMACEUTICAL FORMULATION

Protocol No. 287

Formulation: Pseudoephedrine hydrochloride, Cetirizine hydrochloride

Classification: Respiratory System **Dosage form:** Tablets

Standard preparation: Prepare solutions of both the compounds in methanol to get 10 mg/ml of pseudoephedrine HCl and 1 mg/ml of cetirizine. Further serial dilutions are made to get 10–26 μg/ml of pseudoephedrine HCl and 200–1200 ng/ml of cetirizine.

Sample preparation: Powdered sample equivalent to 25 mg of pseudoephedrine HCl suspended in 20 ml of methanol, sonicated for 15 min, diluted to 25 ml, centrifuged (5000 rpm) for 5 min, and supernatant used for analysis.

Chromatographic equipments:

Sample applicator: Camag Linomat–IV

Development chamber: Camag twin-trough glass chamber, 20 × 20 cm

Densitometric scanner: Camag TLC Scanner–III

Chromatographic conditions:

1. Stationary phase: Silica gel 60F_{254} pre-coated TLC plates, 20 × 10 cm (250 μm) – Merck
2. Mobile phase (MP): Ethyl acetate–methanol–25% ammonia (7 : 1.5 : 1 v/v)
3. Standard/Sample application:
   Band length: 6 mm Volume applied: 1 μl Spacing: 5 mm
4. Chamber saturation: 30 min (MP)
5. RH (%): 55 ± 5
6. Temperature °C: 22 ± 2
7. Separation technique: Ascending
8. Quantity of mobile phase: 15 ml
9. Migration distance: 80 mm
10. Migration time: 30 min

Densitometric evaluation:

Wavelength: UV–240 nm Scanning mode: Reflectance/Absorbance

HRF: Cetirizine HCl—38; Pseudoephedrine HCl—69

Linearity: Pseudoephedrine HCl—10–25 (μg/ml); Cetirizine—200–1200 (ng/ml)

Recovery (%): Pseudoephedrine HCl—99.14; Cetirizine—99.70–101.21

References: Sapna N. Makhija and P.R. Vana, *J. Pharm. and Biomed. Anal.*, **25**, 663–667, 2001.

Comments:

- The method validated for accuracy, precision, linearity, LOD, LOQ, specificity, robustness and ruggedness.
- The method is stability indicating (acid, base, oxidative, thermal, photolytic). The degradation products were separated from main compounds.
- No degradation with acid and alkali.

HPTLC : High Performance Thin Layer Chromatography
HPTLC Densitogram

No. 288

Pseudoephedrine hydrochloride

Loratadine

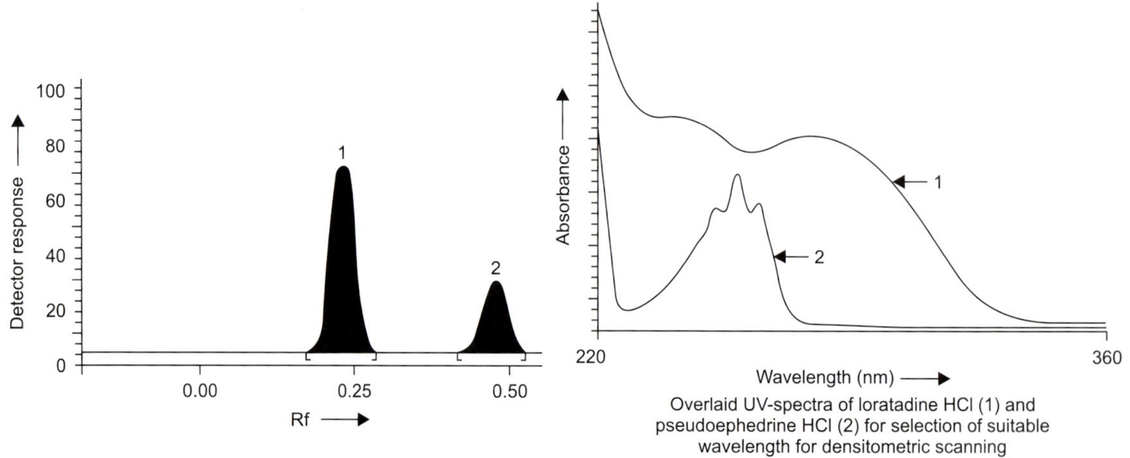

Overlaid UV-spectra of loratadine HCl (1) and pseudoephedrine HCl (2) for selection of suitable wavelength for densitometric scanning

Typical densitogram of the standard containing pseudoephedrine hydrochloride and loratadine hydrochloride. For detailed experimental and chromatographic conditions, refer to Protocol No. 288. Peaks identification: 1. Loratadine HCl; 2. Pseudoephedrine HCl.

PROTOCOL FOR HPTLC ANALYSIS OF PHARMACEUTICAL FORMULATION

Protocol No. 288

Formulation: Pseudoephedrine hydrochloride, Loratadine hydrochloride

Classification: Respiratory System **Dosage form:** Tablets

Standard preparation: Prepare 30 mg/ml solution of pseudoephedrine hydrochloride (PH) and 2 mg/ml of loratadine (LD), both in methanol. Further dilute 0.1–4.2 ml of PH solution and 0.1–3.5 ml of LD solution to 10 ml with methanol and apply 10 µl of each for linearity studies.

Sample preparation: Powdered sample equivalent to 10 mg of loratadine suspended in 50 ml of methanol, shake for 10 min, filter and apply 10 µl for assay.

Chromatographic equipments:

Sample applicator: Camag Linomat–IV

Development chamber: Camag twin-trough glass chamber, 10 × 10 cm

Densitometric scanner: Desaga TLC Scanner

Chromatographic conditions:

1. Stationary phase: Silica gel $60F_{254}$ pre-coated TLC plates, 10 × 10 cm (250 µm) – Merck
2. Mobile phase (MP): n-hexane–dichloromethane–triethylamine (5.5 : 4 : 0.5 v/v)
3. Standard/Sample application:
   Band length: 5 mm Volume applied: 10 µl Spacing: 5 mm
4. Chamber saturation: 10 min (MP)
5. RH (%): 55 ± 5
6. Temperature °C: 22 ± 2
7. Separation technique: Ascending
8. Quantity of mobile phase: 10 ml
9. Migration distance: 80 mm
10. Migration time: 30 min

Densitometric evaluation:

Wavelength: UV–235 nm Scanning mode: Reflectance/Absorbance

HRF: Loratadine HCl—24; Pseudoephedrine HCl—47

Linearity (µg/ml): Pseudoephedrine HCl—12–90; Loratadine HCl—0.8–5

Recovery (%): 99.85–100.06 for both the compounds

References: Sane, R.T. Francis Mary, Khedkar Sachin, Pawar Sagar and Moghe Atul, *Indian Drugs*, **38(8)**, 436–438, 2001.

Comments: The method validated for accuracy, precision, linearity, LOD, LOQ, specificity, robustness and ruggedness.

HPTLC : High Performance Thin Layer Chromatography
HPTLC Densitogram

No. 289

OH H N CH_3 • HCl CH_3

Pseudoephedrine hydrochloride

CH_3 CH_3 COOH H_3C

Ibuprofen

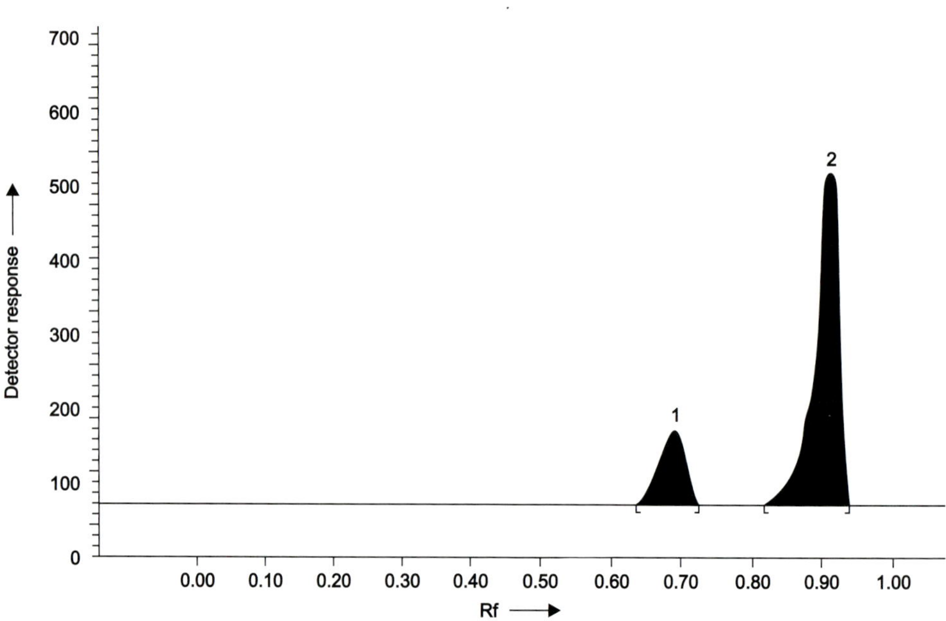

Typical densitogram of the sample containing pseudoephedrine hydrochloride and ibuprofen. For detailed experimental and chromatographic conditions, refer to Protocol No. 289. Peaks identification: 1. Pseudoephedrine HCl; 2. Ibuprofen.

PROTOCOL FOR HPTLC ANALYSIS OF PHARMACEUTICAL FORMULATION

Protocol No. 289

Formulation: Pseudoephedrine hydrochloride, Ibuprofen

Classification: Respiratory System **Dosage form:** Tablets

Standard preparation: Prepare 8 mg/ml solution of ibuprofen and 1.2 mg/ml of pseudoephedrine HCl, both in methanol. Further diluted suitably for analysis. Apply 1–10 μl of each solution for linearity profile.

Sample preparation: Powdered sample equivalent to 200 mg of ibuprofen suspended in 20 ml of methanol, shake for 15 min, diluted to 25 ml, filtered through Whatman No. 1 filter paper and 6 μl of the resulting solution applied for assay.

Chromatographic equipments:

Sample applicator: Camag Linomat–IV

Development chamber: Camag twin-trough glass chamber, 10 × 10 cm

Densitometric scanner: Camag TLC Scanner–III

Chromatographic conditions:

1. Stationary phase: Silica gel $60F_{254}$ pre-coated HPTLC plates, 10 × 10 cm (200 μm) – Merck
2. Mobile phase (MP): t-butanol–ethyl acetate–glacial acetic acid–water (7 : 4 : 2 : 2 v/v)
3. Standard/Sample application:
   Band length: 6 mm Volume applied: 1–10 μl Spacing: 6 mm
4. Chamber saturation: 20 min (MP)
5. RH (%): 55 ± 5
6. Temperature °C: 22 ± 2
7. Separation technique: Ascending
8. Quantity of mobile phase: 15 ml
9. Migration distance: 80 mm
10. Migration time: 30 min

Densitometric evaluation:

Wavelength: UV–254 nm Scanning mode: Reflectance/Absorbance

HRF: Pseudoephedrine HCl—68; Ibuprofen—91

Linearity (μg/ml): Pseudoephedrine HCl—6.8–11.3; Ibuprofen—45.6–75.6

Recovery (%): 100.69–101.3 for both the compounds

References: S.S. Chitlange, D.M. Sarkar, S.B. Wankhede and S.G. Wadodkar, *Indian J. Pharm. Sci.*, **70(3)**, 398–400, 2008.

Comments: The method validated for accuracy, precision, linearity, LOD, LOQ, specificity, robustness and ruggedness.

HPTLC : High Performance Thin Layer Chromatography
HPTLC Densitogram

No. 290

Pseudoephedrine hydrochloride

Guaiphenesin

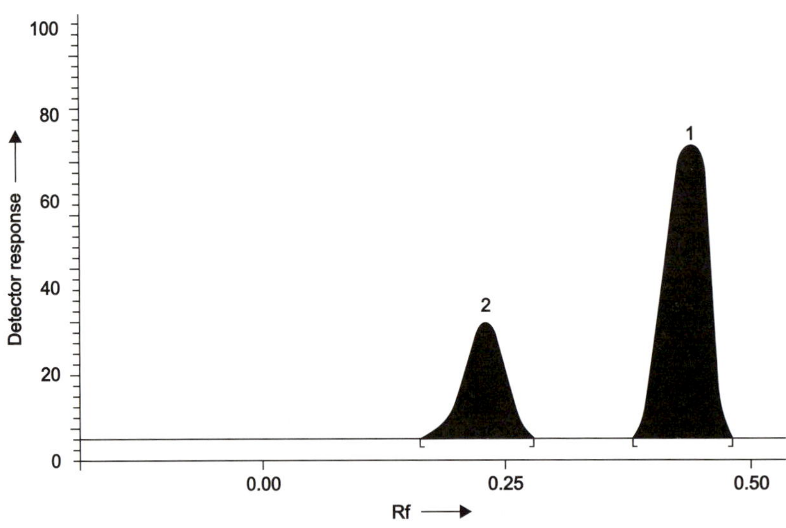

Typical densitogram of the sample containing pseudoephedrine hydrochloride and guaiphenesin. For detailed experimental and chromatographic conditions, refer to Protocol No. 290. Peaks identification: 1. Pseudoephedrine HCl; 2. Guaiphenesin.

PROTOCOL FOR HPTLC ANALYSIS OF PHARMACEUTICAL FORMULATION

Protocol No. 290

Formulation: Pseudoephedrine hydrochloride, Guaiphenesin

Classification: Respiratory System **Dosage form:** Tablets/Syrup

Standard preparation: Prepare solution of both the compounds in methanol to get 50 mg/ml (pseudoephedrine hydrochloride) and 100 mg/ml (guaiphenesin). Further dilutions made to get 5 mg/ml (pseudoephedrine hydrochloride) and 1 mg/ml (guaiphenesin). Apply 2–10 µl for linearity studies.

Sample preparation: The sample equivalent to 600 mg of guaiphenesin suspended in 80 ml of methanol, stirred magnetically for 60 min, filtered through cotton plug, diluted to 100 ml. Further diluted to get 2 mg/ml solution and apply 3 µl for assay.

Chromatographic equipments:

Sample applicator: Camag Linomat–IV

Development chamber: Camag twin-trough glass chamber, 10 × 20 cm, lined with filter paper

Densitometric scanner: Camag TLC Scanner–III

Chromatographic conditions:

1. Stationary phase: Silica gel 60F_{254} pre-coated HPTLC plates, 10 × 20 cm (200 µm) – Merck, pre-washed with dichloromethane–methanol (1 : 1 v/v) and air dried
2. Mobile phase (MP): Ethyl acetate–methanol–25% ammonia (8.5 : 1.0 : 0.5 v/v)
3. Standard/Sample application:
   Band length: 6 mm Volume applied: 3 µl Spacing: 6 mm
4. Chamber saturation: 10 min (MP)
5. RH (%): 55 ± 5
6. Temperature °C: 22 ± 2
7. Separation technique: Ascending
8. Quantity of mobile phase: 10 ml
9. Migration distance: 60 mm
10. Migration time: 12 min

Densitometric evaluation:

Wavelength: UV–210 nm (PH) and 276 nm (G)

Scanning mode: Reflectance/Absorbance

HRF: Pseudoephedrine HCl—23; Guaiphenesin—41

Linearity (µg/ml): Pseudoephedrine HCl—10–40; Guaiphenesin—2–8

Recovery (%): 98.8–99.3 for both the compounds

References: Matthew B. Lippstone, Erin K. Grath and Joseph Sherma, *J. Planar Chromatogr.*, **9(6)**, 456–458, 1996.

Comments: The method validated for accuracy, precision, linearity, LOD, LOQ, specificity, robustness and ruggedness.

HPTLC : High Performance Thin Layer Chromatography
HPTLC Densitogram

No. 291

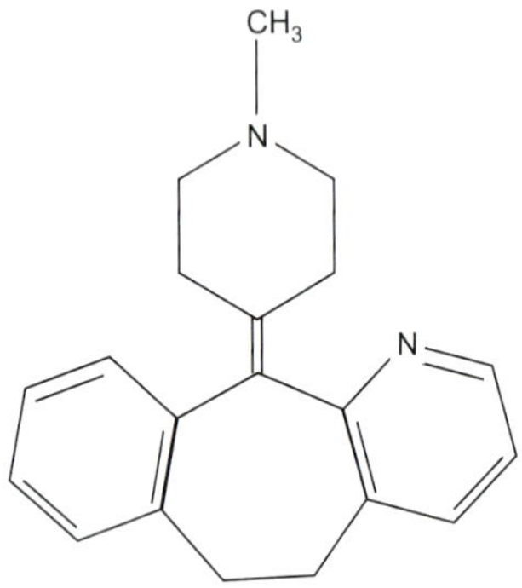

CH_3 N N

Azatadine

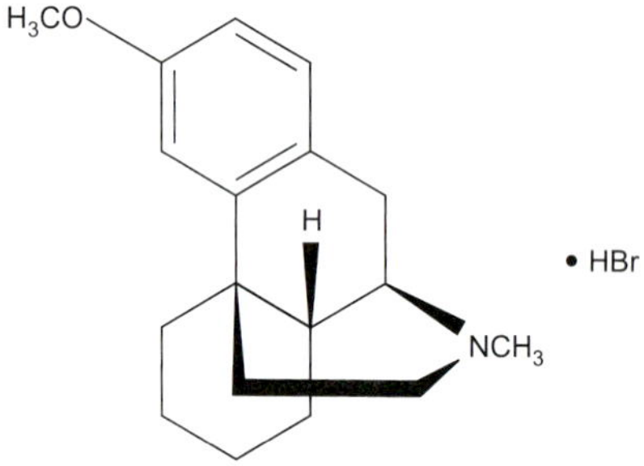

H_3CO H NCH_3 • HBr

Dextromethorphan hydrobromide

Detector response →

1 2 3 4

0.00 0.50 1.00

Rf →

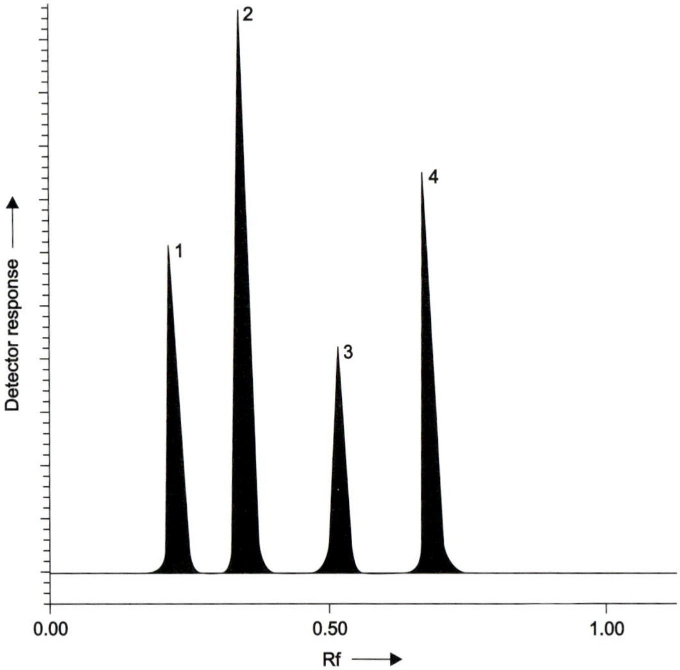

Typical densitogram of the standard containing pseudoephedrine hydrochloride, azatadine maleate and dextromethorphan hydrobromide. For detailed experimental and chromatographic conditions, refer to Protocol No. 291. Peaks identification: 1. Naproxen (IS); 2. Pseudoephedrine HCl; 3. Azatadine maleate; 4. Dextromethorphan HBr.

PROTOCOL FOR HPTLC ANALYSIS OF PHARMACEUTICAL FORMULATION

Protocol No. 291

Formulation: Pseudoephedrine hydrochloride, Dextromethorphan hydrobromide, Azatadine maleate

Classification: Respiratory System **Dosage form:** Tablets

Standard preparation: Prepare mixed standards of all the compounds in methanol to get pseudoephedrine HCl (3750 μg/ml); azatadine maleate (125 μg/ml); dextromethorphan HBr (1500 μg/ml). Dilute 0.8 ml to 8.8 ml of combined standard solution to 10 ml after adding 1 ml of (IS) solution and use for linearity profile.

Sample preparation: Suspend powdered sample equivalent to average of 5 tablets in 20 ml of methanol, sonicate and dilute to 25 ml with methanol. Filter and dilute 4 ml of filtrate to 10 ml after adding 1 ml of (IS) solution. Internal standard (IS): 4000 μg/ml in methanol.

Chromatographic equipments:

Sample applicator: Camag Linomat–IV

Development chamber: Camag twin-trough glass chamber, 10 × 10 cm

Densitometric scanner: Camag TLC Scanner–III

Chromatographic conditions:

1. Stationary phase: Silica gel $60F_{254}$ pre-coated HPTLC plates, 10 × 10 cm (200 μm) – Merck
2. Mobile phase (MP): Dichloromethane–acetone–methanol–triethylamine (7 : 4 : 0.5 : 0.2 v/v)
3. Standard/Sample application:
   Band length: 5 mm Volume applied: 5 μl Spacing: 5 mm
4. Chamber saturation: 10 min (MP)
5. RH (%): 55 ± 5
6. Temperature °C: Ambient
7. Separation technique: Ascending
8. Quantity of mobile phase: 11 ml
9. Migration distance: 70 mm
10. Migration time: 25 min

Densitometric evaluation:

Wavelength: UV–257 nm Scanning mode: Reflectance/Absorbance

HRF: See densitogram

Linearity (μg/band): Pseudoephedrine HCl—6–54; Azatadine maleate—0.05–0.55; Dextromethorphan HBr—1.5–15

Recovery (%): 99.60–100.54 for all the three drugs

References: Renu A. Sodhi, Jyoti L. Chawla and Ramesh T. Sane, *Indian Drugs*, **34(5)**, 433–435, 1997.

Comments: The method validated for accuracy, precision, linearity, LOD, LOQ, specificity, robustness and ruggedness.

HPTLC : High Performance Thin Layer Chromatography
HPTLC Densitogram

No. 293

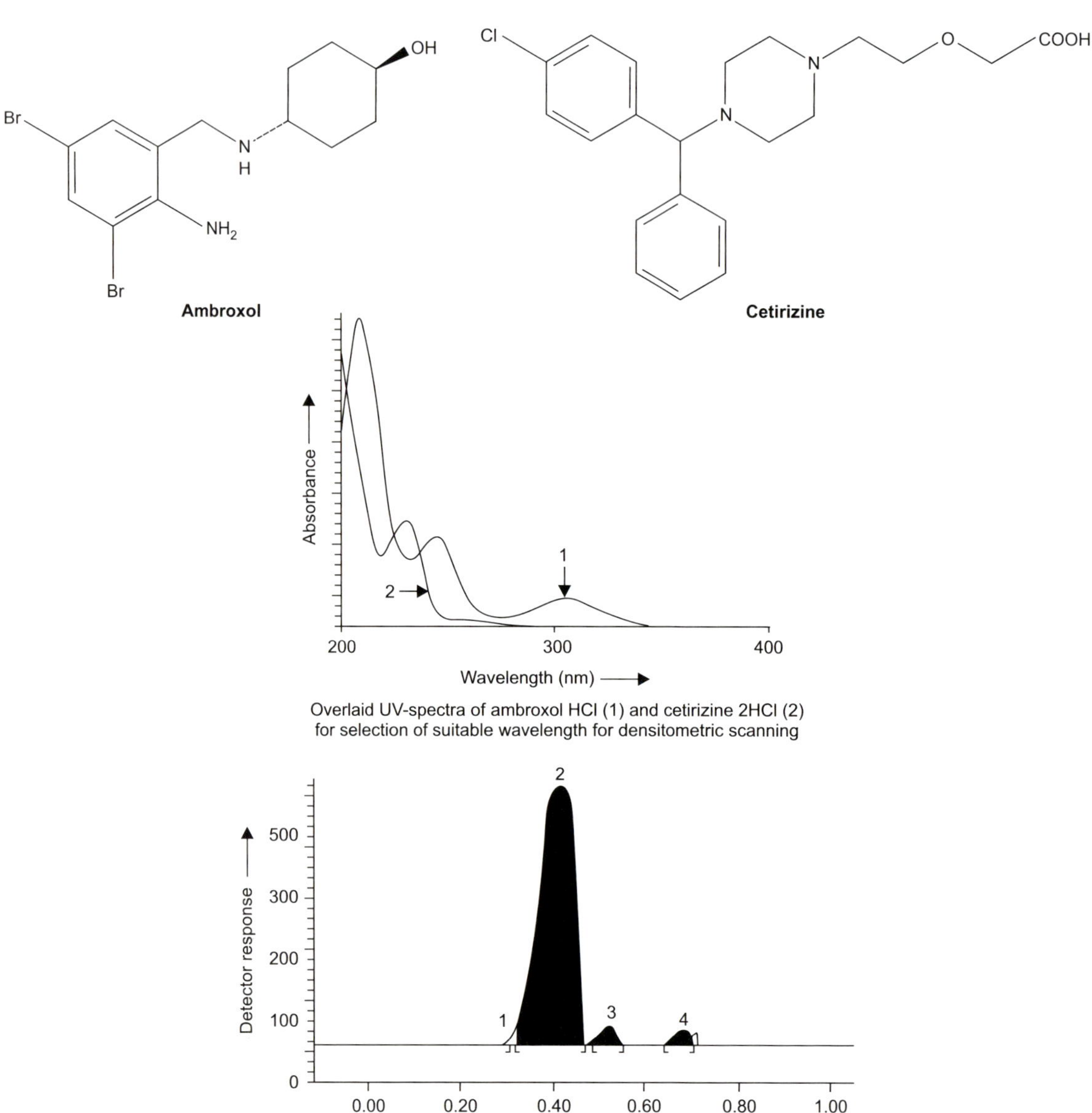

Overlaid UV-spectra of ambroxol HCl (1) and cetirizine 2HCl (2) for selection of suitable wavelength for densitometric scanning

Typical densitogram of the standard containing ambroxol HCl and cetirizine 2HCl. For detailed experimental and chromatographic conditions, refer to Protocol No. 293. Peaks identification: 1. Excipient; 2. Ambroxol HCl; 3. Excipient; 4. Cetirizine 2HCl.

PROTOCOL FOR HPTLC ANALYSIS OF PHARMACEUTICAL FORMULATION

Protocol No. 293

Formulation: Ambroxol hydrochloride, Cetirizine dihydrochloride

Classification: Respiratory System **Dosage form:** Tablets

Standard preparation: Prepare solution of both the compounds in methanol to get 2 mg/ml (cetirizine 2HCl) and 4 mg/ml ambroxol HCl. Further dilutions made suitably with methanol for linearity studies. Apply 10 µl of each solution for analysis.

Sample preparation: An appropriate quantity of the powdered sample suspended in methanol, sonicated, diluted, filtered and the filtrate suitably diluted with methanol for estimation.

Chromatographic equipments:

Sample applicator: Camag Linomat–IV

Development chamber: Camag twin-trough glass chamber, 20 × 20 cm

Densitometric scanner: Camag TLC Scanner–III

Chromatographic conditions:

1. Stationary phase: Silica gel $60F_{254}$ pre-coated TLC plates, 20 × 20 cm (250 µm) – Merck
2. Mobile phase (MP): 0.067 M KH_2PO_4–methanol (6.5 : 3.5 v/v)
3. Standard/Sample application:
   Band length: 10 mm Volume applied: 10 µl Spacing: 15 mm
4. Chamber saturation: 30 min (MP)
5. RH (%): 55 ± 5
6. Temperature °C: Ambient
7. Separation technique: Ascending
8. Quantity of mobile phase: 20 ml
9. Migration distance: 110 mm
10. Migration time: 45 min

Densitometric evaluation:

Wavelength: UV–231 nm Scanning mode: Reflectance/Absorbance

HRF: Ambroxol HCl—40; Cetirizine HCl—70

Linearity (µg/band): Cetirizine 2 HCl—2–16; Ambroxol HCl—200–1600

Recovery (%): Cetirizine 2 HCl—99.7–100.1; Ambroxol HCl—99.8–101.0

References: Lakshmi K and Niraimathi V, *Indian Drugs*, **40(4)**, 227–229, 2003.

Comments: The method validated for accuracy, precision, linearity, LOD, LOQ, specificity, robustness and ruggedness.

HPTLC : High Performance Thin Layer Chromatography
HPTLC Densitogram

No. 294

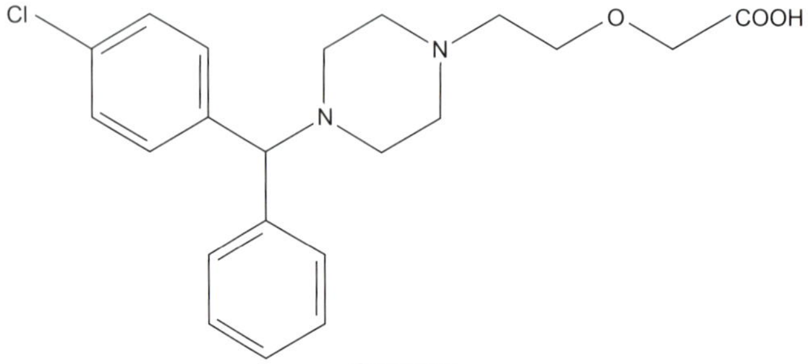

Cl N N O COOH

Cetirizine

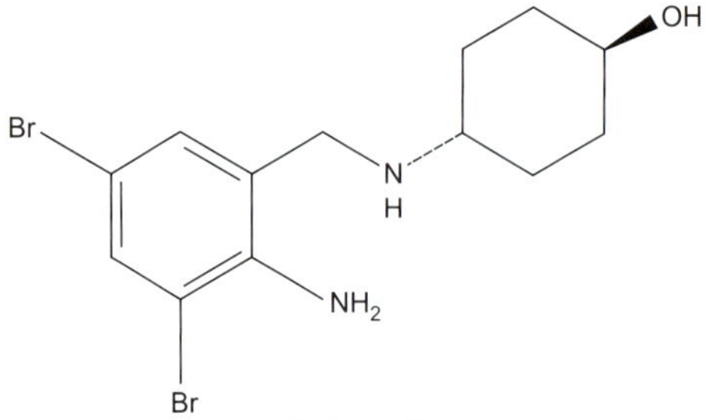

OH Br N H NH_2 Br

Ambroxol

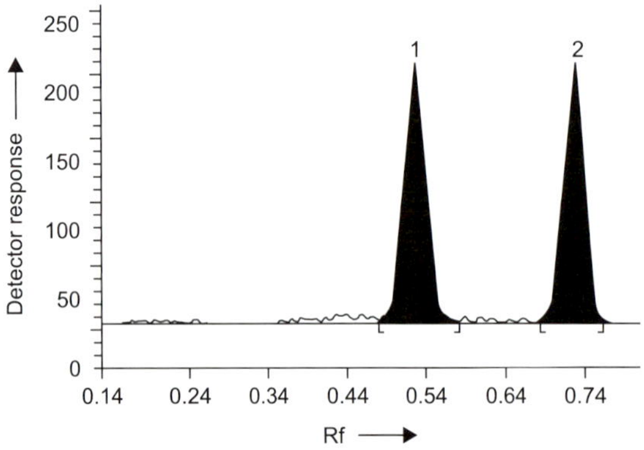

Detector response → 250 200 150 100 50 0

1 2

0.14 0.24 0.34 0.44 0.54 0.64 0.74

Rf →

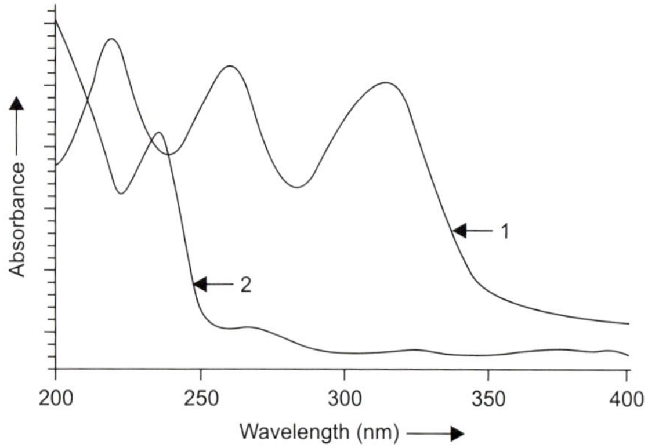

Absorbance →

← 1 ← 2

200 250 300 350 400

Wavelength (nm) →

Overlaid UV-spectra of ambroxol HCl (1) and cetirizine 2HCl (2) for selection of suitable wavelength for densitometric scanning

Typical densitogram of the standard containing ambroxol HCl and cetirizine dihydrochloride. For detailed experimental and chromatographic conditions, refer to Protocol No. 294. Peaks identification: 1. Cetirizine dihydrochloride; 2. Ambroxol hydrochloride.

PROTOCOL FOR HPTLC ANALYSIS OF PHARMACEUTICAL FORMULATION

Protocol No. 294

Formulation: Ambroxol hydrochloride, Cetirizine dihydrochloride

Classification: Respiratory System **Dosage form:** Tablets

Standard preparation: Prepare 1 mg/ml solution of each compound in methanol. Further dilutions made to get 30 μg/ml of ambroxol HCl and 2.5 μg/ml of cetirizine 2HCl. Apply 8–24 μl of each solution for linearity studies.

Sample preparation: Powdered sample equivalent to 30 mg of ambroxol HCl suspended 40 ml of methanol, sonicated for 20 min, diluted to 50 ml, filtered and 1 ml of filtrate diluted to 10 ml with methanol and used for chromatographic evaluation.

Chromatographic equipments:

Sample applicator: Camag Linomat–V

Development chamber: Camag twin-trough glass chamber, 10 × 10 cm

Densitometric scanner: Camag TLC Scanner–III

Chromatographic conditions:

1. Stationary phase: Silica gel $60F_{254}$ pre-coated HPTLC plates, 10 × 10 cm (200 μm) – Merck, activated at 115°C for 30 min prior to use
2. Mobile phase (MP): Carbon tetrachloride–chloroform–methanol (3 : 5 : 2 v/v)
3. Standard/Sample application:
   Band length: 6 mm Volume applied: 8–24 μl Spacing: 10 mm
4. Chamber saturation: 25 min (MP)
5. RH (%): 50 ± 5
6. Temperature °C: 25 ± 2
7. Separation technique: Ascending
8. Quantity of mobile phase: 20 ml
9. Migration distance: 70 mm
10. Migration time: 15 min

Densitometric evaluation:

Wavelength: UV–230 nm Scanning mode: Reflectance/Absorbance

HRF: Cetirizine 2 HCl—50; Ambroxol HCl—74

Linearity (ng/band): Ambroxol HCl—240–720; Cetirizine 2 HCl—20–60

Recovery (%): Ambroxol HCl—99.97–100.02; Cetirizine 2 HCl—99.3–99.97

References: Advaita B. Patel, Sanket G. Patel, Deepa P. Patel, Bhavesh H. Patel and M.M. Patel, *Int. Res. J. of Pharmacy*, **2(3)**, 95–99, 2011.

Comments:

- The method validated for accuracy, precision, linearity, LOD, LOQ, specificity, robustness and ruggedness.
- The method is stability indicating (acid, base, oxidative, thermal, photolytic). The degradation products were separated from main compounds.

HPTLC : High Performance Thin Layer Chromatography
HPTLC Densitogram

No. 295

Br
OH
N
H
NH$_2$
Br
Ambroxol

OH
N
O
N
O
Cl
Levocetirizine

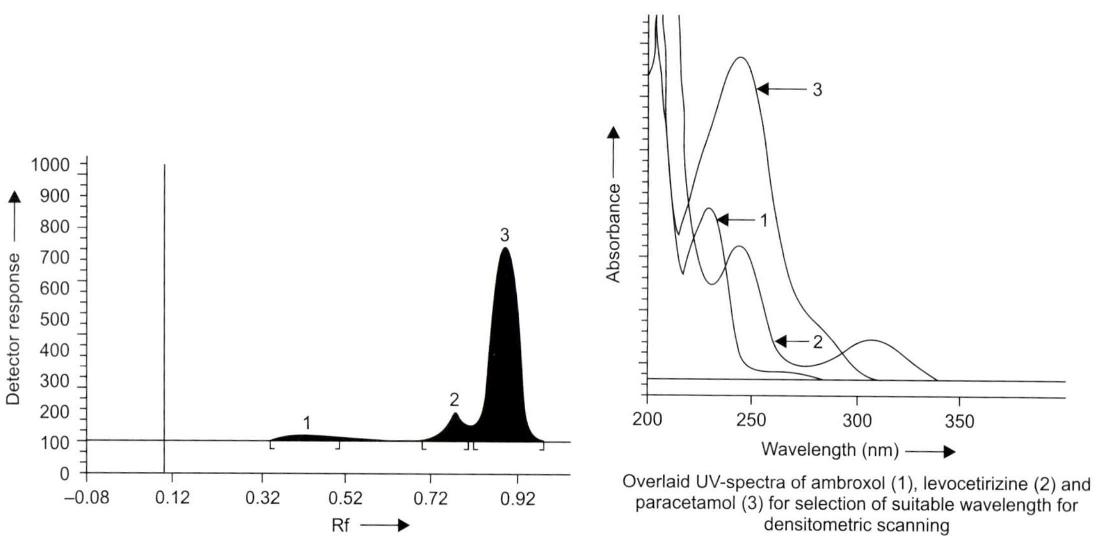

Overlaid UV-spectra of ambroxol (1), levocetirizine (2) and paracetamol (3) for selection of suitable wavelength for densitometric scanning

Typical densitogram of the standard containing ambroxol hydrochloride, levocetirizine dihydrochloride and paracetamol. For detailed experimental and chromatographic conditions, refer to Protocol No. 295. Peaks identification: 1. Ambroxol HCl; 2. Levocetirizine 2HCl; 3. Paracetamol.

PROTOCOL FOR HPTLC ANALYSIS OF PHARMACEUTICAL FORMULATION

Protocol No. 295

Formulation: **Ambroxol hydrochloride, Levocetirizine dihydrochloride, Paracetamol**

Classification: Respiratory System **Dosage form:** Tablets

Standard preparation: Prepare 1 mg/ml solution of each compound in methanol. Further serial dilutions of each solution are made for linearity profile. Apply 3 μl of each solution for chromatographic separation.

Sample preparation: Powdered sample equivalent to 30 mg of ambroxol HCl suspended in 40 ml of methanol, sonicated for 20 min, diluted to 50 ml, filtered and the filtrate suitably diluted with methanol. Apply 3 μl of the resultant solution for assay.

Chromatographic equipments:

Sample applicator: Camag Linomat–IV

Development chamber: Camag twin-trough glass chamber, 20 × 20 cm

Densitometric scanner: Camag TLC Scanner–III

Chromatographic conditions:

1. Stationary phase: Silica gel $60F_{254}$ pre-coated HPTLC plates, 20 × 20 cm (200 μm) – Merck
2. Mobile phase (MP): Methanol–water–methyl ethyl ketone (5 : 14 : 6 v/v)
3. Standard/Sample application:
   Band length: 6 mm Volume applied: 3 μl Spacing: 6 mm
4. Chamber saturation: 30 min (MP)
5. RH (%): 55 ± 5
6. Temperature °C: 22 ± 2
7. Separation technique: Ascending
8. Quantity of mobile phase: 25 ml
9. Migration distance: 55 mm
10. Migration time: 20 min

Densitometric evaluation:

Wavelength: UV–230 nm Scanning mode: Reflectance/Absorbance

HRF: See densitogram

Linearity (ng/band): Ambroxol HCl—600–3000; Levocetirizine 2HCl—50–200; Paracetamol—5–25

Recovery (%): 98.25–99.16 for all the three compounds

References: B. Gouthami, A. Akhilesh Reddy, S. Sagar Alkesh Bhai and N. Krishnaveni, Abstract No. F-273, 63rd IPC, 2011. Analytical details provided by N. Krishnaveni.

Comments: The method validated for accuracy, precision, linearity, LOD, LOQ, specificity, robustness and ruggedness.

HPTLC : High Performance Thin Layer Chromatography
HPTLC Densitogram

No. 296

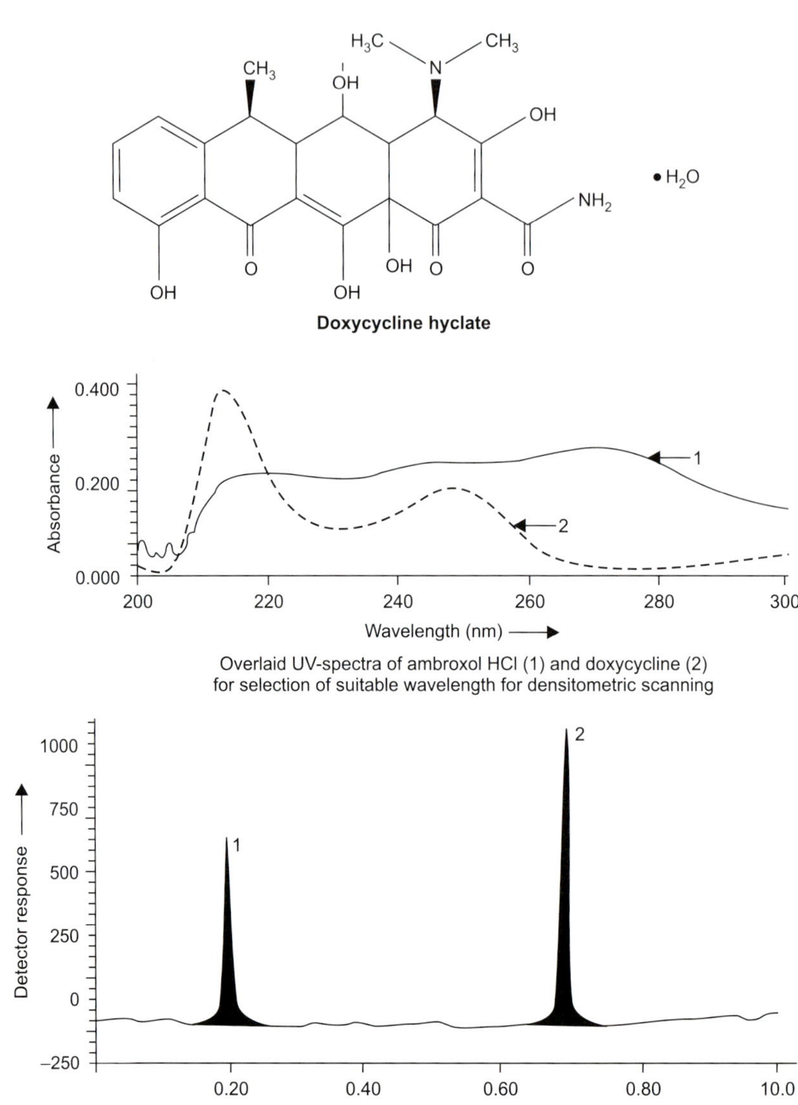

Typical densitogram of the sample containing ambroxol HCl and doxycycline hyclate. For detailed experimental and chromatographic conditions, refer to Protocol No. 296. Peaks identification: 1. Ambroxol HCl; 2. Doxycycline hyclate.

PROTOCOL FOR HPTLC ANALYSIS OF PHARMACEUTICAL FORMULATION

Protocol No. 296

Formulation: Ambroxol hydrochloride, Doxycycline hyclate

Classification: Respiratory System **Dosage form:** Capsules

Standard preparation: Prepare 10 mg/ml solution of each compound in methanol. Further dilutions made with methanol to get different concentrations (1–10 μg/ml). Apply 10 μl of each solution for linearity.

Sample preparation: Powdered sample equivalent to 100 mg of doxycycline suspended in 70 ml of methanol, sonicated for 15 min, diluted to 100 ml with methanol, filtered and the filtrate used for analysis.

Chromatographic equipments:

Sample applicator: 10 μl pipette

Development chamber: Fluka glass chamber, 20 × 20 cm

Densitometric scanner: Shimadzu CS–9301 dual wavelength flying spot densitometer

Chromatographic conditions:

1. Stationary phase: Silica gel $60F_{254}$ pre-coated HPTLC plates, 20 × 20 cm (200 μm) – Fluka
2. Mobile phase (MP): Ethyl acetate–ethanol–glacial acetic acid–water (9 : 4 : 0.5 : 1 v/v)
3. Standard/Sample application:
   Band length: 5 mm Volume applied: 10 μl Spacing: 20 mm
4. Chamber saturation: 60 min (MP)
5. RH (%): 50 ± 5
6. Temperature °C: Ambient
7. Separation technique: Ascending
8. Quantity of mobile phase: 29 ml
9. Migration distance: 160 mm
10. Migration time: 45 min

Densitometric evaluation:

Wavelength: UV–254 nm Scanning mode: Reflectance/Absorbance

HRF: Ambroxol HCl—20; Doxycycline hyclate—70

Linearity: 1–10 μg/ml for both the compounds

Recovery (%): Ambroxol HCl—98.03–101.82; Doxycycline—98.08–101.43

References: Mohammad Abdul-Azim Mohammad and Nagwan Hamdy Zawilla, *J. Planar Chromatogr.*, **22(3)**, 201–206, 2009.

Comments: The method validated for accuracy, precision, linearity, LOD, LOQ, specificity, robustness and ruggedness.

HPTLC : High Performance Thin Layer Chromatography
HPTLC Densitogram

No. 297

Ambroxol

Cefpodoxime

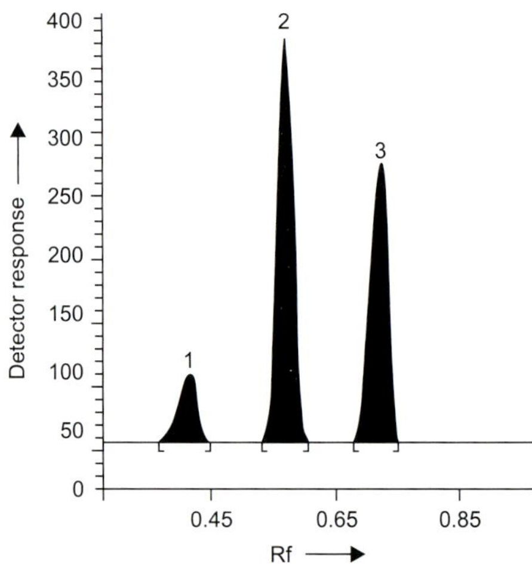

Typical densitogram of the standard containing cefpodoxime proxetil and ambroxol hydrochloride. For detailed experimental and chromatographic conditions, refer to Protocol No. 297. Peaks identification: 1. Paracetamol (IS); 2. Ambroxol HCl; 3. Cefpodoxime proxetil.

PROTOCOL FOR HPTLC ANALYSIS OF PHARMACEUTICAL FORMULATION

Protocol No. 297

Formulation: Ambroxol hydrochloride, Cefpodoxime proxetil

Classification: Respiratory System **Dosage form:** Biological sample

Standard preparation: Prepare 1 mg/ml solution of each compound in methanol. Add 10–60 μl solution of cefpodoxime and 2–12 μl of ambroxol HCl to drug-free plasma. Protein precipitation and extraction was carried out with 3 ml of methanol and 0.1 ml of acetonitrile by vigorous shaking. Centrifuge (5000 rpm) for 10 min, organic phase evaporated, residue taken up in 1 ml of methanol and used for linearity studies.

Sample preparation: —

Chromatographic equipments:

Sample applicator: Camag Linomat–V

Development chamber: Camag twin-trough glass chamber, 20 × 10 cm

Densitometric scanner: Camag TLC Scanner–III

Chromatographic conditions:

1. Stationary phase: Silica gel $60F_{254}$ pre-coated TLC plates (200 μm) – Merck, washed with methanol and activated at 120°C for 20 min prior to use
2. Mobile phase (MP): Chloroform–methanol (9 : 1 v/v)
3. Standard/Sample application:
   Band length: 8 mm Volume applied: — Spacing: 10 mm
4. Chamber saturation: 10 min (MP)
5. RH (%): 55 ± 5
6. Temperature °C: 25 ± 2
7. Separation technique: Ascending
8. Quantity of mobile phase: 20 ml
9. Migration distance: 70 mm
10. Migration time: 15 min

Densitometric evaluation:

Wavelength: UV–240 nm Scanning mode: Reflectance/Absorbance

HRF: Paracetamol—37; Ambroxol HCl—55; Cefpodoxime—69

Linearity (ng/band): Ambroxol HCl—1000–7000; Cefpodoxime—500–3500

Recovery (%): Ambroxol HCl—94.50; Cefpodoxime—74.40

References: Ambadas R. Rote and Sadhana K. Kande, *Pharmaceutical Methods*, **2(6)**, 242–246, Oct–Dec. 2011.

Comments: The method validated for accuracy, precision, linearity, selectivity and stability.

HPTLC : High Performance Thin Layer Chromatography
HPTLC Densitogram

No. 298

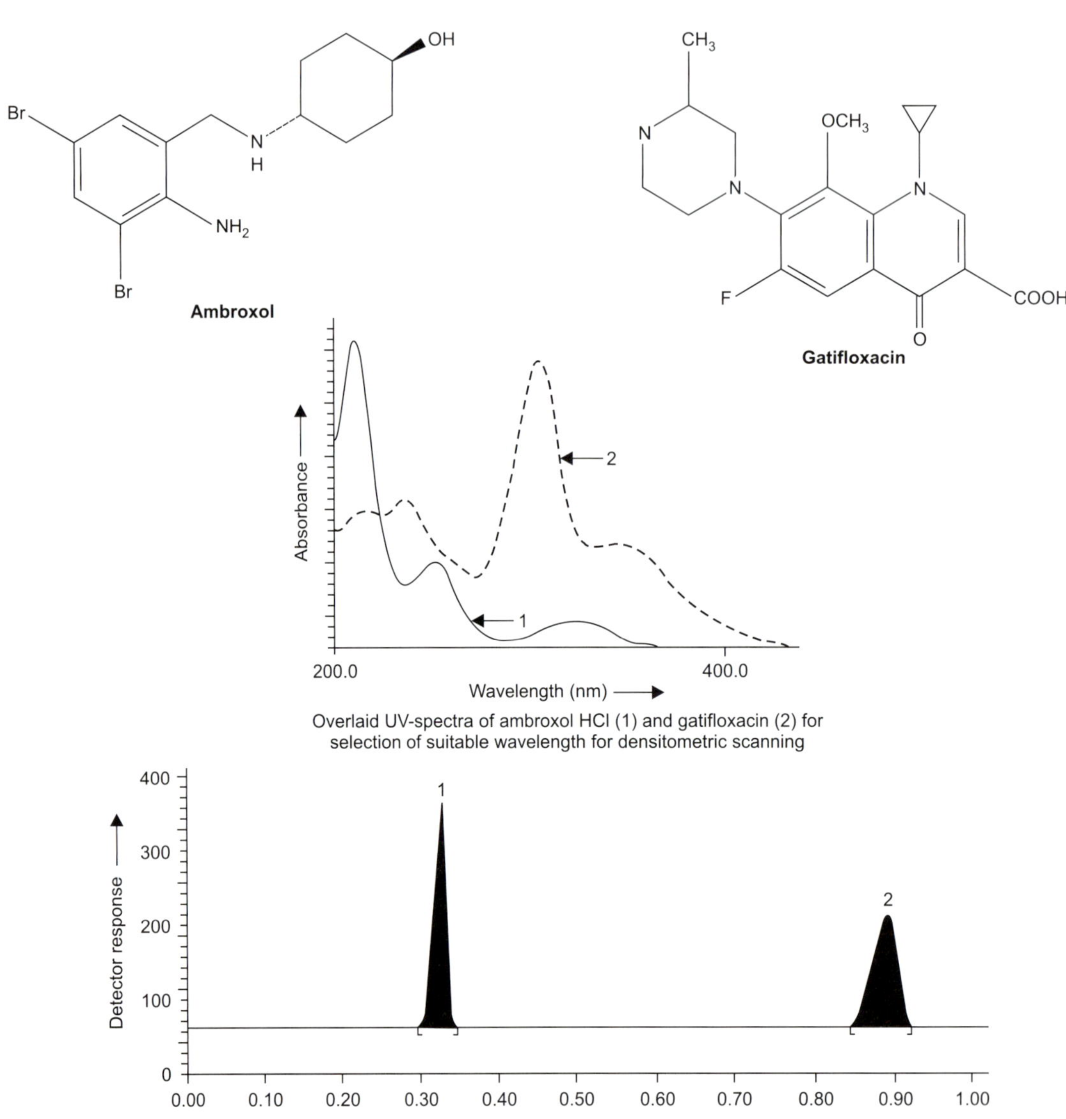

Overlaid UV-spectra of ambroxol HCl (1) and gatifloxacin (2) for selection of suitable wavelength for densitometric scanning

Typical densitogram of the sample containing ambroxol HCl and gatifloxacin. For detailed experimental and chromatographic conditions, refer to Protocol No. 298. Peaks identification: 1. Gatifloxacin; 2. Ambroxol HCl.

PROTOCOL FOR HPTLC ANALYSIS OF PHARMACEUTICAL FORMULATION

Protocol No. 298

Formulation: Ambroxol hydrochloride, Gatifloxacin

Classification: Respiratory System **Dosage form:** Tablets

Standard preparation: Prepare 1 mg/ml solution of each compound in methanol. Further serial dilutions made with mobile phase. Apply 5 µl of each solution for linearity profile.

Sample preparation: Extract powdered sample equivalent to 400 mg of gatifloxacin or 75 mg of ambroxol with 50 ml of mobile phase with sonication, filter and the filtrate suitably diluted with mobile phase. Apply 5 µl for assay.

Chromatographic equipments:

Sample applicator: Camag Linomat–IV

Development chamber: Camag twin-trough glass chamber, 10 × 10 cm

Densitometric scanner: Camag TLC Scanner–IIII

Chromatographic conditions:

1. Stationary phase: Silica gel $60F_{254}$ pre-coated TLC plates, 10 × 10 cm (250 µm) – Merck, pre-washed with methanol, dried at 110°C for 5 min prior to use
2. Mobile phase (MP): n-butanol–water–methanol–25% ammonia (4 : 0.5 : 0.5 : 1 v/v)
3. Standard/Sample application:
   Band length: 6 mm Volume applied: 5 µl Spacing: 5 mm
4. Chamber saturation: 30 min (MP)
5. RH (%): 55 ± 5
6. Temperature °C: 22 ± 2
7. Separation technique: Ascending
8. Quantity of mobile phase: 12 ml
9. Migration distance: 85 mm
10. Migration time: 20 min

Densitometric evaluation:

Wavelength: UV–310 nm Scanning mode: Reflectance/Absorbance

HRF: Gatifloxacin—33; Ambroxol HCl—89

Linearity (ng/band): Gatifloxacin—10–300; Ambroxol HCl—12.5–62.5

Recovery (%): Gatifloxacin—100.01–100.3; Ambroxol HCl—99.50–99.83

References: B. Prathap, G. Nagarjan, C. Roosewelt and V. Gopal, *Scholars Research Library*, **2(3)**, 163–167, 2010.

Comments: The method validated for accuracy, precision, linearity, LOD, LOQ, specificity, robustness and ruggedness.

HPTLC : High Performance Thin Layer Chromatography
HPTLC Densitogram

No. 299

Acebrophylline (Ambroxol and Theophylline-7- acetic acid)

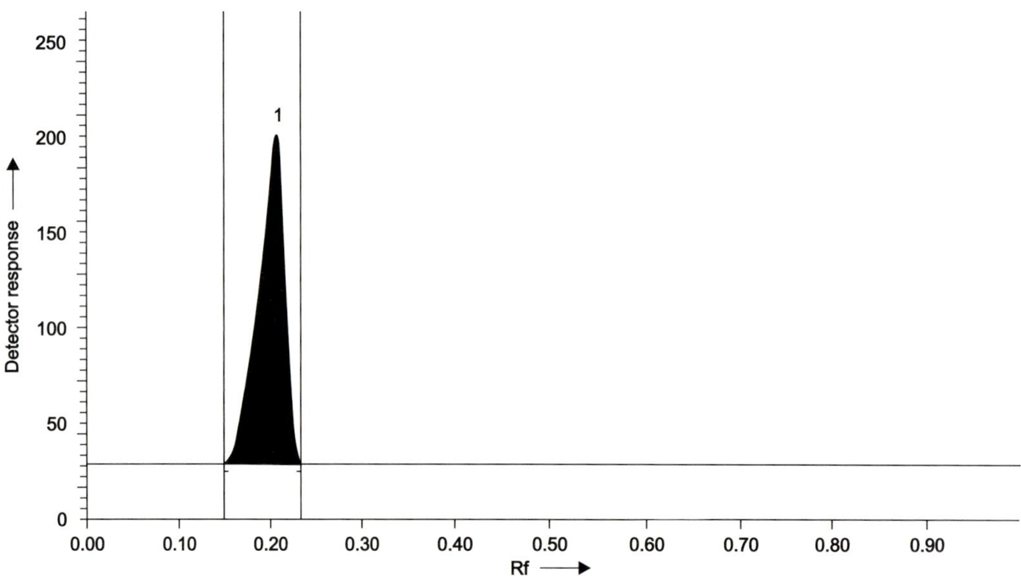

Typical densitogram of the sample containing acebrophylline. For detailed experimental and chromatographic conditions, refer to Protocol No. 299. Peaks identification: 1. Acebrophylline.

PROTOCOL FOR HPTLC ANALYSIS OF PHARMACEUTICAL FORMULATION

Protocol No. 299

Formulation: Acebrophylline (Ambroxol + Theophylline-7-acetic acid)

Classification: Respiratory System **Dosage form:** Capsules

Standard preparation: Prepare 1 mg/ml solution of the compound in water and apply 1–15 µl of the solution for linearity profile.

Sample preparation: Sample equivalent to 100 mg of the substance suspended in methanol–water (1 : 1 v/v), sonicated for 10 min, diluted to 100 ml with water, filtered and used for chromatographic analysis.

Chromatographic equipments:

Sample applicator: Camag Linomat–V

Development chamber: Camag twin-trough glass chamber, 10 × 10 cm

Densitometric scanner: Camag TLC Scanner–III

Chromatographic conditions:

1. Stationary phase: Silica gel $60F_{254}$ pre-coated TLC plates, 10 × 10 cm (250 µm) – Merck
2. Mobile phase (MP): Chloroform–isopropanol–toluene (8 : 1 : 1 v/v)
3. Standard/Sample application:
   Band length: 5 mm Volume applied: 1–5 µl Spacing: 10 mm
4. Chamber saturation: 15 min (MP)
5. RH (%): 55 ± 5
6. Temperature °C: 22 ± 2
7. Separation technique: Ascending
8. Quantity of mobile phase: 10 ml
9. Migration distance: 80 mm
10. Migration time: 18 min

Densitometric evaluation:

Wavelength: UV–254 nm Scanning mode: Reflectance/Absorbance

HRF: Acebrophylline—22

Linearity: 1000–5000 ng/band

Recovery (%): 99.79–101.53

References: W.D. Sam Solomon, M. Manu, S.R. Sivakumar, P.R. Vijai Anand and R. Venkatanarayanan, *J. Pharmacy Research*, **3(11)**, Nov 2010.

Comments: The method validated for accuracy, precision, linearity, LOD, LOQ, specificity, robustness and ruggedness.

HPTLC : High Performance Thin Layer Chromatography
HPTLC Densitogram

No. 300

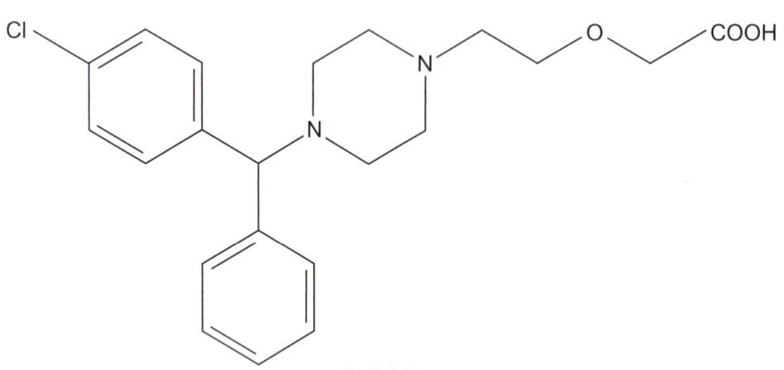

Cetirizine

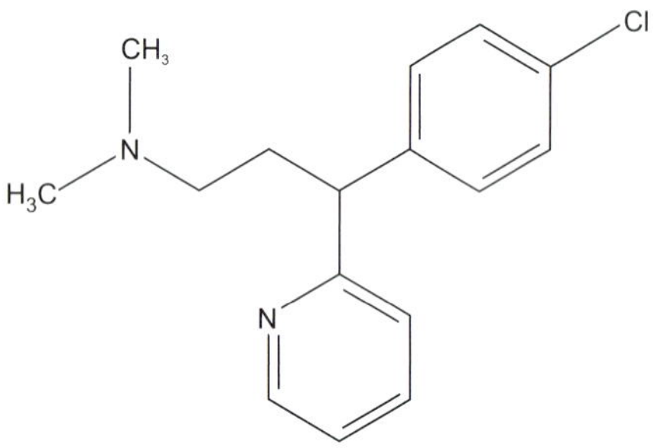

Chlorpheniramine

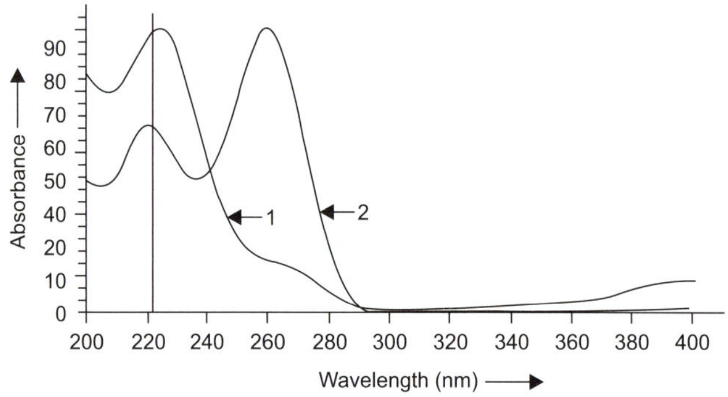

In-situ UV-spectra of cetirizine 2HCl (1) and chlorpheniramine maleate (2) for selection of suitable wavelength for densitometric scanning

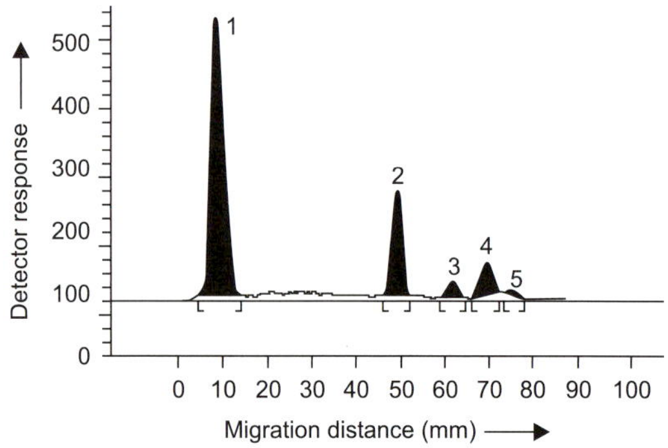

Typical densitogram of the sample containing cetirizine 2HCl and chlorpheniramine maleate. For detailed experimental and chromatographic conditions, refer to Protocol No. 300. Peaks identification: 1. Cetirizine; 2. Chlorpheniramine maleate. Peaks 3, 4 and 5 are of excipients.

PROTOCOL FOR HPTLC ANALYSIS OF PHARMACEUTICAL FORMULATION

Protocol No. 300

Formulation: Chlorpheniramine maleate, Cetirizine dihydrochloride

Classification: Respiratory System **Dosage form:** Tablets

Standard preparation: Prepare 1 mg/ml solution of cetirizine 2HCl and 200 μg/ml solution of chlorpheniramine maleate, both in methanol, and use for analysis.

Sample preparation: Suspend powdered sample equivalent to the weight of one tablet in 100 ml of methanol, sonicate, filter and use the filtrate for assay.

Chromatographic equipments:

Sample applicator: Linomat–IV

Development chamber: Camag twin–trough glass chamber, 10 × 10 cm

Densitometric scanner: Camag TLC scanner–II

Chromatographic conditions:

1. Stationary phase: Silica gel $60F_{254}$ pre-coated HPTLC plates, 10 × 10 cm (200 μm) – Merck
2. Mobile phase (MP): Toluene–ethyl acetate–methanol–25% ammonia (3.5 : 5.0 : 1.5 : 0.3 v/v)
3. Standard/Sample application:
   Band length: 7 mm Volume applied: 5 μl Spacing: 5 mm
4. Chamber saturation: 10 min (MP)
5. RH (%): 55 ± 5
6. Temperature °C: 22 ± 2
7. Separation technique: Ascending
8. Quantity of mobile phase: 10.3
9. Migration distance: 80 mm
10. Migration time: 35 min

Densitometric evaluation:

Wavelength: UV–220 nm Scanning mode: Reflectance/Absorbance

HRF: Cetirizine dihydrochloride—6; Chlorpheniramine maleate—46

Linearity (μg/ml): Cetirizine 2HCl—1–10; Chlorpheniramine maleate—0.5–5

Recovery (%): 98.50–101.25 for both the compounds.

References: —

Comments:

- The method was optimized and analytical work carried out at **Anchrom's HPTLC Application Laboratory**, Mumbai, India.
- Several market samples of similar composition were analysed by the proposed method with reproducible results.

HPTLC : High Performance Thin Layer Chromatography
HPTLC Densitogram

No. 301

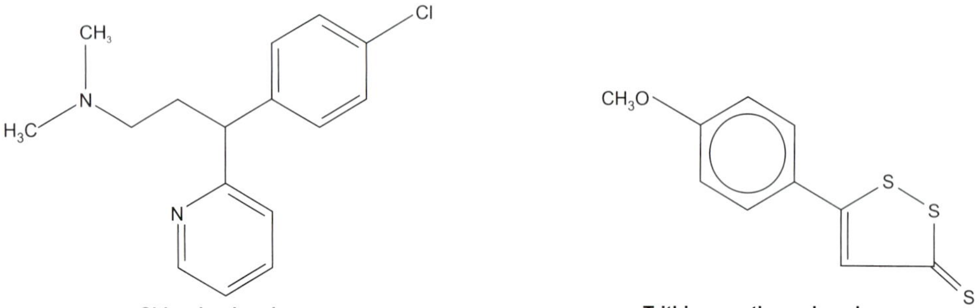

Chlorpheniramine

Trithio-p-methoxyphenylpropene

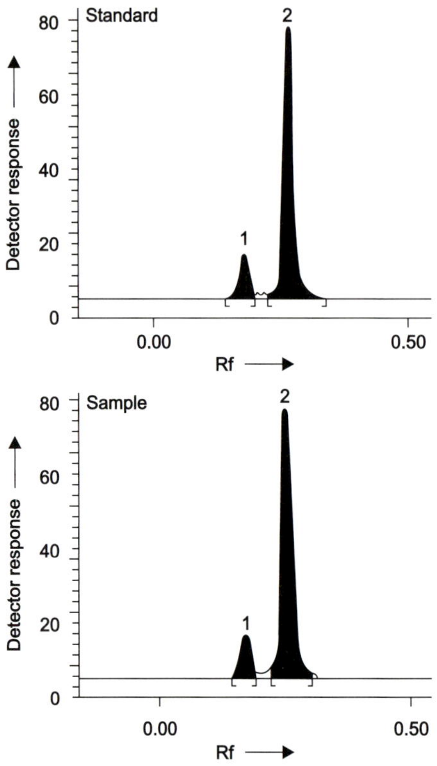

Typical densitogram of the sample and the standard containing chlorpheniramine maleate and trithio-p-methoxy phenylpropene. For detailed experimental and chromatographic conditions, refer to Protocol No. 301. Peaks identification: 1. Chlorpheniramine maleate; 2. Trithio-p-methoxy phenylpropene.

PROTOCOL FOR HPTLC ANALYSIS OF PHARMACEUTICAL FORMULATION

Protocol No. 301

Formulation: Chlorpheniramine maleate, Trithioparamethoxy phenylpropene

Classification: Respiratory System **Dosage form:** Tablets

Standard preparation: Prepare solution of each compound in methanol to get 1.25 mg/ml of trithio-p-methoxy phenylpropene (T) and 1 mg/ml of chlorpheniramine maleate (CPM). Mix 0.5 ml of solution T and 0.25 ml of solution CPM, dilute to 10 ml with methanol and use for analysis.

Sample preparation: Sample equivalent to 25 mg of CPM suspended in 70 ml of methanol, sonicated for 10 min, diluted to 100 ml with methanol, filtered and used for estimation.

Chromatographic equipments:

Sample applicator: Camag Linomat–IV

Development chamber: Camag twin–trough glass chamber, 10 × 10 cm

Densitometric scanner: Camag TLC scanner–II

Chromatographic conditions:

1. Stationary phase: Silica gel 60F_{254} pre-coated HPTLC plates, 10 × 10 cm (200 μm) – Merck, pre-washed with methanol and dried (60°C) for 5 min before use
2. Mobile phase (MP): Cyclohexane–toluene–diethylamine (7.5 : 1.5 : 0.3 v/v)
3. Standard/Sample application:
   Band length: 10 mm Volume applied: 10 μl Spacing: 10 mm
4. Chamber saturation: 20 min (MP)
5. RH (%): 55 ± 5
6. Temperature °C: 22 ± 2
7. Separation technique: Ascending
8. Quantity of mobile phase: 9 ml
9. Migration distance: 50 mm
10. Migration time: 24 min

Densitometric evaluation:

Wavelength: UV–254 nm Scanning mode: Reflectance/Absorbance

HRF: Chlorpheniramine maleate—17; Trithio-p-methoxy phenylpropene—26

Linearity (ng/band): Chlorpheniramine—100–1000; Trithio-p-methoxy phenylpropene—50–500

Recovery (%): 98.90–105.10 for both the compounds

References: —

Comments:

- The method was optimized and analytical work carried out at **Anchrom's HPTLC Application Laboratory**, Mumbai, India.
- Several market samples of similar composition were analysed by the proposed method with reproducible results.

HPTLC : High Performance Thin Layer Chromatography
HPTLC Densitogram

No. 302

Cl N S COONa HO H_3C CH_3

Montelukast sodium

Cl N N O COOH H • 2HCl

Levocetirizine dihydrochloride

1 2 Detector response 0.00 1.00 Rf

Typical densitogram of the sample containing montelukast sodium and levocetirizine dihydrochloride. For detailed experimental and chromatographic conditions, refer to Protocol No. 302. Peaks identification: 1. Montelukast sodium; 2. Levocetirizine dihydrochloride.

PROTOCOL FOR HPTLC ANALYSIS OF PHARMACEUTICAL FORMULATION

Protocol No. 302

Formulation: Montelukast sodium, Levocetirizine dihydrochloride

Classification: Respiratory System **Dosage form:** Tablets

Standard preparation: Prepare 10 mg/ml solution of each compound separately in glacial acetic acid. Further serial dilutions made with methanol to cover linearity range. Apply 5 μl of each solution for linearity studies.

Sample preparation: Powdered sample equivalent to 20 mg of montelukast sodium extracted with 20 × 10 ml of glacial acetic acid by sonication, filtered and filtrate suitably diluted with methanol to get 100 μg/ml solution. Apply 5 μl of the final sample solution for assay.

Chromatographic equipments:

Sample applicator: Camag Linomat–V

Development chamber: Camag twin–trough glass chamber, 10 × 10 cm

Densitometric scanner: Camag TLC scanner–III

Chromatographic conditions:

1. Stationary phase: Silica gel $60F_{254}$ pre-coated HPTLC plates, 10 × 10 cm 200 μm) – Merck
2. Mobile phase (MP): Chloroform–methanol–toluene–glacial acetic acid (10 : 5 : 3 : 0.5 v/v)
3. Standard/Sample application:
   Band length: 5 mm Volume applied: 5 μl Spacing: 15 mm
4. Chamber saturation: 25 min (MP)
5. RH (%): 55 ± 5
6. Temperature °C: 22 ± 2
7. Separation technique: Ascending
8. Quantity of mobile phase: 18.5 ml
9. Migration distance: 60 mm
10. Migration time: 20 min

Densitometric evaluation:

Wavelength: UV–302 nm Scanning mode: Reflectance/Absorbance

HRF: Montelukast sodium—64; Levocetirizine dihydrochloride—89

Linearity (ng/band): Montelukast sodium—600–2400; Levocetirizine 2HCl—500–3500

Recovery (%): Montelukast sodium—99.99–100.03; Levocetirizine 2HCl—99.98–100.09

References: Smita Sharma, M.C. Sharma, D.V. Kohli and A.D. Sharma, *Der Pharmacia Lettre*, **2(1)**, 489–494, 2010.

Comments: The method validated for accuracy, precision, linearity, LOD, LOQ, specificity, robustness and ruggedness.

HPTLC : High Performance Thin Layer Chromatography
HPTLC Densitogram

No. 303

Montelukast sodium

Overlaid UV-spectra of levocetirizine dihydrochloride (1) and montelukast sodium (2) for selection of suitable wavelength for densitometric scanning

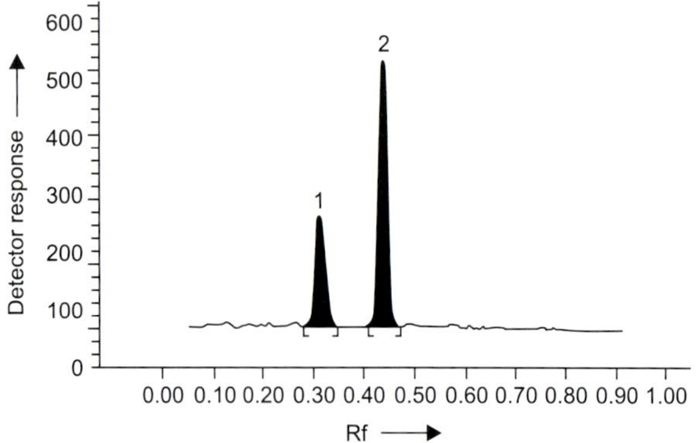

Typical densitogram of the sample containing montelukast sodium and levocetirizine dihydrochloride. For detailed experimental and chromatographic conditions, refer to Protocol No. 303. Peaks identification: 1. Levocetirizine 2HCl; 2. Montelukast Na^{+}.

PROTOCOL FOR HPTLC ANALYSIS OF PHARMACEUTICAL FORMULATION

Protocol No. 303

Formulation: Montelukast sodium, Levocetirizine dihydrochloride

Classification: Respiratory System **Dosage form:** Tablets

Standard preparation: Prepare solution of both the drugs in methanol separately to get 2 mg/ml of montelukast sodium and 1 mg/ml of levocetirizine dihydrochloride. Further dilute to get 500 μg/ml and 1000 μg/ml of levocetirizine dihydrochloride and montelukast sodium respectively. Apply 1–5 μl of each solution for linearity.

Sample preparation: Powdered sample equivalent to 5 mg of levocetirizine and 10 mg of montelukast sodium suspended in 20 ml of methanol, sonicated for 30 min, diluted to 25 ml with methanol. Filter and dilute the filtrate to get 200 μg/ml of levocetirizine and 400 μg/ml of montelukast. Apply 4 μl of the resulting solution and carry out the chromatographic analysis.

Chromatographic equipments:

Sample applicator: Camag Linomat–IV

Development chamber: Camag twin–trough glass chamber, 20 × 10 cm

Densitometric scanner: Camag TLC scanner–III

Chromatographic conditions:

1. Stationary phase: Silica gel $60F_{254}$ pre-coated TLC plates, 10 × 10 cm (250 μm) – Merck, pre-washed with methanol, activated at 110°C for 5 min prior to use
2. Mobile phase (MP): Toluene–ethyl acetate–methanol–25% ammonia (2.5 : 7 : 2.5 : 1 v/v)
3. Standard/Sample application:
   Band length: 6 mm Volume applied: 1–5 μl Spacing: 10 mm
4. Chamber saturation: 30 min (MP)
5. RH (%): 60 ± 5
6. Temperature °C: 25 ± 2
7. Separation technique: Ascending
8. Quantity of mobile phase: 26 ml
9. Migration distance: 80 mm
10. Migration time: 25 min

Densitometric evaluation:

Wavelength: UV–230 nm (iso-absorption point)

Scanning mode: Reflectance/Absorbance

HRF: Levocetirizine 2HCl—31; Montelukast Na^+—44

Linearity (ng/band): Montelukast Na^+—1000–5000; Levocetirizine 2HCl—500–2500

Recovery (%): Montelukast Na^+—100.40–102.66; Levocetirizine 2HCl—100.12–100.94

References: Atul S. Rathore, L. Sathiyanarayanan and K.R. Mahadik, *Pharmaceutica Analytica Acta*, **1(1)**, 1–6, 2010.

Comments:

- The method validated for accuracy, precision, linearity, LOD, LOQ, specificity, robustness and ruggedness.
- The sample was also analysed by RP-HPLC, the results were comparable by both the methods.

HPTLC : High Performance Thin Layer Chromatography
HPTLC Densitogram

No. 304

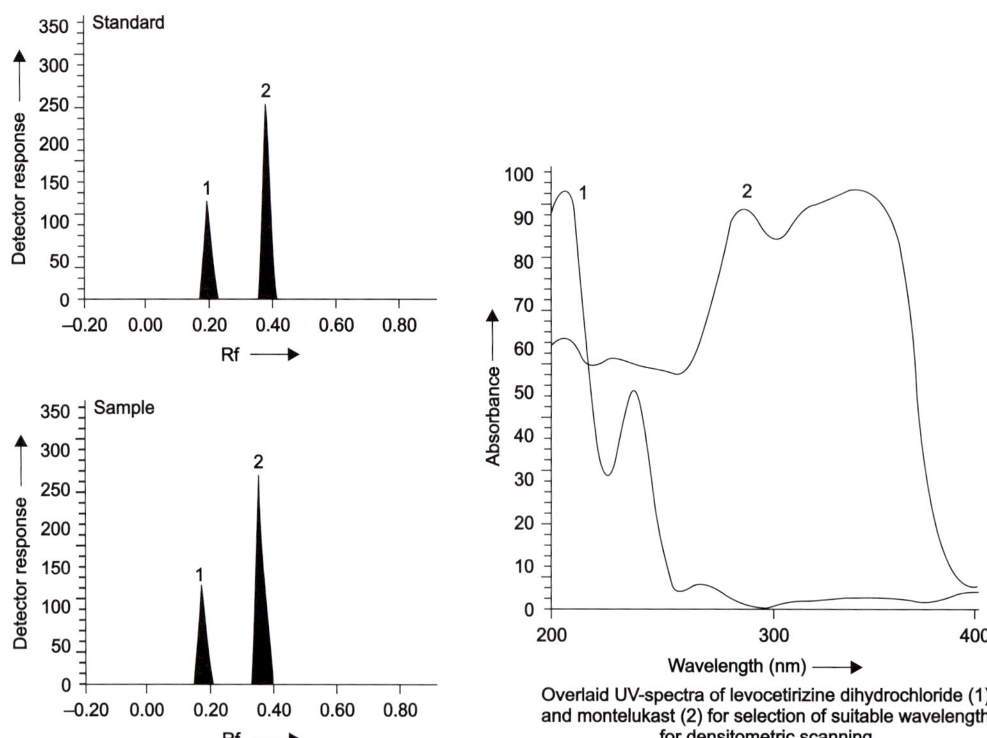

Overlaid UV-spectra of levocetirizine dihydrochloride (1) and montelukast (2) for selection of suitable wavelength for densitometric scanning

Typical densitogram of the standard and the sample containing levocetirizine dihydrochloride and montelukast Na^+. For detailed experimental and chromatographic conditions, refer to Protocol No. 304. Peaks identification: 1. Levocetirizine dihydrochloride; 2. Montelukast Na^+.

PROTOCOL FOR HPTLC ANALYSIS OF PHARMACEUTICAL FORMULATION

Protocol No. 304

Formulation: Montelukast sodium, Levocetirizine dihydrochloride

Classification: Respiratory System **Dosage form:** Tablets

Standard preparation: Prepare 100 μg/ml solution of each compound in methanol. Further serial dilutions are suitably made with methanol for linearity studies.

Sample preparation: Powdered sample equivalent to 5 mg of montelukast sodium is suspended in methanol, sonicated for 15 min, diluted to 25 ml. Further dilutions made suitably with methanol for chromatographic analysis.

Chromatographic equipments:

Sample applicator: Camag Linomat–V

Development chamber: Camag ADC–2, saturated with Camag saturation pad

Densitometric scanner: Camag TLC scanner–III

Chromatographic conditions:

1. Stationary phase: Silica gel 60F_{254} pre-coated TLC plates, 10 × 10 cm (250 μm) – Merck
2. Mobile phase (MP): Ethyl acetate–methanol–25% ammonia (7 : 1.4 : 0.7 v/v)
3. Standard/Sample application:
   Band length: 8 mm Volume applied: 10 μl Spacing: 10 mm
4. Chamber saturation: 20 min (MP)
5. RH (%): 55 ± 5
6. Temperature °C: 25 ± 2
7. Separation technique: Ascending
8. Quantity of mobile phase: 20 ml
9. Migration distance: 80 mm
10. Migration time: 15 min

Densitometric evaluation:

Wavelength: UV–231 nm Scanning mode: Reflectance/Absorbance

HRF: Levocetirizine dihydrochloride—19; Montelukast sodium—36

Linearity (ng/band): Montelukast sodium—500–2500; Cetirizine 2HCl—400–3200

Recovery (%): —

References: —

Comments: The method was optimized and analytical work carried out at **Anchrom's HPTLC Application Laboratory**, Mumbai, India.

HPTLC : High Performance Thin Layer Chromatography
HPTLC Densitogram

No. 305

Levocetirizine dihydrochloride

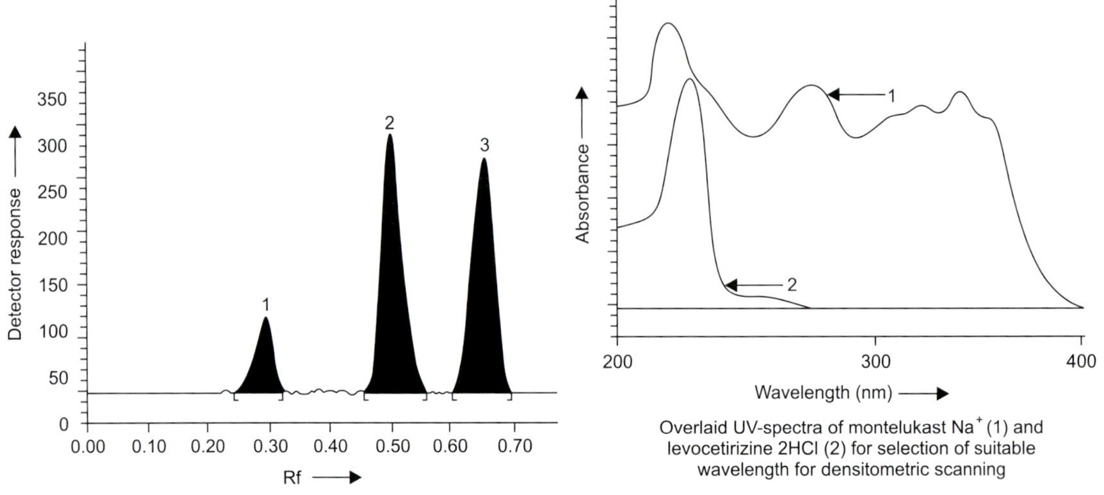

Overlaid UV-spectra of montelukast Na^+ (1) and levocetirizine 2HCl (2) for selection of suitable wavelength for densitometric scanning

Typical densitogram of the standard containing montelukast Na^+ and levocetirizine 2HCl. For detailed experimental and chromatographic conditions, refer to Protocol No. 305. Peaks identification: 1. Levocetirizine 2HCl; 2. Montelukast Na^+; 3. Paracetamol (IS).

PROTOCOL FOR HPTLC ANALYSIS OF PHARMACEUTICAL FORMULATION

Protocol No. 305

Formulation: Montelukast sodium, Levocetirizine dihydrochloride
Classification: Respiratory System **Dosage form:** Tablets
Standard preparation: Prepare solution of each compound in methanol to get 1 mg/ml of montelukast sodium, 0.5 mg/ml of levocetirizine dihydrochloride and 1 mg/ml of paracetamol (IS). Apply varying volumes of each solution for linearity profile.
Sample preparation: Powdered sample equivalent to 10 mg of montelukast sodium suspended in 8 ml of methanol, sonicated, diluted to 10 ml and filtered. Apply 0.5 μl of the resultant solution keeping concentration of (IS) at 600 ng/band and carry out the chromatographic separation and evaluation.
Chromatographic equipments:
Sample applicator: Camag Linomat–V
Development chamber: Camag twin-trough glass chamber, 20 × 10 cm
Densitometric scanner: Camag TLC scanner–III
Chromatographic conditions:
1. Stationary phase: Silica gel $60F_{254}$ pre-coated TLC plates, 20 × 10 cm (250 μm), pre-washed with methanol and activated at 120°C for 20 min prior to chromatographic development
2. Mobile phase (MP): Ethyl acetate–methanol–triethylamine (5 : 5 : 0.02 v/v)
3. Standard/Sample application:
   Band length: 6 mm Volume applied: 0.5 μl Spacing: 8.9 mm
4. Chamber saturation: 20 min (MP)
5. RH (%): 60 ± 5
6. Temperature °C: 23 ± 2
7. Separation technique: Ascending
8. Quantity of mobile phase: 20 ml
9. Migration distance: 70 mm
10. Migration time: 7 min

Densitometric evaluation:
Wavelength: UV–240 nm Scanning mode: Reflectance/Absorbance
HRF: Levocetirizine 2HCl—29; Montelukast Na^+—50; Paracetamol (IS)—65
Linearity (ng/band): Montelukast Na^+—400–1200; Levocetirizine 2HCl—200–600
Recovery (%): Montelukast Na^+—97.91–101.80; Levocetirizine 2HCl—97.98–100.74
References: Ambadas R. Rote and Vaishali S. Niphade, *J. Liq. Chromatogr. and Related Technologies*, **34**, 155–167, 2011.
Comments:
- The method was validated for accuracy, precision, linearity, LOD, LOQ, specificity and robustness.
- The sample was simultaneously analysed by first-derivative spectroscopy for comparable results.

HPTLC : High Performance Thin Layer Chromatography
HPTLC Densitogram

No. 306

H3C N O N O N CH3 N N OH

Etofylline

H3C N O N O N CH3 H N N

Theophylline

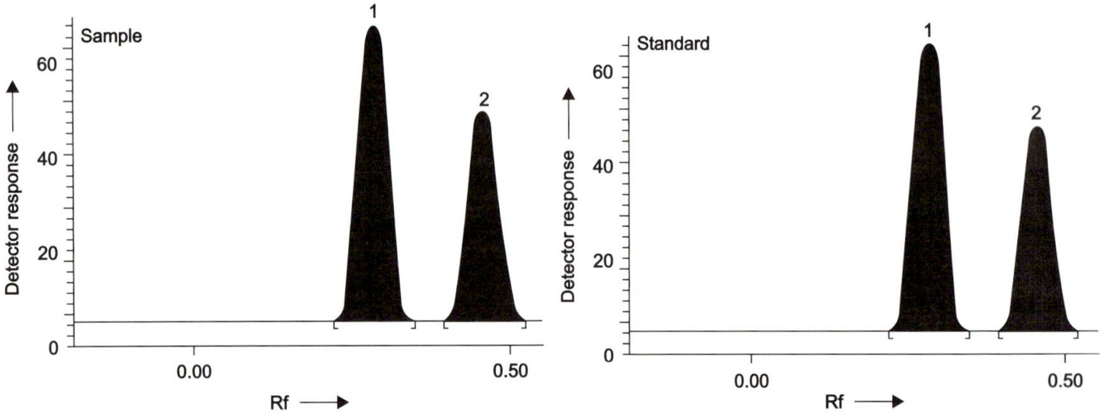

Typical densitogram of the sample and the standard containing etofylline and theophylline. For detailed experimental and chromatographic conditions, refer to Protocol No. 306. Peaks identification: 1. Etofylline; 2. Theophylline.

PROTOCOL FOR HPTLC ANALYSIS OF PHARMACEUTICAL FORMULATION

Protocol No. 306

Formulation: **Theophylline, Etofylline**
Classification: Respiratory System **Dosage form:** Tablets, Syrup, Injection
Standard preparation: Weigh accurately 35 mg of theophylline (T) and 115 mg of etofylline, add 20 ml of water, 2 ml of 25% ammonia, dilute to 100 ml with methanol. Dilute 1 ml of resulting solution to 10 ml with methanol and use for analysis.
Sample preparation: Sample equivalent to 115 mg of etofylline suspended in 20 ml of water and 2 ml of ammonia, vortexed for 10 min, diluted to 100 ml with methanol, filtered and 1 ml of the filtrate diluted to 10 ml with methanol and used for estimation.
Chromatographic equipments:
Sample applicator: Camag Linomat–IV
Development chamber: Camag twin–trough glass chamber, 10 × 10 cm
Densitometric scanner: Camag TLC scanner–II
Chromatographic conditions:
1. Stationary phase: Silica gel $60F_{254}$ pre-coated HPTLC plates, 7 × 10 cm (200 μm) – Merck
2. Mobile phase (MP): (i) Chloroform–acetone–glacial acetic acid (8 : 2 : 0.2 v/v); (ii) Chloroform–ethyl acetate–formic acid (19 : 1 : 2 v/v)
3. Standard/Sample application:
Band length: 10 mm Volume applied: 5 μl Spacing: 10 mm
4. Chamber saturation: 20 min (MP)
5. RH (%): 55 ± 5
6. Temperature °C: 22 ± 2
7. Separation technique: Ascending
8. Quantity of mobile phase: 10 ml
9. Migration distance: 50 mm
10. Migration time: 15–20 min

Densitometric evaluation:
Wavelength: UV–275 nm Scanning mode: Reflectance/Absorbance
HRF: Etofylline—28; Theophylline—45
Linearity: 40–200 ng/band for both the drugs
Recovery (%): 102.30–103.40 for both the drugs
References: —
Comments:
- The method was optimized and analytical work carried out at **Anchrom's HPTLC Application Laboratory**, Mumbai, India.
- Several market samples of similar composition were analysed by the proposed method with reproducible results.
- The method is suitable for dissolution profile of sustained release formulations as well.

HPTLC : High Performance Thin Layer Chromatography
HPTLC Densitogram

No. 307

Etofylline

Theophylline

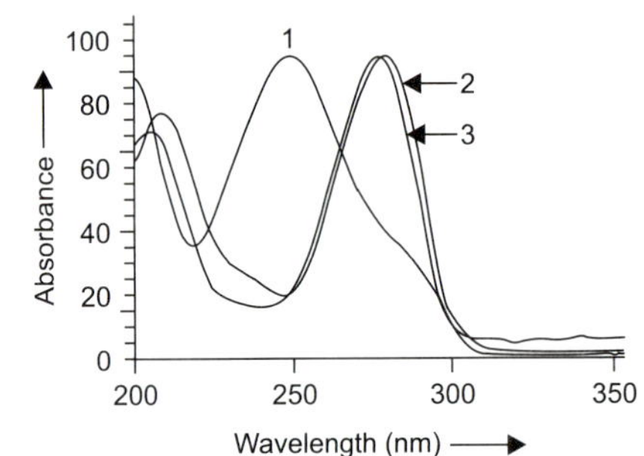

In-situ overlaid UV-spectra of paracetamol (1), etofylline (2) and theophylliine (3) for selection of suitable wavelength for densitometric scanning

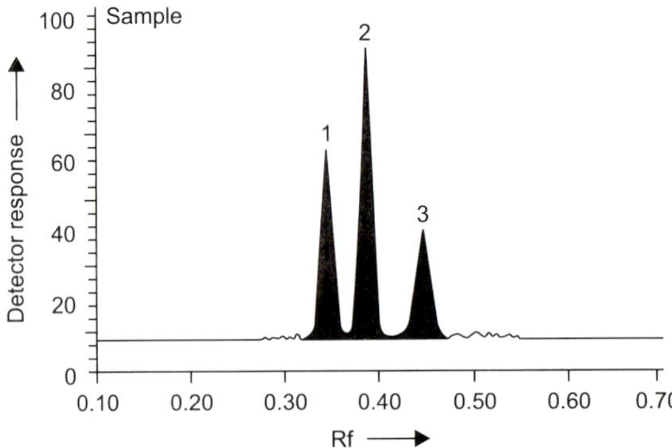

Typical densitogram of the sample containing theophylline and etofylline. For detailed experimental and chromatographic conditions, refer to Protocol No. 307. Peaks identification: 1. Paracetamol (IS); 2. Etofylline; 3. Theophylline.

PROTOCOL FOR HPTLC ANALYSIS OF PHARMACEUTICAL FORMULATION

Protocol No. 307

Formulation: Theophylline, Etofylline

Classification: Respiratory System **Dosage form:** Tablets, Syrup, Injection

Standard preparation: Prepare standard solution of both the drugs in methanol to get 20 μg/ml (theophylline) and 60 μg/ml (etofylline) and use for analysis.

Sample preparation: Powdered sample of tablets was extracted with methanol by sonication whereas samples of syrups and injections were directly diluted with methanol to get required concentration of each drug and used for estimation.

Chromatographic equipments:

Sample applicator: Camag Linomat–IV

Development chamber: Camag twin–trough glass chamber, 10 × 10 cm

Densitometric scanner: Camag TLC scanner–II

Chromatographic conditions:

1. Stationary phase: Silica gel 60F_{254} pre-coated HPTLC plates, 10 × 10 cm
2. Mobile phase (MP): Chloroform–methanol–25% ammonia (9 : 1 : 0.1 v/v)
3. Standard/Sample application:
   Band length: 7 mm Volume applied: 10 μl Spacing: 7 mm
4. Chamber saturation: 20 min (MP)
5. RH (%): 55 ± 5
6. Temperature °C: 22 ± 2
7. Separation technique: Ascending
8. Quantity of mobile phase: 10 ml
9. Migration distance: 50 mm
10. Migration time: 20 min

Densitometric evaluation:

Wavelength: UV–278 nm Scanning mode: Reflectance/Absorbance

HRF: Retention order; paracetamol (IS); etofylline; theophylline

Linearity (ng/band): Theophylline—20–80; Etofylline—60–240

Recovery (%): 99.18–99.74 for both the drugs

References: V.M. Shinde, N.M. Tendulkar and B.S. Desai, *J. Planar Chromatogr.*, **7**, 133–136, 1994.

Comments: The method suitable for dissolution profile of sustained release formulations.

HPTLC : High Performance Thin Layer Chromatography
HPTLC Densitogram

No. 308

Etofylline

Theophylline

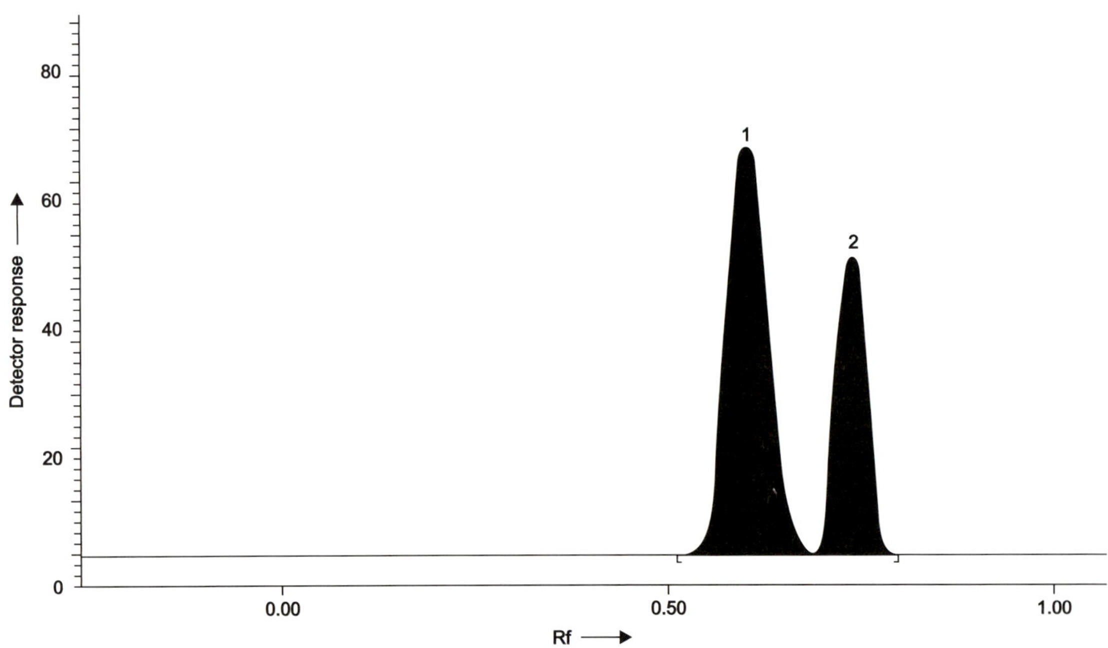

Typical densitogram of the standard containing etofylline and theophylline. For detailed experimental and chromatographic conditions, refer to Protocol No. 308. Peaks identification: 1. Etofylline; 2. Theophylline.

PROTOCOL FOR HPTLC ANALYSIS OF PHARMACEUTICAL FORMULATION

Protocol No. 308

Formulation: Theophylline, Etofylline

Classification: Respiratory System **Dosage form:** Tablets

Standard preparation: Prepare 100 μg/ml solution of each drug in isopropyl alcohol and use for chromatographic analysis.

Sample preparation: Powdered sample equivalent to 10 mg of etofylline suspended in isopropanol, sonicated for 10 min, diluted to get 100 μg/ml of each, filtered and used for chromatographic evaluation.

Chromatographic equipments:

Sample applicator: Camag Linomat–V

Development chamber: Camag twin–trough glass chamber, 10 × 10 cm

Densitometric scanner: Camag TLC scanner–III

Chromatographic conditions:

1. Stationary phase: Silica gel 60F_{254} pre-coated TLC plates, 10 × 10 cm (250 μm) – Merck, pre-washed with isopropylalcohol, activated at 50°C for 5 min prior to use
2. Mobile phase (MP): Toluene–isopropyl alcohol–acetic acid (6 : 6 : 0.5 v/v)
3. Standard/Sample application:

   Band length: 10 mm Volume applied: 2–8 μl Spacing: 10 mm
4. Chamber saturation: 30 min (MP)
5. RH (%): 55 ± 5
6. Temperature °C: 22 ± 2
7. Separation technique: Ascending
8. Quantity of mobile phase: 12.5 ml
9. Migration distance: 90 min
10. Migration time: 25 min

Densitometric evaluation:

Wavelength: UV–261 nm Scanning mode: Reflectance/Absorbance

HRF: Etofylline—63; Theophylline—75

Linearity (ng/band): Etofylline—200–400; Theophylline—60–80

Recovery (%): Etofylline—99.10–100.87; Theophylline—99.92–102.06

References: V. Venkatesh, A. Elphine Prabahav, P. Venkata Suresh, Uma Maheshwari and N. Rama Rao, *Asian J. Chem.*, **23(1)**, 309–311, 2011.

Comments: The method validated for accuracy, precision, linearity, LOD, LOQ, specificity, robustness and ruggedness.

HPTLC : High Performance Thin Layer Chromatography
HPTLC Densitogram

No. 309

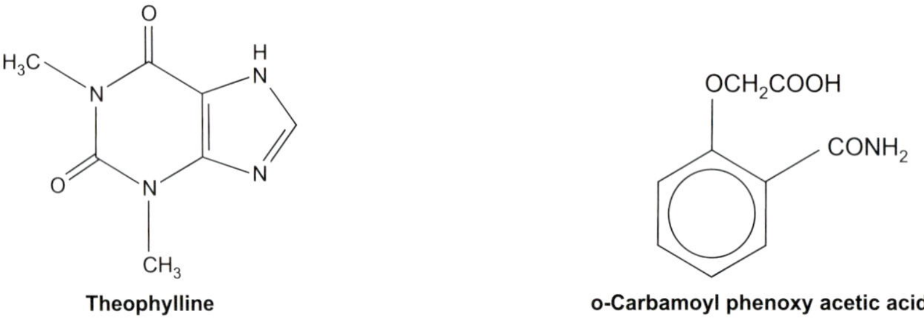

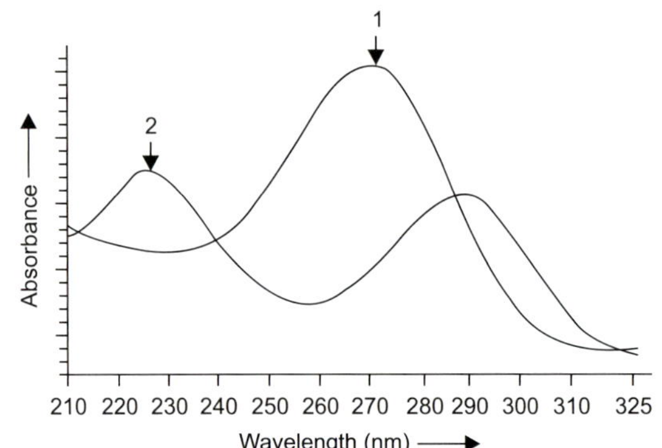

In-situ overlaid UV-spectra of theophylline (1) and o-carbamoyl phenoxy acetic acid (2) for selection of suitable wavelength for densitometric scanning

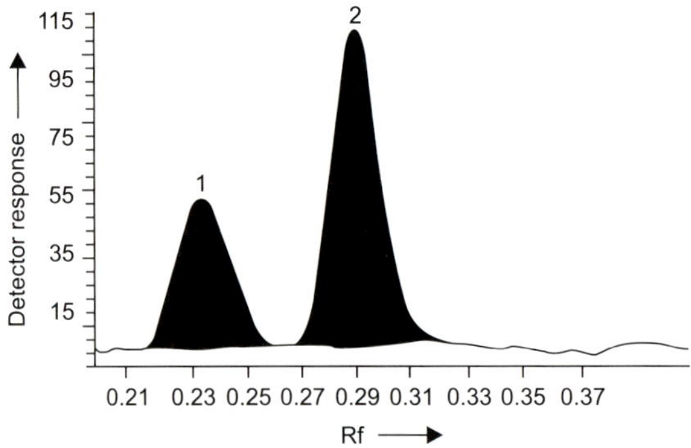

Typical densitogram of the sample containing theophylline and o-carbamoyl phenoxy acetic acid. For detailed experimental and chromatographic conditions, refer to Protocol No. 309. Peaks identification: 1. o-Carbamoyl phenoxy acetic acid; 2. Theophylline.

PROTOCOL FOR HPTLC ANALYSIS OF PHARMACEUTICAL FORMULATION

Protocol No. 309

Formulation: Theophylline, o-Carbamoyl phenoxy acetic acid

Classification: Respiratory System **Dosage form:** Drops

Standard preparation: Dissolve 10 mg of theophylline and 20 mg of amide in diluent to produce 10 ml. Further dilute 1 ml of the resultant solution to 10 ml with diluent and use for analysis.

Sample preparation: Dilute 0.5 ml of the drops to 25 ml with diluent. Further dilute 0.5 ml of the resultant solution to 10 ml with diluent and use for chromatographic estimation.

Diluent: Ethyl alcohol–water (1 : 1 v/v).

Chromatographic equipments:

Sample applicator: Desaga TLC-applicator AS–30

Development chamber: Desaga HPTLC chamber

Densitometric scanner: Desaga CD–60

Chromatographic conditions:

1. Stationary phase: Silica gel 60–NH_2 F_{254s} pre-coated HPTLC plates, 10 × 10 cm (200 μm) – Merck
2. Mobile phase (MP): Ethyl alcohol–50% aq. diethylamine (9.5 : 0.5 v/v)
3. Standard/Sample application:
   Band length: 5 mm Volume applied: 2 μl Spacing: 5 mm
4. Chamber saturation: 30 min (MP)
5. RH (%): 55 ± 5
6. Temperature °C: 22 ± 2
7. Separation technique: Ascending
8. Quantity of mobile phase: 10 ml
9. Migration distance: 60 mm
10. Migration time: 12 min

Densitometric evaluation:

Wavelength: UV–225 nm (o-Carbamoyl phenoxy acetic acid), UV–275 nm (Theophylline)

Scanning mode: Reflectance/Absorbance

HRF: o-Carbamoyl phenoxy acetic acid—23; Theophylline—29

Linearity (ng/band): 20–60

Recovery (%): 100.40–100.75 for both the compounds

References: C. Weings and H. York, Application Notes.

Comments: Due to poor water solubility of theophylline, o-carbamoyl phenoxy acetic acid (amide) is added as solubilizing agent.

HPTLC : High Performance Thin Layer Chromatography
HPTLC Densitogram

No. 310

Theophylline

Etofylline

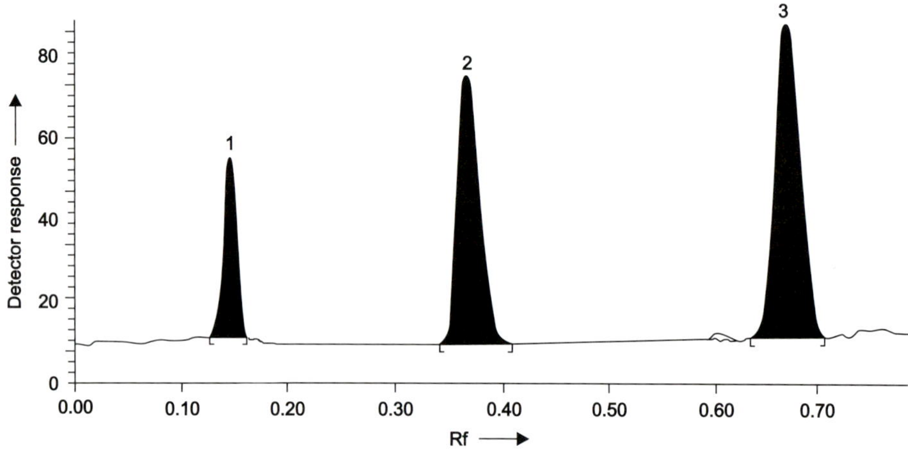

Typical densitogram of the standard containing theophylline, etofylline and caffeine. For detailed experimental and chromatographic conditions, refer to Protocol No. 310. Peaks identification: 1. Theophylline; 2. Etofylline; 3. Caffeine.

PROTOCOL FOR HPTLC ANALYSIS OF PHARMACEUTICAL FORMULATION

Protocol No. 310

Formulation: Theophylline, Etofylline, Caffeine citrate

Classification: Respiratory System **Dosage form:** Tablets

Standard preparation: Prepare 400 μg/ml solution of each compound in methanol for analysis.

Sample preparation: The powdered sample extracted with methanol by shaking to produce 400 μg/ml solution, filtered and used for estimation.

Chromatographic equipments:

Sample applicator: Camag Linomat–IV

Development chamber: All glass chamber, 20 × 20 cm

Densitometric scanner: Camag TLC Scanner–II

Chromatographic conditions:

1. Stationary phase: Silica gel $60F_{254}$ pre-coated HPTLC plates, 10 × 10 cm (250 μm) – Merck
2. Mobile phase (MP): Acetone–ethyl acetate–25% ammonia (7.5 : 2.3 : 0.2 v/v)
3. Standard/Sample application:
   Band length: 5 mm Volume applied: 5 μl Spacing: 5 mm
4. Chamber saturation: —
5. RH (%): 55 ± 5
6. Temperature °C: 22 ± 2
7. Separation technique: Ascending
8. Quantity of mobile phase: 30 ml
9. Migration distance: 60 mm
10. Migration time: 15 min

Densitometric evaluation:

Wavelength: UV–273 nm; Vis–500 nm Scanning mode: Reflectance/Absorbance

HRF: Theophylline—15; Etofylline—38; Caffeine citrate—68

Linearity: —

Recovery (%): 98.75–102.25 for all the three compounds

References: Meter, B. Wagner and J.H. York, Training Course No. 301.

Comments:

- After development, the plate dried in stream of dry air and scanned at 273 nm (caffeine) and dipped in the reagent for 2 s and scanned at 500 nm (theophylline and etofylline).
- The method was suitable for detection of caffeine ($\ngtr$ 1% of caffeine).
- Reagent: Dissolve 0.8 g of KI and 0.8 g I_2 in 40 ml of ethyl alcohol, add 10 ml of HCl.

HPTLC : High Performance Thin Layer Chromatography
HPTLC Densitogram

No. 311

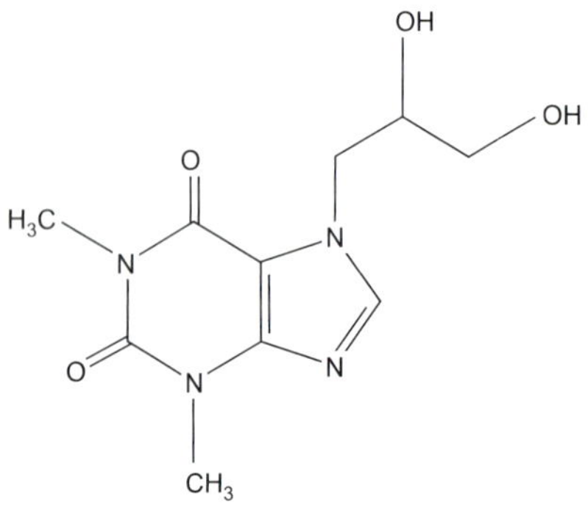

Diprophylline

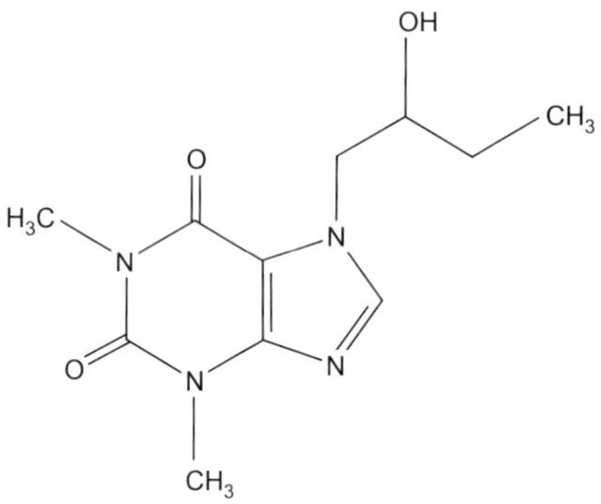

Proxyphylline

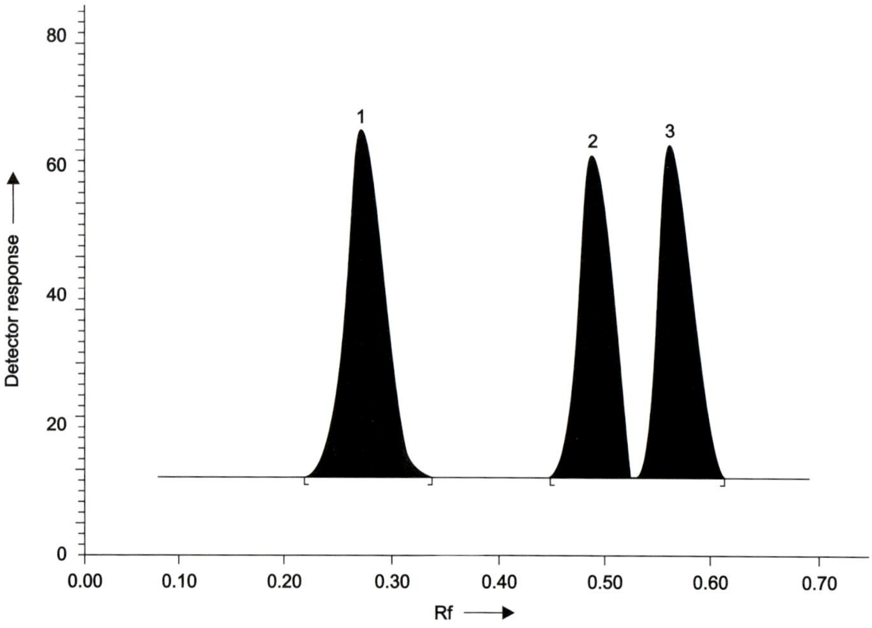

Typical densitogram of the standard containing theophylline, diprophylline and proxyphylline. For detailed experimental and chromatographic conditions, refer to Protocol No. 311. Peaks identification: 1. Theophylline; 2. Diprophylline; 3. Proxyphylline.

PROTOCOL FOR HPTLC ANALYSIS OF PHARMACEUTICAL FORMULATION

Protocol No. 311

Formulation: Theophylline, Diprophylline, Proxyphylline

Classification: Respiratory System

Dosage form: Tablets (sustained release)

Standard preparation: Prepare standard solution of each compound in methanol to get 75 μg/ml (theophylline); 112.5 μg/ml (diprophylline and proxyphylline) and use for analysis.

Sample preparation: Powdered sample equivalent to 75 mg of theophylline shaken with 70 ml of methanol, diluted to 100 ml, filtered and 1 ml of the filtrate diluted to 10 ml for estimation.

Chromatographic equipments:

Sample applicator: Camag Linomat–IV

Development chamber: Camag twin-trough glass chamber, 10 × 10 cm

Densitometric scanner: Camag TLC Scanner–II

Chromatographic conditions:

1. Stationary phase: Silica gel $60F_{254}$ pre-coated HPTLC plates, 10 × 10 cm (200 μm) – Merck
2. Mobile phase (MP): Chloroform–ethanol–formic acid (8.5 : 0.5 : 1.0 v/v)
3. Standard/Sample application:
   Band length: 5 mm Volume applied: 1 μl Spacing: 5 mm
4. Chamber saturation: —
5. RH (%): 55 ± 5
6. Temperature °C: 22 ± 2
7. Separation technique: Ascending
8. Quantity of mobile phase: 10 ml
9. Migration distance: 50 mm
10. Migration time: 25 min

Densitometric evaluation:

Wavelength: UV–275 nm Scanning mode: Reflectance/Absorbance

HRF: Theophylline—28; Diprophylline—48; Proxyphylline—58

Linearity (ng/band): Theophylline—40–200; Diprophylline and Proxyphylline—60–300

Recovery (%): 99.5–101.5 for all the three compounds

References: D. Agbaba, D. Zivanor-Stakic and N. Vakicevic, *Biomed. Chromatogr.*, **6**, 141–142, 1992.

Comments: The method validated for accuracy, precision, linearity, LOD, LOQ, specificity, robustness and ruggedness.

HPTLC : High Performance Thin Layer Chromatography
HPTLC Densitogram

No. 312

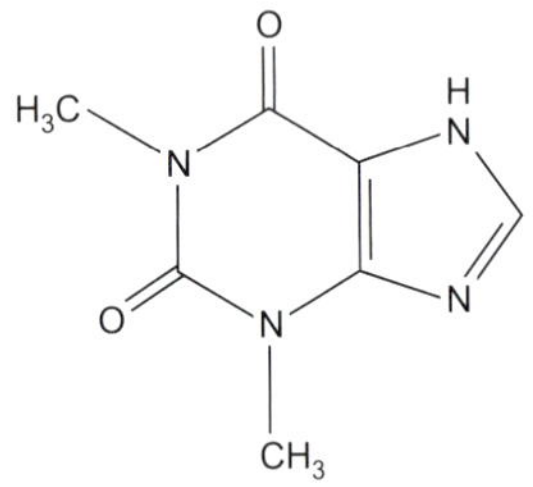

Theophylline

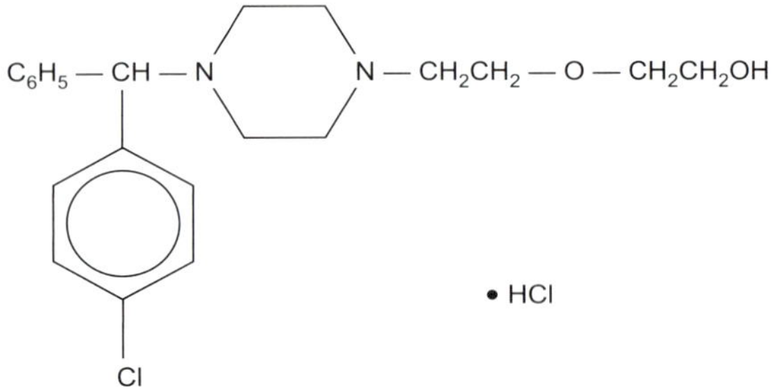

Hydroxyzine hydrochloride

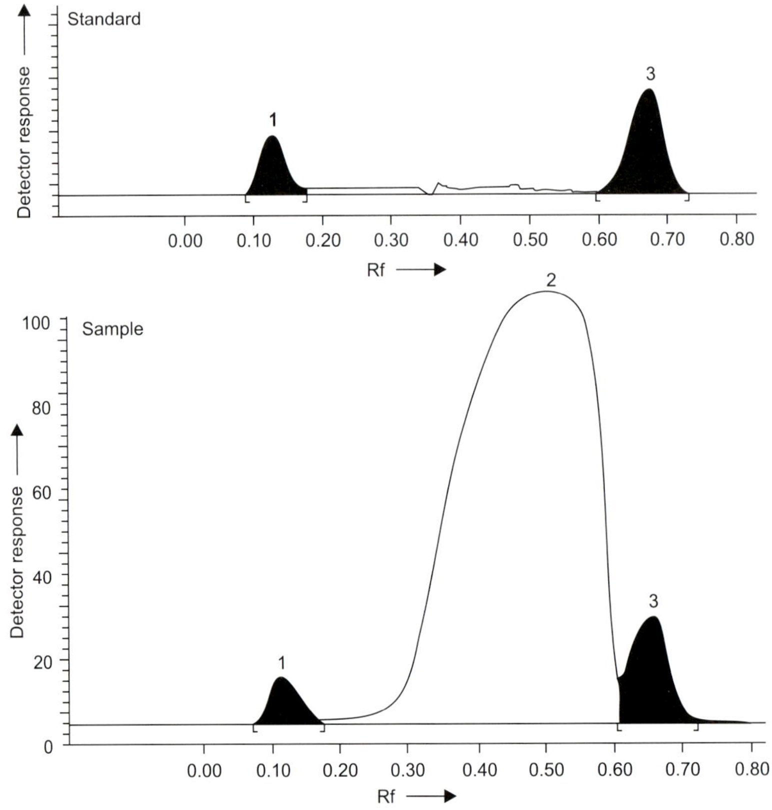

Typical densitogram of the sample and standard containing ephedrine hydrochloride, theophylline and hydroxyzine hydrochloride. For detailed experimental and chromatographic conditions, refer to Protocol No. 312. Peaks identification: 1. Ephedrine HCl; 2. Theophylline; 3. Hydroxyzine HCl.

PROTOCOL FOR HPTLC ANALYSIS OF PHARMACEUTICAL FORMULATION

Protocol No. 312

Formulation: Theophylline, Ephedrine hydrochloride, Hydroxyzine hydrochloride

Classification: Respiratory System **Dosage form:** Tablets, Capsules

Standard preparation: Dissolve 10 mg of hydroxyzine hydrochloride (HH) and 25 mg of ephedrine hydrochloride (EH) in methanol to produce 10 ml. Weigh 65 mg of theophylline (T), add 5 ml of 25% ammonia to dissolve, dilute to 10 ml with methanol. Mix 0.1 ml of (HH) solution, 0.2 ml of (EH) and 2 ml of (T) solution, dilute to 10 ml with methanol for analysis.

Sample preparation: To powdered sample, equivalent to 20 mg of hydroxyzine HCl, add 3 ml of ammonia and 5 ml of water, vortex for 10 min, dilute to 25 ml with methanol, filter and dilute 0.5 ml to 50 ml with methanol and use for analysis.

Chromatographic equipments:

Sample applicator: Camag Linomat–IV
Development chamber: Camag twin-trough glass chamber, 10 × 10 cm
Densitometric scanner: Camag TLC Scanner–II

Chromatographic conditions:

1. Stationary phase: Silica gel 60F_{254} pre-coated HPTLC plates, 10 × 10 cm (200 μm) – Merck
2. Mobile phase (MP): Ethyl acetate–methanol–25% ammonia (10 : 1.5 : 0.05 v/v)
3. Standard/Sample application:
   Band length: — Volume applied: — Spacing: —
4. Chamber saturation: 20 min (MP)
5. RH (%): 55 ± 5
6. Temperature °C: 22 ± 2
7. Separation technique: Ascending
8. Quantity of mobile phase: 10 ml
9. Migration distance: 50 mm
10. Migration time: 15 min

Densitometric evaluation:

Wavelength: UV–254 nm (EH and HH), UV–272 nm (T)
Scanning mode: Reflectance/Absorbance
HRF: Ephedrine HCl—12; Theophylline—42; Hydroxyzine HCl—67
Linearity: —
Recovery (%): 98.44–103.3 for all three drugs

References: —

Comments:

- The method was optimized and analytical work carried out at **Anchrom's HPTLC Application Laboratory**, Mumbai, India.
- Theophylline, being the major compound, could not be simultaneously estimated. For that, dilute solution of the sample needs to be applied for chromatographic separation and then scanned at 272 nm for estimation.
- Several market samples of similar composition were analysed by the proposed method with reproducible results.

HPTLC : High Performance Thin Layer Chromatography
HPTLC Densitogram

No. 313

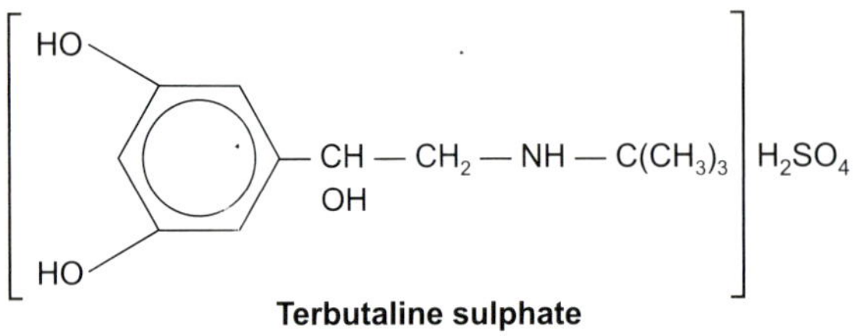

HO, HO — [benzene ring] — CH — CH_2 — NH — $C(CH_3)_3$ H_2SO_4
OH

Terbutaline sulphate

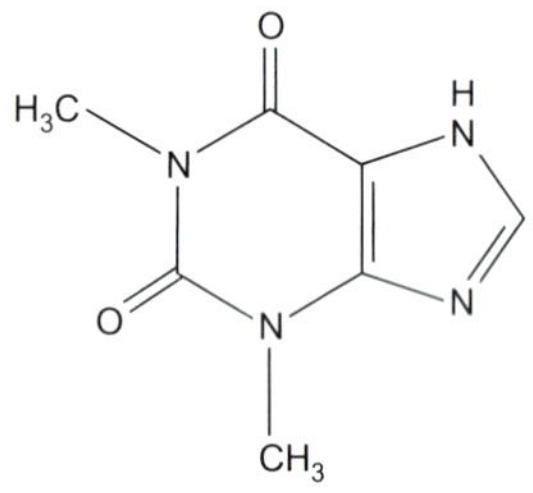

H_3C, O, N, H, N, O, N, N, CH_3

Theophylline

Standard

Detector response ⟶ 0, 20, 40, 60, 80

Peaks: 1, 2

Rf ⟶ 0.00, 0.10, 0.20, 0.30, 0.40, 0.50, 0.60

Sample

Detector response ⟶ 0, 20, 40, 60, 80

Peaks: 1, 2

Rf ⟶ 0.00, 0.10, 0.20, 0.30, 0.40, 0.50, 0.60

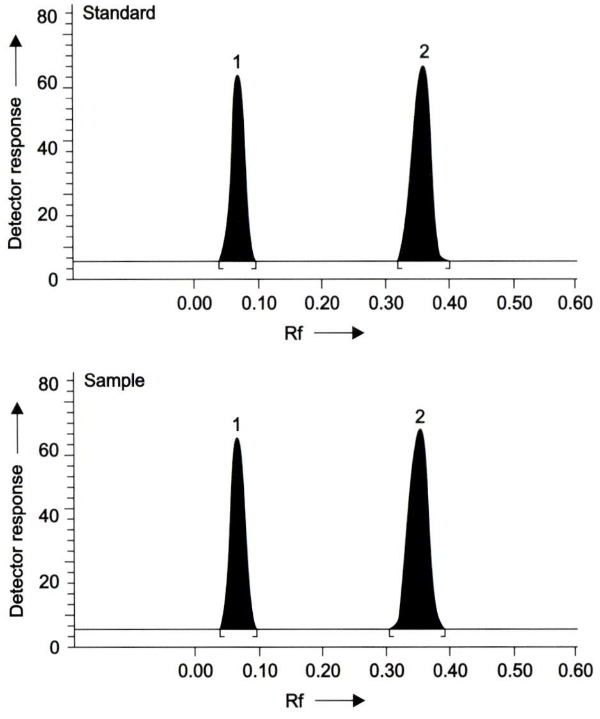

Typical densitogram of the sample and standard containing terbutaline sulphate and theophylline. For detailed experimental and chromatographic conditions, refer to Protocol No. 313. Peaks identification: 1. Terbutaline sulphate; 2. Theophylline.

PROTOCOL FOR HPTLC ANALYSIS OF PHARMACEUTICAL FORMULATION

Protocol No. 313

Formulation: **Terbutaline sulphate, Theophylline**
Classification: Respiratory System **Dosage form:** Tablets
Standard preparation: Weigh 10 mg of terbutaline sulphate (TS), add 1 ml of water and dilute to 10 ml with methanol. Weigh 40 mg of theophylline (T), add 1 ml of TS solution, dilute to 10 ml with methanol. Further dilute 0.2 ml of this solution to 10 ml with methanol and use for analysis.
Sample preparation: Weigh powdered sample equivalent to 100 mg of theophylline, add 3 ml of water, 1.5 ml of 25% ammonia and 15 ml of methanol, sonicate for 10 min, dilute to 25 ml with methanol, filter and dilute 0.2 ml of filtrate to 10 ml with methanol and use for estimation.
Chromatographic equipments:
Sample applicator: Camag Linomat–IV
Development chamber: Camag twin-trough glass chamber, 10 × 10 cm
Densitometric scanner: Camag TLC Scanner–II
Chromatographic conditions:
1. Stationary phase: Silica gel $60F_{254}$ pre-coated HPTLC plates, 7 × 10 cm (200 μm) – Merck, pre-washed with methanol, dried (60°) for 5 min prior to use
2. Mobile phase (MP): Chloroform–acetone–methanol–25% ammonia (8 : 2 : 1 : 0.2 v/v)
3. Standard/Sample application:
 Band length: 5 mm Volume applied: 5 μl, 10 μl Spacing: 5 mm
4. Chamber saturation: 20 min (MP)
5. RH (%): 55 ± 5
6. Temperature °C: 22 ± 2
7. Separation technique: Ascending
8. Quantity of mobile phase: 11 ml
9. Migration distance: 50 mm
10. Migration time: 15 min

Densitometric evaluation:
Wavelength: UV–205 nm (TS); UV–275 nm (T)
Scanning mode: Reflectance/Absorbance
HRF: Terbutaline sulphate—08; Theophylline—35
Linearity (ng/band): Theophylline—100–500; Terbutaline sulphate—10–50
Recovery (%): 99.25–102 for both the compounds
References: —
Comments:
- The method was optimized and analytical work carried out at **Anchrom's HPTLC Application Laboratory**, Mumbai, India.
- Since the amount of theophylline is 40 times the level of TS, both compounds could not be simultaneously scanned in single track, hence applied different concentrations in different tracks and scanned at 205 nm (TS) and 275 nm (T).
- Several market samples of similar composition were analysed by the proposed method with reproducible results.

HPTLC : High Performance Thin Layer Chromatography
HPTLC Densitogram

No. 314

[HO, HO-substituted benzene ring — $CH - CH_2 - NH - C(CH_3)_3$ with OH] H_2SO_4

Terbutaline sulphate

Theophylline

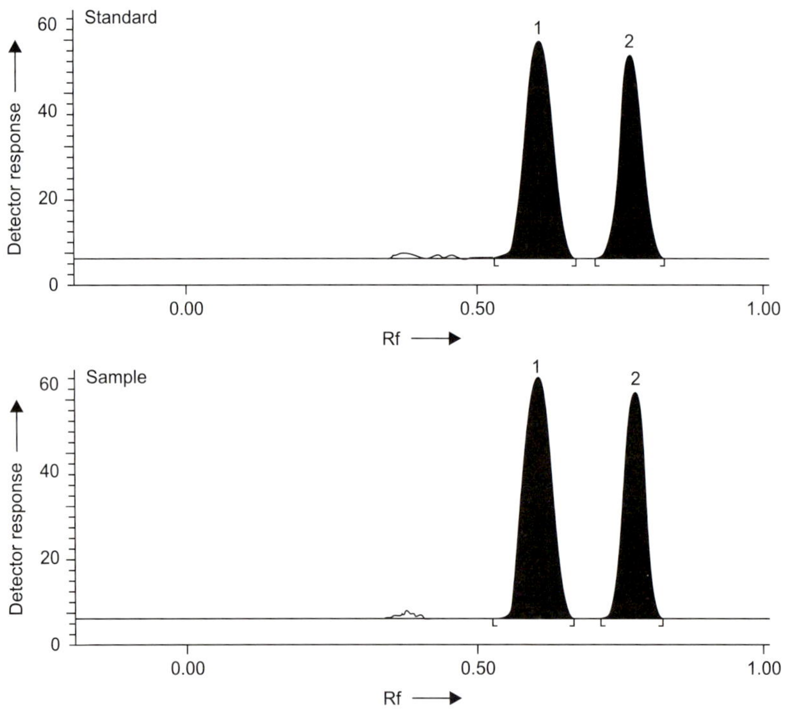

Typical densitogram of the sample and standard containing terbutaline sulphate and theophylline. For detailed experimental and chromatographic conditions, refer to Protocol No. 314. Peaks identification: 1. Theophylline; 2. Terbutaline sulphate.

PROTOCOL FOR HPTLC ANALYSIS OF PHARMACEUTICAL FORMULATION

Protocol No. 314

Formulation: **Terbutaline sulphate, Theophylline**
Classification: Respiratory System **Dosage form:** Tablets
Standard preparation: Weigh 10 mg of terbutaline sulphate (TS), add 1 ml of water and dilute to 10 ml with methanol. Weigh 40 mg of theophylline (T), add 1 ml of TS solution, dilute to 10 ml with methanol. Further dilute 0.2 ml of this solution to 10 ml with methanol and use for analysis.
Sample preparation: Weigh powdered sample equivalent to 100 mg of theophylline, add 3 ml of water, 1.5 ml of 25% ammonia and 15 ml of methanol, sonicate for 10 min, dilute to 25 ml with methanol, filter and dilute 0.2 ml of the filtrate to 10 ml with methanol and use for estimation.
Chromatographic equipments:
Sample applicator: Camag Linomat–IV
Development chamber: Camag twin-trough glass chamber, 10 × 10 cm
Densitometric scanner: Camag TLC Scanner–II
Chromatographic conditions:
1. Stationary phase: Silica gel 60 RP-18F_{254s} pre-coated HPTLC plates, 5 × 7.5 cm (200 μm) – Merck
2. Mobile phase (MP): 0.5 M sod. chloride–methanol–glacial acetic acid (12 : 8 : 0.01 v/v)
3. Standard/Sample application:
   Band length: 7 mm Volume applied: 5 μl, 10 μl Spacing: 10 mm
4. Chamber saturation: 20 min (MP)
5. RH (%): 55 ± 5
6. Temperature °C: 22 ± 2
7. Separation technique: Ascending
8. Quantity of mobile phase: 20 ml
9. Migration distance: 50 mm
10. Migration time: 40 min

Densitometric evaluation:
Wavelength: UV–205 nm (TS); UV–275 nm (T)
Scanning mode: Reflectance/Absorbance
HRF: Theophylline—60; Terbutaline sulphate—80;
Linearity (ng/band): Theophylline—100–500; Terbutaline sulphate—10–50
Recovery (%): 98.95–99.0 for both the drugs
References: —
Comments:
- The method was optimized and analytical work carried out at **Anchrom's HPTLC Application Laboratory**, Mumbai, India.
- As the amount of theophylline is 40 times higher than TS in formulations, both the compounds could not be scanned simultaneously on single track, hence different concentrations applied in different tracks and scanned at 205 nm (TS) and 275 nm (T).
- Several market samples of similar composition were analysed by the proposed method with reproducible results.
- Reversal of retention order in RP-chromatography as compared to NP-chromatography.

HPTLC : High Performance Thin Layer Chromatography
HPTLC Densitogram

No. 315

Terbutaline sulphate

Etofylline

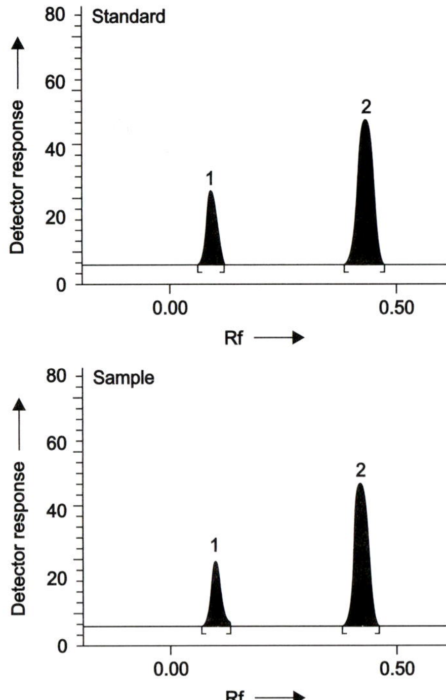

Typical densitogram of the sample and standard containing terbutaline sulphate and etofylline. For detailed experimental and chromatographic conditions, refer to Protocol No. 315. Peaks identification: 1. Terbutaline sulphate; 2. Etofylline.

PROTOCOL FOR HPTLC ANALYSIS OF PHARMACEUTICAL FORMULATION

Protocol No. 315

Formulation: **Terbutaline sulphate, Etofylline**
Classification: Respiratory System **Dosage form:** Tablets
Standard preparation: Weigh 10 mg of terbutaline sulphate (TS), add 1 ml of water, dilute to 10 ml with methanol. Weigh 40 mg of etofylline (E), add 1 ml of TS solution, 0.5 ml of ammonia and 1 ml of water and dilute to 10 ml with methanol. Further dilute 0.2 ml to 10 ml with methanol and use for analysis.
Sample preparation: To powdered sample, equivalent to 100 mg of etofylline, add 3 ml of water and 1.5 ml 25% ammonia, shake for 10 min, dilute to 25 ml with methanol. Filter and dilute 0.2 ml of the filtrate to 10 ml with methanol and use for estimation.
Chromatographic equipments:
Sample applicator: Camag Linomat–IV
Development chamber: Camag twin-trough glass chamber, 10 × 10 cm
Densitometric scanner: Camag TLC Scanner–II
Chromatographic conditions:

1. Stationary phase: Silica gel $60F_{254}$ pre-coated HPTLC plates, 7 × 10 cm (200 μm) – Merck, pre-washed with methanol, dried (60°C) for 5 min prior to use
2. Mobile phase (MP): Chloroform–acetone–methanol–25% ammonia (8 : 2 : 1 : 0.2 v/v)
3. Standard/Sample application:
   Band length: 5 mm Volume applied: 5 μl, 10 μl Spacing: 5 mm
4. Chamber saturation: 20 min (MP)
5. RH (%): 55 ± 5
6. Temperature °C: 22 ± 2
7. Separation technique: Ascending
8. Quantity of mobile phase: 11 ml
9. Migration distance: 50 mm
10. Migration time: 15 min

Densitometric evaluation:
Wavelength: UV–205 nm (TS); UV–275 nm (E)
Scanning mode: Reflectance/Absorbance
HRF: Terbutaline sulphate (TS)—10; Etofylline (E)—44
Linearity (ng/band): Terbutaline sulphate (TS)—10–50; Etofylline (E)—100–500
Recovery (%): 98.30–101.6 for both the compounds
References: —
Comments:

- The method was optimized and analytical work carried out at **Anchrom's HPTLC Application Laboratory**, Mumbai, India.
- Several market samples of similar composition were analysed by the proposed method with reproducible results.

HPTLC : High Performance Thin Layer Chromatography
HPTLC Densitogram

No. 316

Terbutaline sulphate

Etofylline

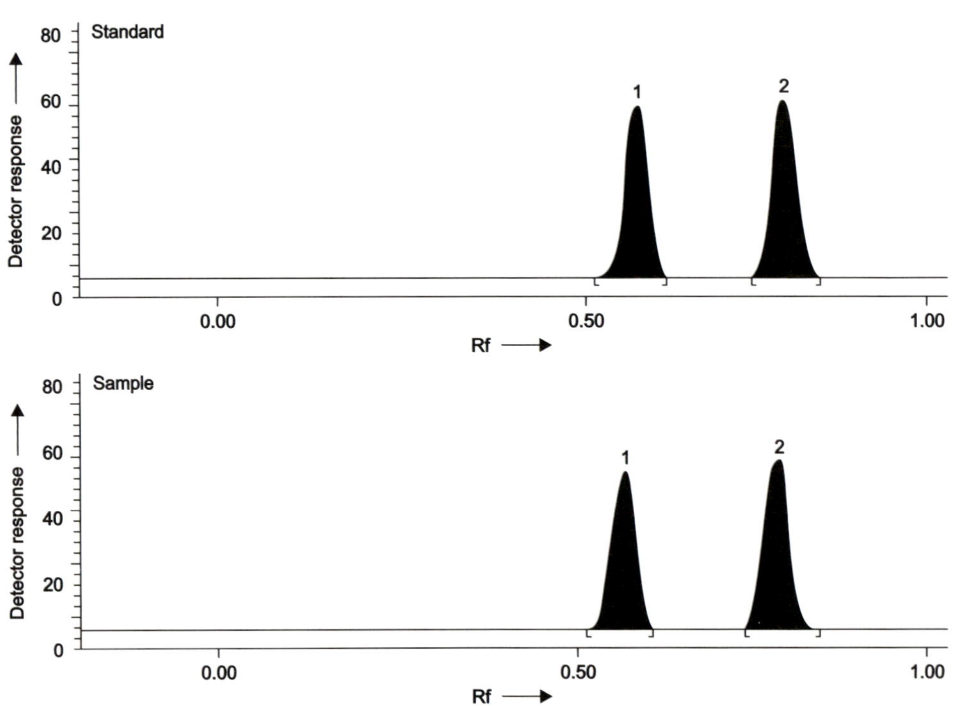

Typical densitogram of the sample and standard containing terbutaline sulphate and etofylline For detailed experimental and chromatographic conditions, refer to Protocol No. 316. Peaks identification: 1. Etofylline; 2. Terbutaline sulphate.

PROTOCOL FOR HPTLC ANALYSIS OF PHARMACEUTICAL FORMULATION

Protocol No. 316

Formulation: Terbutaline sulphate, Etofylline

Classification: Respiratory System **Dosage form:** Tablets

Standard preparation: Weigh 10 mg of terbutaline sulphate (TS), add 1 ml of water, dilute to 10 ml with methanol. To 40 mg of etofylline, add 1 ml of 'TS' solution, 1 ml of water and 0.5 ml of ammonia, shake, dilute to 10 ml with methanol. Further dilute 0.2 ml to 10 ml with methanol and use for analysis.

Sample preparation: To powdered sample, equivalent to 100 mg of etofylline, add 3 ml of water and 1.5 ml 25% ammonia and 15 ml of methanol, shake, dilute to 25 ml, filter and dilute 0.2 ml of filtrate to 10 ml with methanol and use for estimation.

Chromatographic equipments:

Sample applicator: Camag Linomat–IV

Development chamber: Camag twin-trough glass chamber, 10 × 10 cm

Densitometric scanner: Camag TLC Scanner–II

Chromatographic conditions:

1. Stationary phase: Silica gel 60 RP-18F_{254s} pre-coated HPTLC plates, 10 × 10 cm (200 μm) – Merck
2. Mobile phase (MP): 0.5 M sod. chloride–methanol–glacial acetic acid (12 : 8 : 0.01 v/v)
3. Standard/Sample application:
   Band length: 5 mm Volume applied: 5 μl, 10 μl Spacing: 5 mm
4. Chamber saturation: 20 min (MP)
5. RH (%): 55 ± 5
6. Temperature °C: 22 ± 2
7. Separation technique: Ascending
8. Quantity of mobile phase: 20 ml
9. Migration distance: 50 mm
10. Migration time: 40 min

Densitometric evaluation:

Wavelength: UV–205 nm (TS); UV–275 nm (E)

Scanning mode: Reflectance/Absorbance

HRF: Etofylline (E)—60; Terbutaline sulphate (TS)—80

Linearity (ng/band): Etofylline (E)—100–500; Terbutaline sulphate (TS)—10–50

Recovery (%): 98.75–99.0 for both the compounds

References: —

Comments:

- The method was optimized and analytical work carried out at **Anchrom's HPTLC Application Laboratory**, Mumbai, India.
- Several market samples of similar composition were analysed by the proposed method with reproducible results.
- RP-chromatography resulted in reversal of retention order as compared to NP-chromatography.

HPTLC : High Performance Thin Layer Chromatography
HPTLC Densitogram

No. 317

$[(HO)_2C_6H_3-CH(OH)-CH_2-NH-C(CH_3)_3]\ H_2SO_4$

Terbutaline sulphate

Guaiphenesin

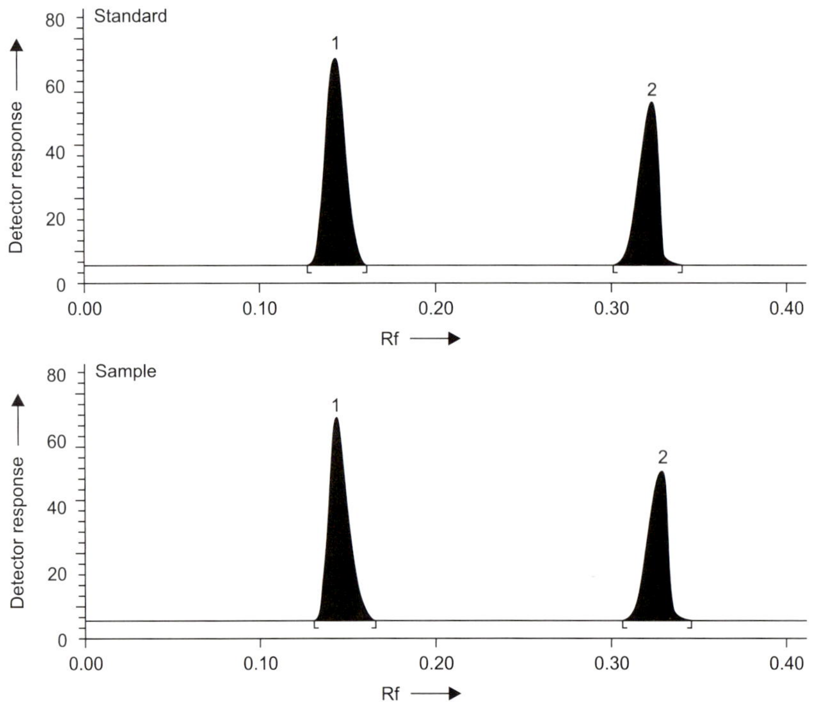

Typical densitogram of the sample and standard containing terbutaline sulphate and guaiphenesin. For detailed experimental and chromatographic conditions, refer to Protocol No. 317. Peaks identification: 1. Terbutaline sulphate; 2. Guaiphenesin.

PROTOCOL FOR HPTLC ANALYSIS OF PHARMACEUTICAL FORMULATION

Protocol No. 317

Formulation: Terbutaline sulphate, Guaiphenesin

Classification: Respiratory System **Dosage form:** Tablets, Syrup

Standard preparation: Prepare 1 mg/ml solution of terbutaline sulphate (TS) in methanol. Take 40 mg of guaiphenesin, add 1 ml of 'TS' solution, dilute to 10 ml with methanol.

Dilute solution: Dilute 0.5 ml to 10 ml with methanol and use both stock solution and dilute solution for analysis.

Sample preparation: Weigh sample equivalent to 100 mg of guaiphenesin, add 3 ml of water, 15 ml of methanol, vortex for 10 min, dilute to 25 ml with methanol, filter (stock solution). Dilute 0.5 ml to 10 ml with methanol. Use both dilute and stock solutions for analysis.

Chromatographic equipments:

Sample applicator: Camag Linomat–IV

Development chamber: Camag twin-trough glass chamber, 10 × 10 cm

Densitometric scanner: Camag TLC Scanner–II

Chromatographic conditions:

1. Stationary phase: Silica gel $60F_{254}$ pre-coated HPTLC plates, 10 × 10 cm (200 μm) – Merck
2. Mobile phase (MP): (i) Chloroform–acetone–methanol–25% ammonia (8 : 2 : 1 : 0.2 v/v); (ii) Toluene–methanol–25% ammonia (5 : 5 : 0.5 v/v)
3. Standard/Sample application:
   Band length: 10 mm
   Volume applied: 10 μl (both dilute and stock solution) Spacing: 10 mm
4. Chamber saturation: 20 min (MP)
5. RH (%): 55 ± 5
6. Temperature °C: 22 ± 2
7. Separation technique: Ascending
8. Quantity of mobile phase: 11 ml
9. Migration distance: 50 mm
10. Migration time: 15 min/12 min

Densitometric evaluation:

Wavelength: UV–205 nm (TS); UV–275 nm (TS and G)

Scanning mode: Reflectance/Absorbance

HRF: Terbutaline sulphate (TS)—15; Guaiphenesin—33

Linearity (ng/band): Terbutaline sulphate (TS)—10–50; Guaiphenesin—100–500

Recovery (%): 98.75–99.0 for both the compounds

References: —

Comments:

- The method was optimized and analytical work carried out at **Anchrom's HPTLC Application Laboratory**, Mumbai, India.
- Several market samples of similar composition were analysed by the proposed method with reproducible results.

HPTLC : High Performance Thin Layer Chromatography
HPTLC Densitogram

No. 318

[HO-, HO-substituted benzene ring]-CH(OH)-CH_2-NH-$C(CH_3)_3$ H_2SO_4

Terbutaline sulphate

OH, O, OH, OCH_3

Guaiphenesin

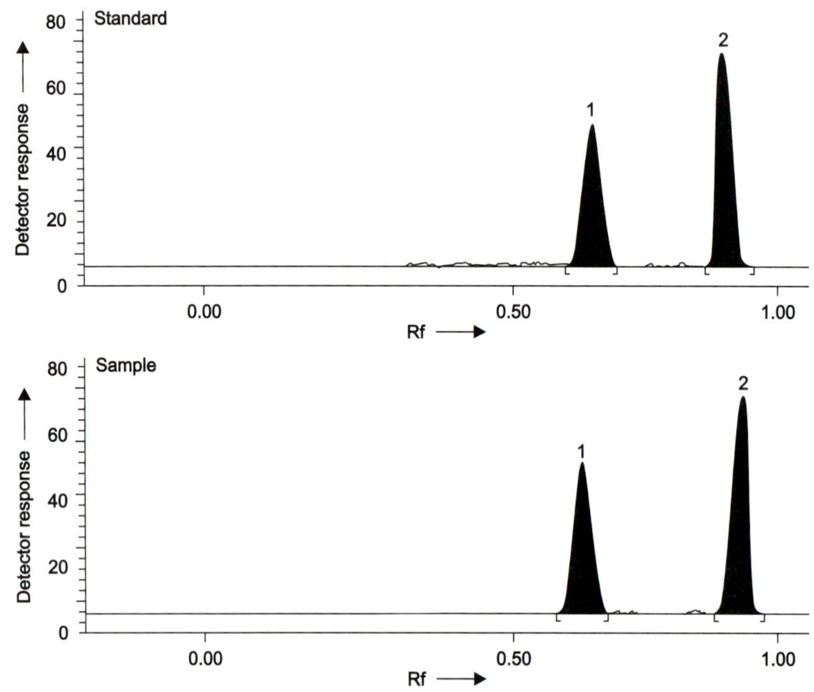

Typical densitogram of the sample and standard containing terbutaline sulphate and guaiphenesin. For detailed experimental and chromatographic conditions, refer to Protocol No. 318. Peaks identification: 1. Guaiphenesin; 2. Terbutaline sulphate.

PROTOCOL FOR HPTLC ANALYSIS OF PHARMACEUTICAL FORMULATION

Protocol No. 318

Formulation: **Terbutaline sulphate, Guaiphenesin**

Classification: Respiratory System **Dosage form:** Tablets, Syrup

Standard preparation: Prepare 1 mg/ml solution of terbutaline sulphate (TS) in methanol. Take 40 mg of guaiphenesin, add 1 ml of 'TS' solution, dilute to 10 ml with methanol. Dilute solution: Dilute 0.5 ml to 10 ml with methanol and use both stock solution and dilute solution for analysis.

Sample preparation: Weigh sample equivalent to 100 mg of guaiphenesin, add 3 ml of water, 15 ml of methanol, vortex for 10 min, dilute to 25 ml with methanol, filter. Dilute solution: Dilute 0.5 ml to 10 ml with methanol and use both stock solution and dilute solution for analysis.

Chromatographic equipments:

Sample applicator: Camag Linomat–IV

Development chamber: Camag twin-trough glass chamber, 10 × 10 cm

Densitometric scanner: Camag TLC Scanner–II

Chromatographic conditions:

1. Stationary phase: Silica gel RP-18F_{254s} pre-coated HPTLC plates, 10 × 10 cm (200 μm) – Merck
2. Mobile phase (MP): 0.5 M sod. chloride-methanol–glacial acetic acid (12 : 8 : 0.01 v/v)
3. Standard/Sample application:
   Band length: 10 mm Volume applied: 10 μl Spacing: 10 mm
4. Chamber saturation: 20 min (MP)
5. RH (%): 55 ± 5
6. Temperature °C: 22 ± 2
7. Separation technique: Ascending
8. Quantity of mobile phase: 20 ml
9. Migration distance: 50 mm
10. Migration time: 40 min

Densitometric evaluation:

Wavelength: UV–275 nm (TS and G) Scanning mode: Reflectance/Absorbance

HRF: Guaiphenesin—60; Terbutaline SO_4—82

Linearity (ng/band): Terbutaline SO_4—10–50; Guaiphenesin—100–500

Recovery (%): 98.90–101.60 for both the compounds

References: —

Comments:

- The method was optimized and analytical work carried out at **Anchrom's HPTLC Application Laboratory**, Mumbai, India.
- RP-chromatography resulted in reversal of retention order as compared to NP-chromatography.
- Several market samples of similar composition were analysed by the proposed method with reproducible results.

HPTLC : High Performance Thin Layer Chromatography
HPTLC Densitogram

No. 319

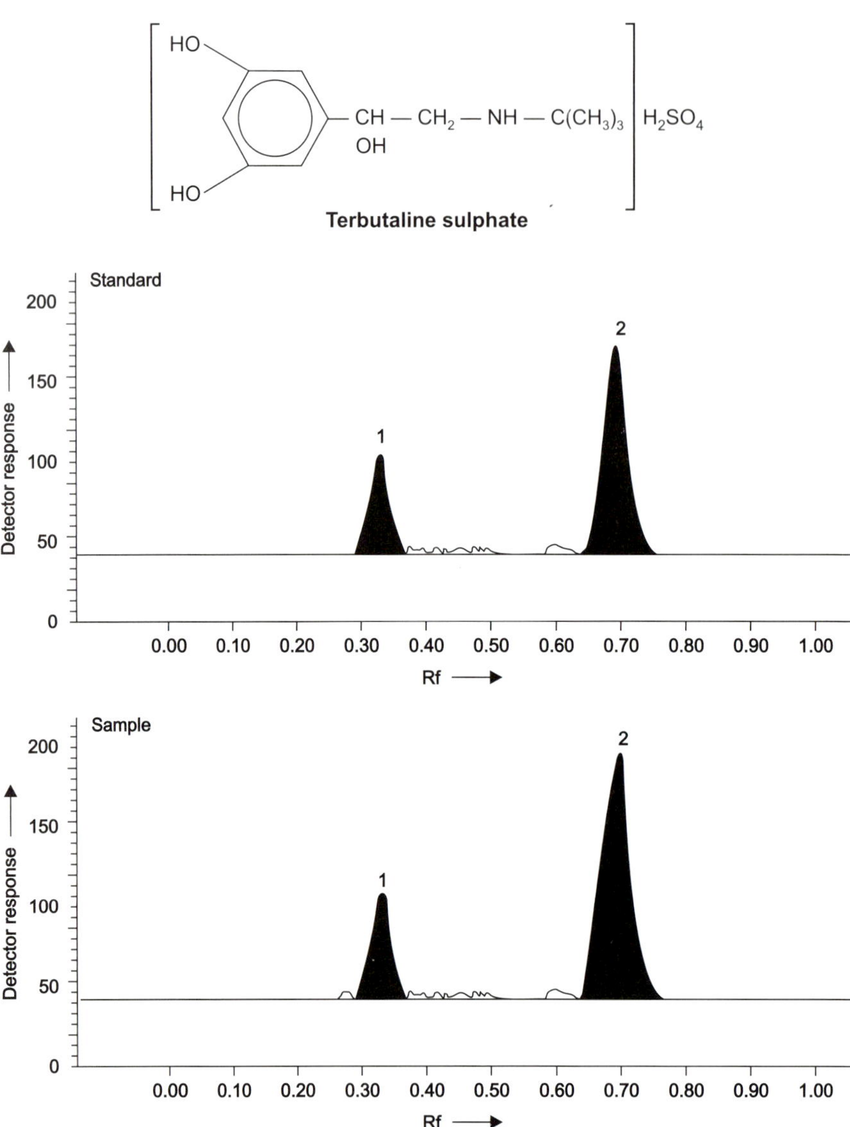

Typical densitogram of the sample and standard containing bromhexine hydrochloride and terbutaline sulphate. For detailed experimental and chromatographic conditions, refer to Protocol No. 319. Peaks identification: 1. Terbutaline sulphate; 2. Bromhexine hydrochloride.

PROTOCOL FOR HPTLC ANALYSIS OF PHARMACEUTICAL FORMULATION

Protocol No. 319

Formulation: Terbutaline sulphate, Bromhexine hydrochloride

Classification: Respiratory System **Dosage form:** Tablets

Standard preparation: Prepare solution of both the drugs in methanol to get 250 µg/ml (terbutaline sulphate) and 800 µg/ml (bromhexine hydrochloride). Further suitable dilutions made with methanol for chromatographic analysis.

Sample preparation: Powdered sample equivalent to 8 mg of bromhexine HCl suspended in methanol, sonicated for 10 min, diluted to 10 ml with methanol. Filtered and 1 ml of filtrate diluted to 10 ml with methanol and used for chromatographic analysis.

Chromatographic equipments:

Sample applicator: Camag Linomat–IV

Development chamber: Camag twin-trough glass chamber, 20 × 10 cm

Densitometric scanner: Camag TLC Scanner–III

Chromatographic conditions:

1. Stationary phase: Silica gel $60F_{254}$ pre-coated HPTLC plates, 20 × 10 cm (200 µm) – Merck, pre-washed with methanol, activated at 105°C for 10 min prior to use
2. Mobile phase (MP): Methanol–water–25% ammonia (19 : 2 : 0.3 v/v)
3. Standard/Sample application:
   Band length: 8 mm Volume applied: 15 µl Spacing: 10 mm
4. Chamber saturation: 20 min (MP)
5. RH (%): 55 ± 5
6. Temperature °C: 25 ± 2
7. Separation technique: Ascending
8. Quantity of mobile phase: 21 ml
9. Migration distance: 80 mm
10. Migration time: 16 min

Densitometric evaluation:

Wavelength: UV–210 nm Scanning mode: Reflectance/Absorbance

HRF: Terbutaline sulphate—34; Bromhexine hydrochloride—69

Linearity: —

Recovery (%): —

References: —

Comments:

- The method was optimized and analytical work carried out at **Anchrom's HPTLC Application Laboratory**, Mumbai, India.
- The method is suitable for content-uniformity of both the drugs.
- Several market samples of similar composition were analysed by the proposed method with reproducible results.

HPTLC : High Performance Thin Layer Chromatography
HPTLC Densitogram

No. 320

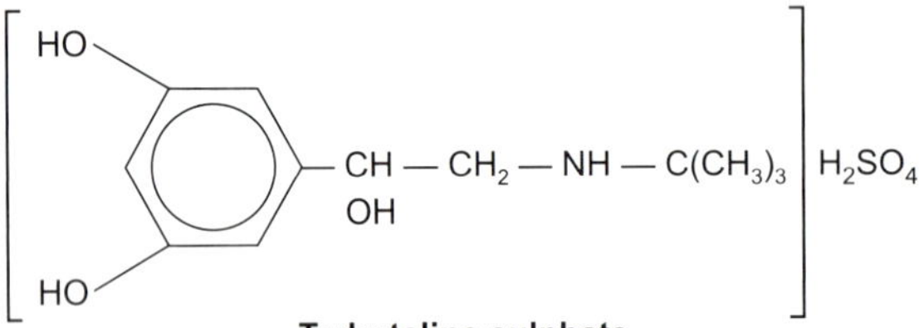

Terbutaline sulphate

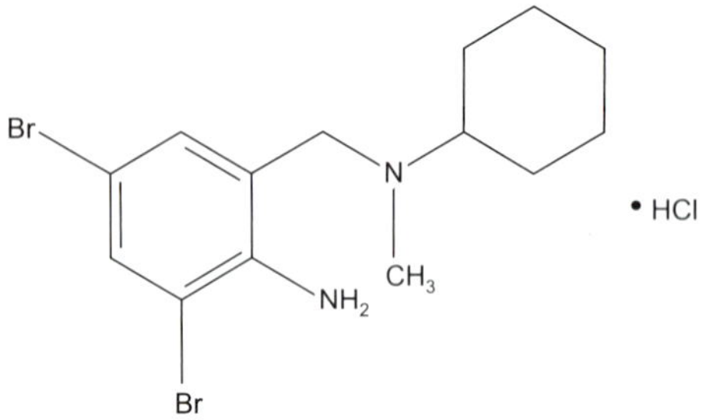

Bromhexine hydrochloride

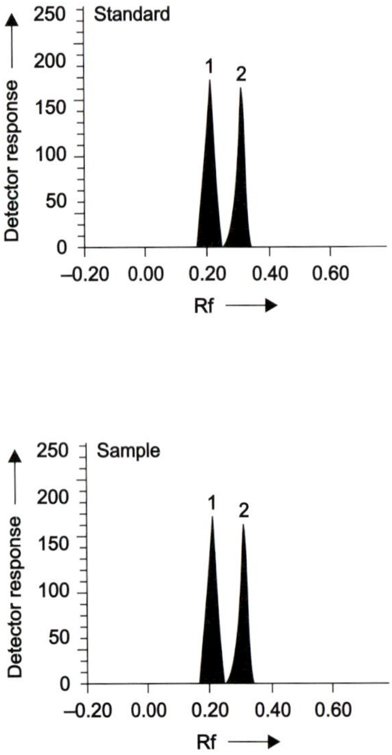

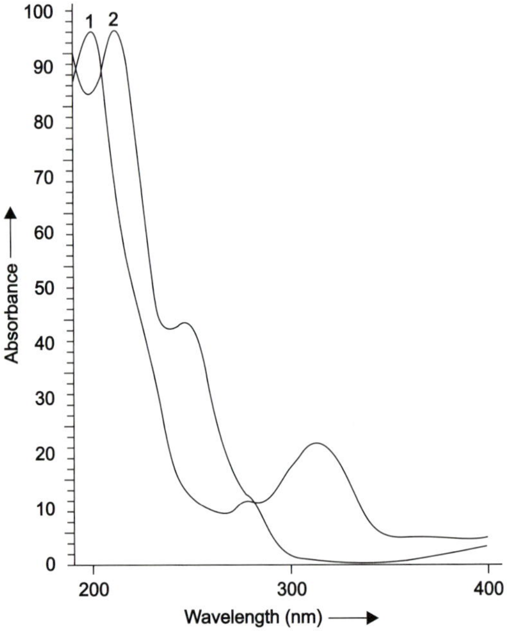

Overlaid UV-spectra of bromhexine hydrochloride (1) and terbutaline sulphate (2) for selection of suitable wavelength for densitometric scanning

Typical densitogram of the standard and sample containing bromhexine hydrochloride and terbutaline sulphate. For detailed experimental and chromatographic conditions, refer to Protocol No. 320. Peaks identification: 1. Bromhexine hydrochloride; 2. Terbutaline sulphate.

PROTOCOL FOR HPTLC ANALYSIS OF PHARMACEUTICAL FORMULATION

Protocol No. 320

Formulation: Terbutaline sulphate, Bromhexine hydrochloride

Classification: Respiratory System **Dosage form:** Tablets

Standard preparation: Prepare 1 mg/ml solution of terbutaline sulphate and 2 mg/ml solution of bromhexine hydrochloride, both in methanol. Further serial dilutions made with methanol for linearity studies. Apply 10 µl of each solution for analysis.

Sample preparation: Powdered sample equivalent to 2.5 mg of terbutaline sulphate suspended in 8 ml of methanol, sonicated for 10 min, diluted to 10 ml, filtered and 1 ml of filtrate diluted to 10 ml with methanol and used for chromatographic analysis by applying 10 µl.

Chromatographic equipments:

Sample applicator: Camag Linomat–V

Development chamber: Camag ADC–2, saturated with Camag saturation pad

Densitometric scanner: Camag TLC Scanner–III

Chromatographic conditions:

1. Stationary phase: Silica gel $60F_{254}$ pre-coated TLC plates, 20 × 10 cm (200 µm) – Merck
2. Mobile phase (MP): Isopropanol–cyclohexane–formic acid (6.5 : 2.5 : 0.1 v/v)
3. Standard/Sample application:
   Band length: 8 mm Volume applied: 10 µl Spacing: 10 mm
4. Chamber saturation: 20 min (MP)
5. RH (%): 55 ± 5
6. Temperature °C: 25 ± 1
7. Separation technique: Ascending
8. Quantity of mobile phase: 18 ml
9. Migration distance: 70 mm
10. Migration time: 15 min

Densitometric evaluation:

Wavelength: UV–200 nm Scanning mode: Reflectance/Absorbance

HRF: Bromhexine hydrochloride—20; Terbutaline sulphate—31

Linearity (ng/band): Bromhexine HCl—200–1600; Terbutaline—100–1000

Recovery (%): —

References: —

Comments:

- The method was optimized and the analytical work was carried out at **Anchrom HPTLC Application Laboratory**, Mumbai, India.
- The method is suitable for content uniformity.

HPTLC : High Performance Thin Layer Chromatography
HPTLC Densitogram

No. 321

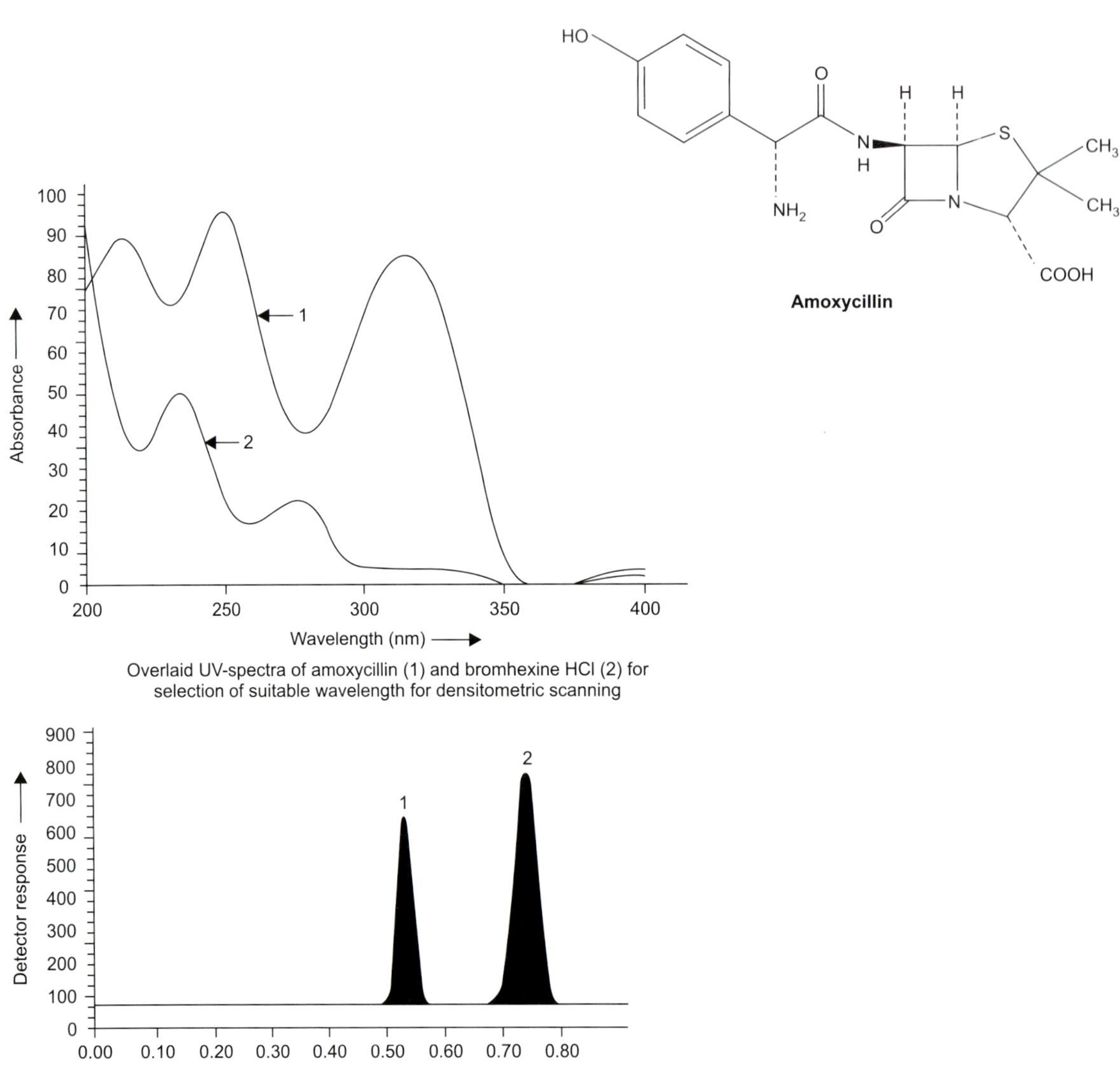

Overlaid UV-spectra of amoxycillin (1) and bromhexine HCl (2) for selection of suitable wavelength for densitometric scanning

Typical densitogram of the standard containing amoxycillin and bromhexine HCl. For detailed experimental and chromatographic conditions, refer to Protocol No. 321. Peaks identification: 1. Amoxycillin; 2. Bromhexine hydrochloride.

PROTOCOL FOR HPTLC ANALYSIS OF PHARMACEUTICAL FORMULATION

Protocol No. 321

Formulation: Amoxycillin, Bromhexine hydrochloride

Classification: Respiratory System **Dosage form:** Capsules

Standard preparation: Prepare 1 mg/ml solution of amoxycillin and 100 μg/ml of bromhexine, both in methanol. Apply 10–30 μl of amoxycillin solution and 2–10 μl of bromhexine solution for linearity studies.

Sample preparation: Sample equivalent to 10 mg of amoxycillin suspended in 5 ml of methanol, sonicated for 10 min, diluted to 10 ml with methanol, filter and apply volume equivalent to 400 ng of bromhexine and 12.5 μg/band of amoxycillin and carry out chromatographic analysis.

Chromatographic equipments:

Sample applicator: Camag Linomat–V

Development chamber: Camag twin-trough glass chamber, 10 × 10 cm

Densitometric scanner: Camag TLC Scanner–III

Chromatographic conditions:

1. Stationary phase: Silica gel 60F_{254} pre-coated TLC plates, 10 × 10 cm (250 μm) – Merck
2. Mobile phase (MP): Butyl acetate–methanol–water–glacial acetic acid (5 : 2.5 : 2.5 : 1 v/v)
3. Standard/Sample application:
   Band length: 6 mm Volume applied: — Spacing: 10 mm
4. Chamber saturation: 20 min (MP)
5. RH (%): 55 ± 5
6. Temperature °C: 22 ± 2
7. Separation technique: Ascending
8. Quantity of mobile phase: 11 ml
9. Migration distance: 90 mm
10. Migration time: 40 min

Densitometric evaluation:

Wavelength: UV–235 nm (bromhexine), 320 nm for amoxycillin or 235 nm for both the drugs

Scanning mode: Reflectance/Absorbance

HRF: Amoxycillin—51; Bromhexine HCl—74

Linearity: Amoxycillin—10–30 μg/band; Bromhexine HCl—200–1000 ng/band

Recovery (%): Amoxycillin—99.68–101.35; Bromhexine HCl—100.14–100.60

References: M.V. Dhoka, V.T. Gawande and P.P. Joshi, *J. Pharm. Sci. and Res.*, **2(8)**, 477–483, 2010.

Comments: The method validated for accuracy, precision, linearity, LOD, LOQ, specificity, robustness and ruggedness.

HPTLC : High Performance Thin Layer Chromatography
HPTLC Densitogram

No. 322

Salbutamol

Guaiphenesin

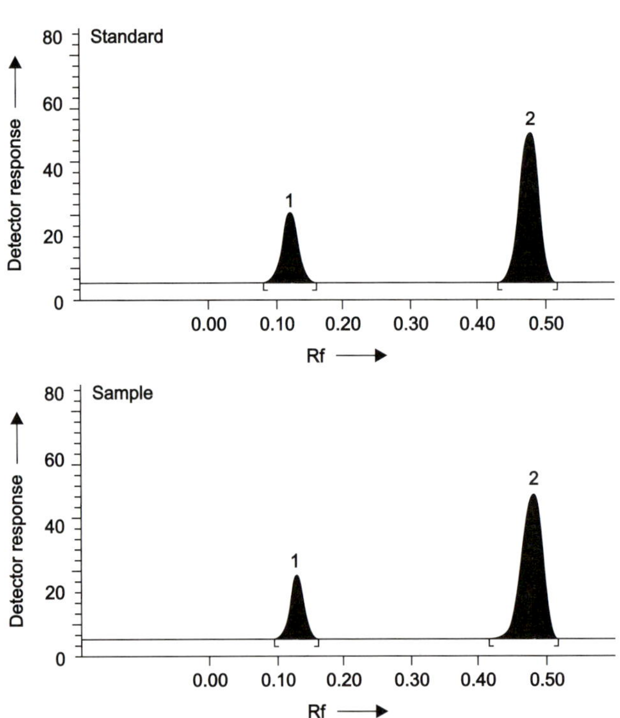

Typical densitogram of the sample and standard containing salbutamol sulphate and guaiphenesin. For detailed experimental and chromatographic conditions, refer to Protocol No. 322. Peaks identification: 1. Salbutamol sulphate; 2. Guaiphenesin.

PROTOCOL FOR HPTLC ANALYSIS OF PHARMACEUTICAL FORMULATION

Protocol No. 322

Formulation: Salbutamol sulphate, Guaiphenesin

Classification: Respiratory System **Dosage form:** Syrup

Standard preparation: Weigh 12 mg of the salbutamol sulphate (SS), add 2 ml of ammonia, dilute to 10 ml with water. Take 25 mg of guaiphenesin, add 0.5 ml of SS solution, 0.5 ml of ammonia and dilute to 10 ml with methanol. Further dilute 1 ml to 10 ml for analysis.

Sample preparation: To 2.5 ml of the sample, add 0.2 ml of ammonia, dilute to 10 ml with methanol. Dilute further 1 ml to 10 ml with methanol, filter and the filtrate used for estimation.

Chromatographic equipments:

Sample applicator: Camag Linomat–IV

Development chamber: Camag twin-trough glass chamber, 10 × 10 cm

Densitometric scanner: Camag TLC Scanner–II

Chromatographic conditions:

1. Stationary phase: Silica gel $60F_{254}$ pre-coated HPTLC plates, 10 × 10 cm (200 μm) – Merck
2. Mobile phase (MP): Chloroform–acetone–methanol–25% ammonia (8 : 2 : 1 : 0.2 v/v)
3. Standard/Sample application:
   Band length: 5 mm Volume applied: 10 μl Spacing: 5 mm
4. Chamber saturation: 20 min (MP)
5. RH (%): 55 ± 2
6. Temperature °C: 22 ± 2
7. Separation technique: Ascending
8. Quantity of mobile phase: 11 ml
9. Migration distance: 50 mm
10. Migration time: 15 min

Densitometric evaluation:

Wavelength: UV–280 nm Scanning mode: Reflectance/Absorbance

HRF: Salbutamol sulphate—12; Guaiphenesin—48

Linearity (μg/ml): Salbutamol sulphate—1–10; Guaiphenesin—10–200

Recovery (%): 97.5–101.69 for both the compounds

References: —

Comments:

- The method was optimized and analytical work carried out at **Anchrom's HPTLC Application Laboratory**, Mumbai, India.
- Several market samples of similar composition were analysed by the proposed method with reproducible results.

HPTLC : High Performance Thin Layer Chromatography
HPTLC Densitogram

No. 323

OH, H, N, HO, $C(CH_3)_3$, HO

Salbutamol

OH, O, OH, OCH_3

Guaiphenesin

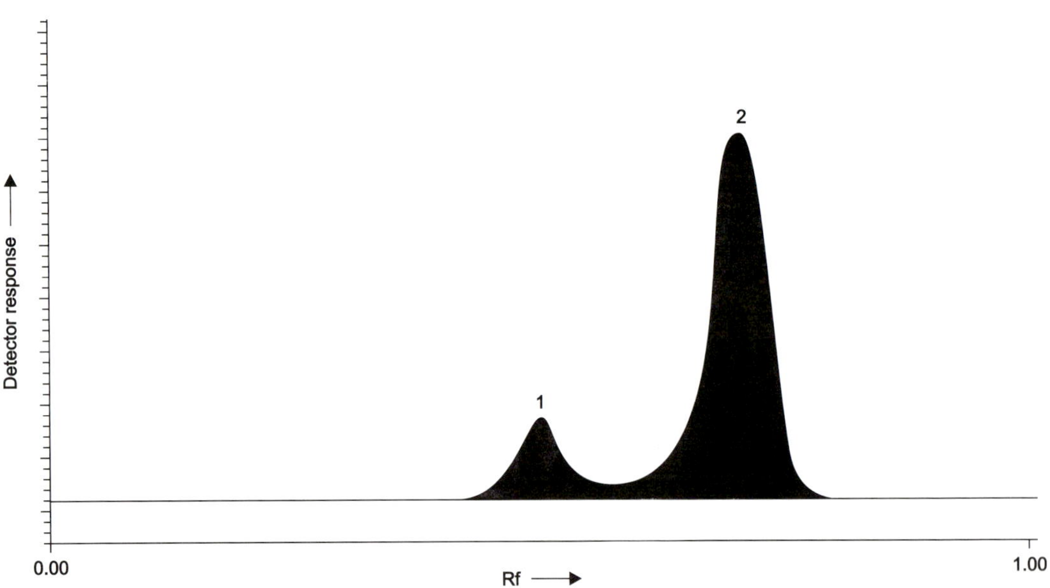

Typical densitogram of the sample containing salbutamol sulphate and guaiphenesin. For detailed experimental and chromatographic conditions, refer to Protocol No. 323. Peaks identification: 1. Salbutamol sulphate; 2. Guaiphenesin.

PROTOCOL FOR HPTLC ANALYSIS OF PHARMACEUTICAL FORMULATION

Protocol No. 323

Formulation: Salbutamol sulphate, Guaiphenesin

Classification: Respiratory System **Dosage form:** Syrup

Standard preparation: Prepare stock solution of salbutamol sulphate (200 μg/ml) and guaiphenesin (10 mg/ml) with methanol. Dilute appropriately with methanol to get final solution of 20 μg/ml (salbutamol sulphate) and 1 mg/ml (guaiphenesin). Apply different volumes for linearity studies.

Sample preparation: Dilute the sample (syrup) appropriately with methanol, filter and use for assay.

Chromatographic equipments:

Sample applicator: Camag Linomat–IV

Development chamber: Camag twin-trough glass chamber, 10 × 10 cm

Densitometric scanner: Camag TLC Scanner–III

Chromatographic conditions:

1. Stationary phase: Silica gel $60F_{254}$ pre-coated HPTLC plates, 10 × 10 cm (200 μm) – Merck
2. Mobile phase (MP): Ethyl acetate–methanol–25% ammonia (7.5 : 1.5 : 1 v/v)
3. Standard/Sample application:
   Band length: 10 mm Volume applied: 15 μl Spacing: 5 mm
4. Chamber saturation: 30 min (MP)
5. RH (%): 55 ± 5
6. Temperature °C: 25 ± 2
7. Separation technique: Ascending
8. Quantity of mobile phase: 10 ml
9. Migration distance: 45 mm
10. Migration time: 20 min

Densitometric evaluation:

Wavelength: UV–280 nm Scanning mode: Reflectance/Absorbance

HRF: See densitogram

Linearity: Salbutamol sulphate—200–1600 ng/band; Guaiphenesin—10–50 μg/band

Recovery (%): 98.36–100.66 for both the compounds

References: Kruti D. Bhalaria, D.D. Bhalara, I.S. Rathod and Sindhu Ezhava, Personal communication.

Comments: The method validated for accuracy, precision, linearity, LOD, LOQ, specificity, robustness and ruggedness.

HPTLC : High Performance Thin Layer Chromatography
HPTLC Densitogram

No. 324

OH, H, N, HO, HO, $C(CH_3)_3$

Salbutamol

OH, O, OH, OCH_3

Guaiphenesin

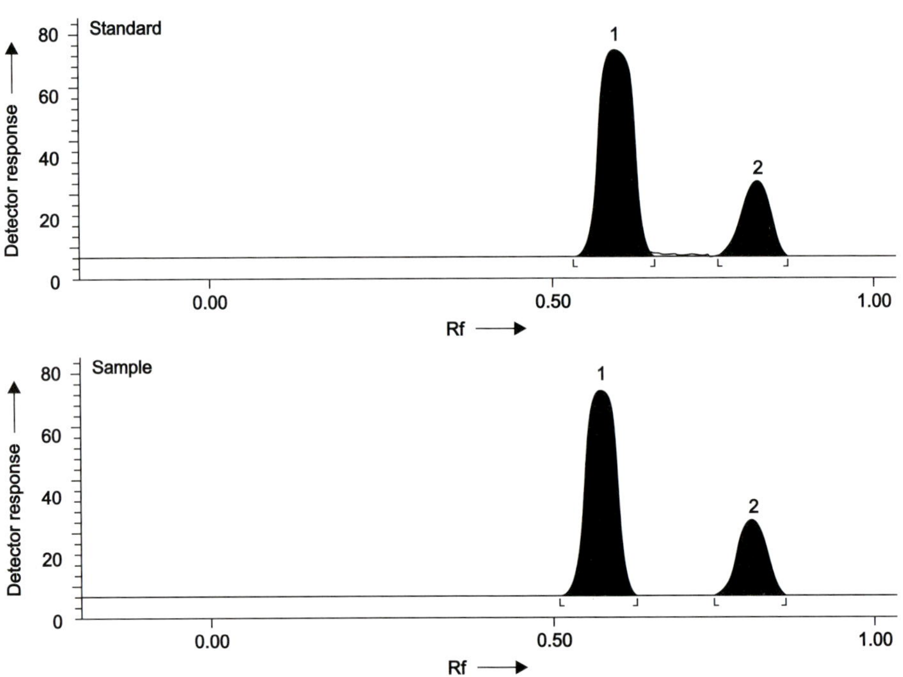

Typical densitogram of the sample and standard containing salbutamol sulphate and guaiphenesin. For detailed experimental and chromatographic conditions, refer to Protocol No. 324. Peaks identification: 1. Guaiphenesin; 2. Salbutamol sulphate.

PROTOCOL FOR HPTLC ANALYSIS OF PHARMACEUTICAL FORMULATION

Protocol No. 324

Formulation: Salbutamol sulphate, Guaiphenesin

Classification: Respiratory System **Dosage form:** Syrup

Standard preparation: Weigh 12 mg of salbutamol sulphate, add 2 ml of ammonia, dilute to 10 ml with water. Take 25 mg of guaiphenesin, add 0.5 ml solution and 0.5 ml of ammonia, dilute to 10 ml with methanol. Further dilute 1 ml to 10 ml with methanol for analysis.

Sample preparation: To 2.5 ml of the sample add 0.2 ml of ammonia, dilute to 10 ml with methanol. Dilute further 1 ml to 10 ml with methanol, filter and use the filtrate for estimation.

Chromatographic equipments:

Sample applicator: Camag Linomat–IV
Development chamber: Camag twin-trough glass chamber, 10 × 10 cm
Densitometric scanner: Camag TLC Scanner–II

Chromatographic conditions:

1. Stationary phase: Silica gel RP-18F_{254s} pre-coated HPTLC plates, 10 × 10 cm (200 μm) – Merck
2. Mobile phase (MP): 0.5 M sod. chloride–methanol–glacial acetic acid (12 : 8 : 0.01 v/v)
3. Standard/Sample application:
   Band length: 5 mm Volume applied: 10 μl Spacing: 5 mm
4. Chamber saturation: 30 min (MP)
5. RH (%): 55 ± 5
6. Temperature °C: 22 ± 2
7. Separation technique: Ascending
8. Quantity of mobile phase: 20 ml
9. Migration distance: 50 mm
10. Migration time: 40 min

Densitometric evaluation:

Wavelength: UV–280 nm Scanning mode: Reflectance/Absorbance
HRF: Guaiphenesin—60; Salbutamol sulphate—82
Linearity (μg/ml): Salbutamol sulphate—1–10; Guaiphenesin—10–200
Recovery (%): 100.15–101.10 for both the compounds

References: —

Comments:

- The method was optimized and analytical work carried out at **Anchrom's HPTLC Application Laboratory**, Mumbai, India.
- RP-chromatography resulted in reversal of retention order as compared to NP-chromatography.
- Several market samples of similar composition were analysed by the proposed method with reproducible results.

HPTLC : High Performance Thin Layer Chromatography
HPTLC Densitogram

No. 325

OH NH$_2$ CH$_3$ • HCl

Phenylpropanolamine hydrochloride

OH O OH OCH$_3$

Guaiphenesin

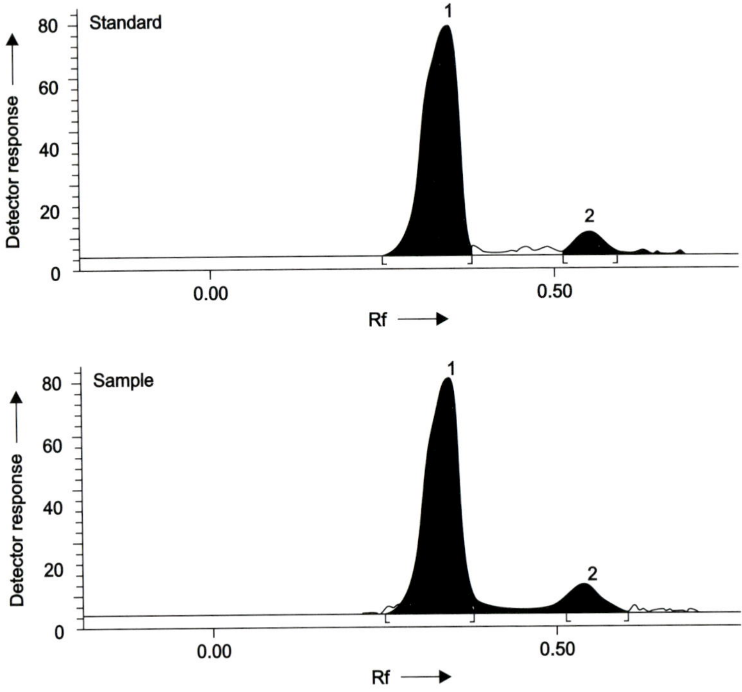

Typical densitogram of the sample and standard containing phenylpropanolamine hydrochloride and guaiphenesin. For detailed experimental and chromatographic conditions, refer to Protocol No. 325. Peaks identification: 1. Guaiphenesin; 2. Phenylpropanolamine hydrochloride.

PROTOCOL FOR HPTLC ANALYSIS OF PHARMACEUTICAL FORMULATION

Protocol No. 325

Formulation: Phenylpropanolamine hydrochloride, Guaiphenesin

Classification: Respiratory System **Dosage form:** Tablets, Syrup

Standard preparation: Dissolve 20 mg of guaiphenesin in methanol with shaking for 5 min, and dilute to 10 ml. To 5 ml of this solution, add 12.5 mg of phenylpropanolamine HCl and make up to 10 ml with methanol and use for analysis.

Sample preparation: Sample equivalent to 50 mg of guaiphenesin suspended in 30–35 ml of methanol, shake for 5 min, dilute to 50 ml, filter and use for analysis.

Chromatographic equipments:

Sample applicator: Camag Linomat–IV

Development chamber: Camag twin-trough glass chamber, 10 × 10 cm

Densitometric scanner: Camag TLC Scanner–II

Chromatographic conditions:

1. Stationary phase: Silica gel $60F_{254}$ pre-coated HPTLC plates, 10 × 10 cm (200 μm) – Merck
2. Mobile phase (MP): Toluene–acetone–25% ammonia (5 : 5 : 0.2 v/v)
3. Standard/Sample application:
   Band length: 10 mm Volume applied: 10 μl Spacing: 20 mm
4. Chamber saturation:
5. RH (%): 55 ± 5
6. Temperature °C: 22 ± 2
7. Separation technique: Ascending
8. Quantity of mobile phase: 10 ml
9. Migration distance: 70 mm
10. Migration time: 15 min

Densitometric evaluation:

Wavelength: UV–254 nm Scanning mode: Reflectance/Absorbance

HRF: Guaiphenesin—32; Phenylpropanolamine HCl—58

Linearity (μg/ml): Phenylpropanolamine HCl—50–1500; Guaiphenesin—250–1250

Recovery (%): 99.31–99.72 for both the drugs

References: —

Comments:

- The method was optimized and analytical work carried out at **Anchrom's HPTLC Application Laboratory**, Mumbai, India.
- Several market samples of similar composition were analysed by the proposed method with reproducible results.

HPTLC : High Performance Thin Layer Chromatography
HPTLC Densitogram

No. 326

Phenylpropanolamine hydrochloride

Guaiphenesin

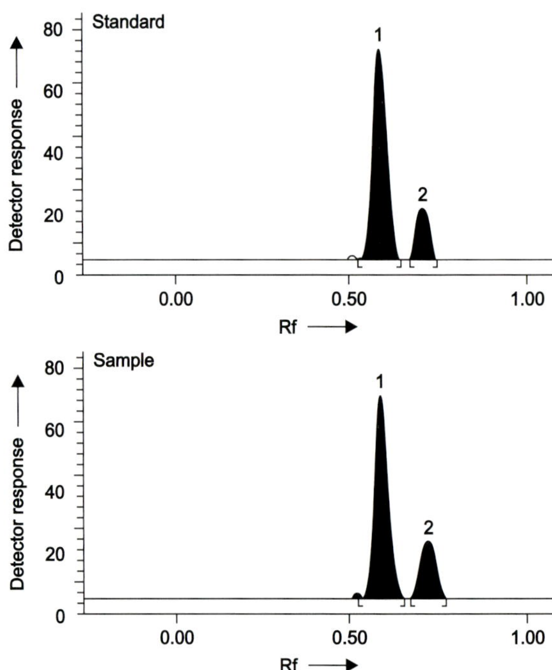

Typical densitogram of the sample and standard containing phenylpropanolamine hydrochloride and guaiphenesin. For detailed experimental and chromatographic conditions, refer to Protocol No. 326. Peaks identification: 1. Guaiphenesin; 2. Phenylpropanolamine hydrochloride.

PROTOCOL FOR HPTLC ANALYSIS OF PHARMACEUTICAL FORMULATION

Protocol No. 326

Formulation: Phenylpropanolamine hydrochloride, Guaiphenesin

Classification: Respiratory System **Dosage form:** Tablets, Syrup

Standard preparation: Dissolve 20 mg of guaiphenesin in methanol with shaking to produce 10 ml. To 5 ml of this solution, add 12.5 mg of phenylpropanolamine HCl, dilute to 10 ml with methanol and use for analysis.

Sample preparation: Sample equivalent to 50 mg of guaiphenesin suspended in 30–40 ml of methanol, shake for 5 min, dilute to 50 ml, filter and use for chromatographic application.

Chromatographic equipments:

Sample applicator: Camag Linomat–IV

Development chamber: Camag twin-trough glass chamber, 10 × 10 cm

Densitometric scanner: Camag TLC Scanner–II

Chromatographic conditions:

1. Stationary phase: Silica gel 60 RP-18F_{254s} pre-coated HPTLC plates, 10 × 10 cm (200 μm) – Merck
2. Mobile phase (MP): 0.5 M sod. chloride–methanol–glacial acetic acid (12 : 8 : 0.01 v/v)
3. Standard/Sample application:
   Band length: 10 mm Volume applied: 10 μl Spacing: 10 mm
4. Chamber saturation: 30 min (MP)
5. RH (%): 55 ± 5
6. Temperature °C: 22 ± 2
7. Separation technique: Ascending
8. Quantity of mobile phase: 20 ml
9. Migration distance: 50 mm
10. Migration time: 40 min

Densitometric evaluation:

Wavelength: UV–254 nm Scanning mode: Reflectance/Absorbance

HRF: Guaiphenesin—60; Phenylpropanolamine HCl—72

Linearity (μg/ml): Phenylpropanolamine HCl—50–1500; Guaiphenesin—250–1250

Recovery (%): 100.75–104.35 for both the drugs

References: —

Comments:

- The method was optimized and analytical work carried out at **Anchrom's HPTLC Application Laboratory**, Mumbai, India.
- Several market samples of similar composition were analysed by the proposed method with reproducible results.

HPTLC : High Performance Thin Layer Chromatography
HPTLC Densitogram

No. 327

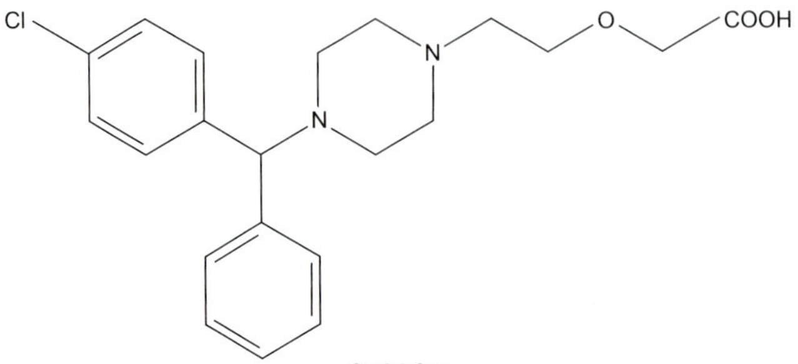

Cetirizine

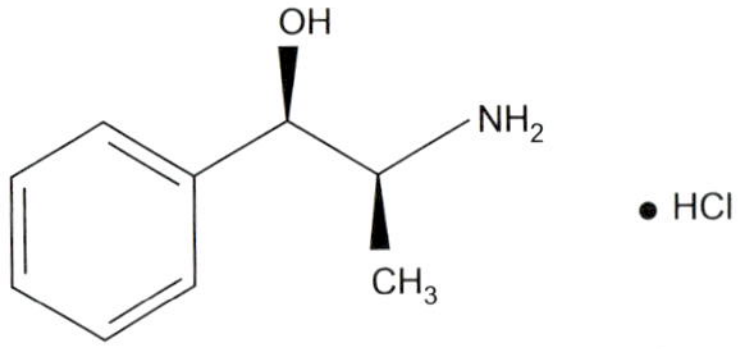

Phenylpropanolamine hydrochloride

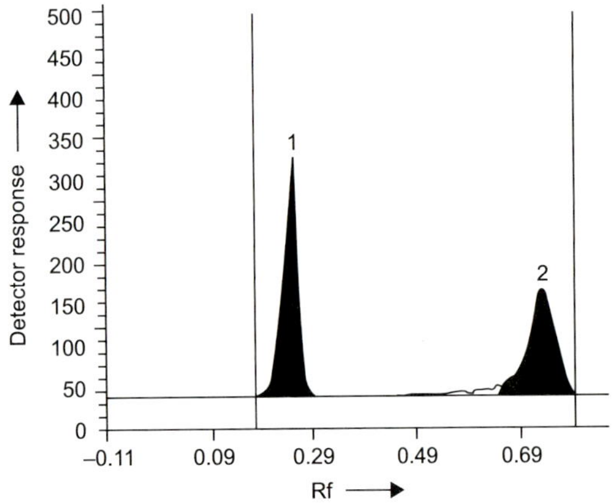

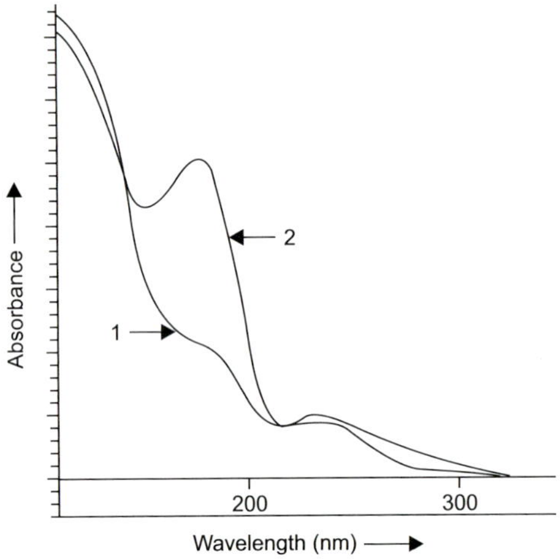

Overlaid UV-spectra of cetirizine HCl (1) and phenylpropanolamine HCl (2) for selection of suitable wavelength for densitometric scanning

Typical densitogram of the standard containing cetirizine hydrochloride and phenylpropanolamine hydrochloride. For detailed experimental and chromatographic conditions, refer to Protocol No. 327. Peaks identification: 1. Cetirizine HCl; 2. Phenylpropanolamine HCl.

PROTOCOL FOR HPTLC ANALYSIS OF PHARMACEUTICAL FORMULATION

Protocol No. 327

Formulation: Phenylpropanolamine hydrochloride, Cetirizine hydrochloride

Classification: Respiratory System **Dosage form:** Tablets

Standard preparation: Prepare solution of both the compounds separately in methanol to get 250 μg/ml of cetirizine hydrochloride and 5000 μg/ml of phenylpropanolamine hydrochloride. Apply varying volumes of each solution for linearity profile.

Sample preparation: Powdered sample equivalent 5 mg of cetirizine hydrochloride or 25 mg of phenylpropanolamine hydrochloride suspended in 5 ml of methanol, sonicated for 5 min, filtered and diluted to 10 ml with methanol. The final solution applied for linearity profile.

Chromatographic equipments:

Sample applicator: Camag Linomat–V

Development chamber: Camag twin-trough glass chamber, 10 × 10 cm

Densitometric scanner: Camag TLC Scanner–III

Chromatographic conditions:

1. Stationary phase: Silica gel $60F_{254}$ pre-coated HPTLC plates, 10 × 10 cm (200 μm) – Merck
2. Mobile phase (MP): Ethyl acetate–methanol (5.5 : 4.5 v/v)
3. Standard/Sample application:
   Band length: 6 mm Volume applied: 10 μl Spacing: 5 mm
4. Chamber saturation: 30 min (MP)
5. RH (%): 55 ± 5
6. Temperature °C: 22 ± 2
7. Separation technique: Ascending
8. Quantity of mobile phase: 10 ml
9. Migration distance: 80 mm
10. Migration time: 20 min

Densitometric evaluation:

Wavelength: UV–254 nm Scanning mode: Reflectance/Absorbance

HRF: Cetirizine hydrochloride—25; Phenylpropanolamine hydrochloride—72

Linearity (μg/band): Cetirizine hydrochloride—7.5–17.5; Phenylpropanolamine hydrochloride—37.5–87.5

Recovery (%): Cetirizine HCl—98.6–103.0; Phenylpropanolamine HCl—98.5–100.46

References: Pinak Patel, Falgun Mehta and Swayam Prakash Patel, *Int. J. Pharmacy and Pharmaceutical Sci.*, **3(2)**, 251–255, 2011.

Comments: The method validated for accuracy, precision, linearity, LOD, LOQ, specificity, robustness and ruggedness.

HPTLC : High Performance Thin Layer Chromatography
HPTLC Densitogram

No. 328

Cl COOH N N O

Cetirizine

OH NH_2 • HCl CH_3

Phenylpropanolamine hydrochloride

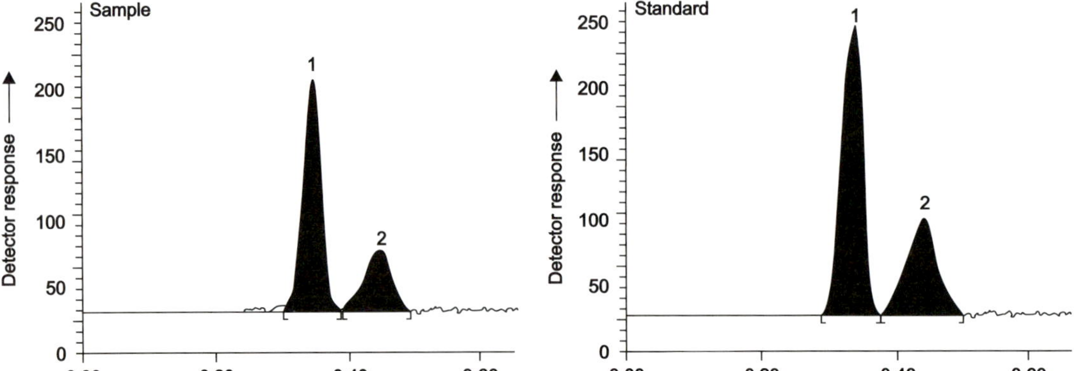

Typical densitogram of the sample and standard containing phenylpropanolamine HCl and cetirizine HCl. For detailed experimental and chromatographic conditions, refer to Protocol No. 328. Peaks identification: 1. Cetirizine HCl; 2. Phenylpropanolamine HCl.

PROTOCOL FOR HPTLC ANALYSIS OF PHARMACEUTICAL FORMULATION

Protocol No. 328

Formulation: Phenylpropanolamine hydrochloride, Cetirizine hydrochloride

Classification: Respiratory System **Dosage form:** Tablets

Standard preparation: Prepare solution of each compound separately in methanol to get 50 μg/ml of phenylpropanolamine hydrochloride and 10 μg/ml of cetirizine hydrochloride. Further dilute suitably for linearity profile.

Sample preparation: Powdered sample equivalent to 5 mg of cetirizine hydrochloride or 25 mg of phenylpropanolamine hydrochloride suspended in 30 ml of methanol, sonicated for 15 min, diluted to 50 ml, filtered and filtrate suitably diluted for assay.

Chromatographic equipments:

Sample applicator: Camag Linomat–V

Development chamber: Camag twin-trough glass chamber, 20 × 10 cm

Densitometric scanner: Camag TLC Scanner–III

Chromatographic conditions:

1. Stationary phase: Silica gel $60F_{254}$ pre-coated HPTLC plates, 10 × 10 cm (200 μm) – Merck, pre-washed with methanol, activated at 50°C for 10 min prior to use
2. Mobile phase (MP): Ethyl acetate–methanol–formic acid (7.5 : 1.5 : 0.5 v/v)
3. Standard/Sample application:
   Band length: 8 mm Volume applied: 5 μl Spacing: 10 mm
4. Chamber saturation: 10 min (MP)
5. RH (%): 55 ± 5
6. Temperature °C: 22 ± 2
7. Separation technique: Ascending
8. Quantity of mobile phase: 19 ml
9. Migration distance: 50 mm
10. Migration time: 10 min

Densitometric evaluation:

Wavelength: UV–254 nm Scanning mode: Reflectance/Absorbance

HRF: Cetirizine HCl—34; Phenylpropanolamine HCl—45

Linearity (ng/band): Phenylpropanolamine HCl—50–175; Cetirizine HCl—20–120

Recovery (%): 99.68–100.11 for both the compounds

References: P.S. Dhongle, S.J. Sahare, S.S. Dhongle, A.S. Mundhey and S.P. Wate, *Der Pharmacia Lettre*, **3(4)**, 111–119, 2011.

Comments: The method validated for accuracy, precision, linearity, LOD, LOQ, specificity and robustness.

HPTLC : High Performance Thin Layer Chromatography
HPTLC Densitogram

No. 329

Dextromethorphan hydrobromide

Doxylamine

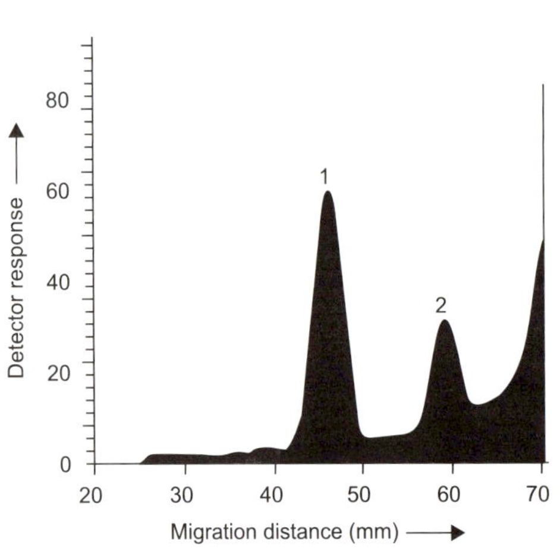

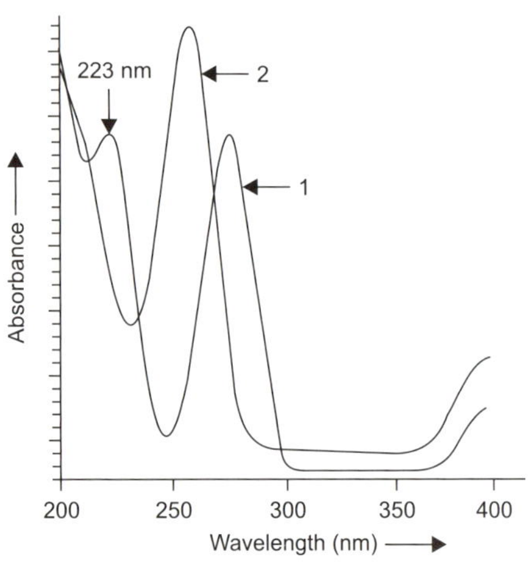

Overlaid UV-spectra of dextromethorphan base (1) and doxylamine succinate (2) for selection of suitable wavelength for densitometric scanning

Typical densitogram of the sample containing dextromethorphan hydrobromide and doxylamine succinate. For detailed experimental and chromatographic conditions, refer to Protocol No. 329. Peaks identification: 1. Dextromethorphan HBr; 2. Doxylamine succinate.

PROTOCOL FOR HPTLC ANALYSIS OF PHARMACEUTICAL FORMULATION

Protocol No. 329

Formulation: Dextromethorphan hydrobromide, Doxylamine succinate

Classification: Respiratory System **Dosage form:** Syrup

Standard preparation: Prepare 500 µg/ml solution of each compound in water. Then transfer 5 ml of dextromethorphan HBr and 3 ml of doxylamine succinate solutions, dilute to 10 ml with water. Apply 1–5 µl of the final solution for linearity.

Sample preparation: The sample (syrup) was basified with 25% ammonia, extracted with n-hexane (3 × 3 ml), total n-hexane evaporated to dryness under N_2, the residue taken up in n-hexane and 2 µl spotted for estimation.

Chromatographic equipments:

Sample applicator: Camag Nanomat–III

Development chamber: Camag twin-trough glass chamber, 20 × 10 cm

Densitometric scanner: Camag TLC Scanner–II

Chromatographic conditions:

1. Stationary phase: Silica gel $60F_{254}$ pre-coated TLC plates, 10 × 10 cm (250 µm) – Merck, pre-washed with methanol and dried (60°C) for 5 min prior to use
2. Mobile phase (MP): Methanol–25% ammonia (14 : 1 v/v)
3. Standard/Sample application:
   Band length: 5 mm Volume applied: 2 µl Spacing: 10 mm
4. Chamber saturation: 20 min (MP)
5. RH (%): 55 ± 5
6. Temperature °C: 25 ± 2
7. Separation technique: Ascending
8. Quantity of mobile phase: 15 ml
9. Migration distance: 80 mm
10. Migration time: 20 min

Densitometric evaluation:

Wavelength: UV–223 nm Scanning mode: Reflectance/Absorbance

HRF: Dextromethorphan HBr—54; Doxylamine succinate—74

Linearity (µg/band): Dextromethorphan HBr—2.4–12.2; Doxylamine succinate—1.5–7.4

Recovery (%): 98.2–102.1 for both the drugs

References: Gunawan Indrayanto, *J. Planar Chromatogr.*, **9(4)**, 282–286, 1996.

Comments: The method validated for accuracy, precision, linearity, LOD, LOQ, specificity, robustness and ruggedness.

Index

D

K

L

M

N

O

P

Q

R

S

T

V

Z